# Evidence Based Practice in Pediatric Radiation Oncology

Renu Madan • Shikha Goyal
Supriya Mallick
Editors

# Evidence Based Practice in Pediatric Radiation Oncology

Springer

*Editors*
Renu Madan
Department of Radiotherapy and Oncology
Postgraduate Institute of Medical Education
and Research
Chandigarh, India

Shikha Goyal
Department of Radiotherapy and Oncology
Postgraduate Institute of Medical Education
and Research
Chandigarh, India

Supriya Mallick
Department of Radiation Oncology
National Cancer Institute
Jhajjar, Haryana, India

2nd Campus AIIMS
New Delhi, Delhi, India

ISBN 978-981-96-4871-9 ISBN 978-981-96-4872-6 (eBook)
https://doi.org/10.1007/978-981-96-4872-6



This Springer imprint is published by the registered company Springer Nature Singapore Pte Ltd.
The registered company address is: 152 Beach Road, #21-01/04 Gateway East, Singapore 189721, Singapore

# Foreword

The editors of *Evidence Based Practice in Pediatric Radiation Oncology* are to be congratulated for compiling a succinct and informative book that efficiently conveys the essentials of evidence-based practice in this critical field. This textbook presents a multidisciplinary approach to pediatric cancers, including radiology, pathology, and clinical expertise for optimum patient care.

Pediatric radiation oncology is a rapidly evolving field that requires a deep understanding of the complex interplay between radiation therapy, pediatric oncology, and the unique needs of children with cancer. The evolving understanding of pediatric cancers underscores the need for innovative, empathetic care that prioritizes the unique needs of children and families affected.

This textbook, *Evidence Based Practice in Pediatric Radiation Oncology*, brings together the expertise of renowned specialists in the field of pediatric oncology, radiation oncology, radiologist, pathologist, neurosurgeon, and pediatric surgeon to provide a comprehensive resource for healthcare professionals caring for children with cancer. This textbook is designed to serve as a comprehensive resource, aggregating the latest evidence and expert consensus to guide treatment decisions and aims to synthesize the current literature on pediatric radiation oncology.

Within these pages, readers will find in-depth coverage of the biology and management of childhood cancers, including brain tumors, leukemia, lymphoma, and solid tumors. The authors have also shared their insights on topics, such as epidemiology, cancer genetics, acute and late effects of radiation, radiotherapy planning aspect, need for the daily anesthesia, and challenges in low middle income countries. The authors have also discussed their expertise in radiosurgery and proton therapy.

This textbook is designed to serve as a valuable resource for radiation oncologists, pediatric oncologists, medical students, medical physicists, nurses, and other healthcare professionals caring for children with cancer seeking to stay up-to-date on the latest advances in pediatric radiation oncology.

We hope that this comprehensive guide will contribute to improving outcomes and bring hope for children and families affected by cancer.

Department of Radiation Oncology
Ex Chief DR.B.R.A.I.R.C.H
AIIMS, New Delhi, India

Ex-head National Cancer Institute
(2nd Campus AIIMS), Jhajjar, Haryana, India

G. K. Rath

# Preface

Introducing *Evidence Based Practice in Pediatric Radiation Oncology*, which offers a comprehensive review of the current evidence-based practices in pediatric radiation oncology. As a rapidly evolving field, pediatric radiation oncology demands a profound comprehension of the distinct needs and challenges that arise when treating children with cancer. The unique physiology and developmental stages of pediatric patients introduce complexities that necessitate specialized knowledge and expertise. This textbook covers the fundamentals of radiation oncology, genetics, imaging, pathology, and multidisciplinary management of pediatric cancers with a focus on radiation therapy. It also highlights the unique challenges in children with cancer, including the need for daily anesthesia, treatment-related side effects, and survivorship concerns. We hope that this textbook will provide a valuable resource to students, radiation oncologists, pediatric oncologists, pediatric surgeons, and other healthcare professionals involved in pediatric cancer management.

The journey commenced in 2022, and it took 3 years to reach a satisfying milestone. We are grateful to our authors and contributors for their hard work and dedication to this project. We also wish to acknowledge the courage and resilience of the children and families who inspire us to continue advancing the field of pediatric radiation oncology.

This book has been prepared to the best of our knowledge, but there may be mistakes and shortcomings. But we invite all readers to come up with constructive criticism so that we can rectify such weaknesses and make this book an all-time reference.


| | |
|---|---|
| Chandigarh, India | Renu Madan |
| Chandigarh, India | Shikha Goyal |
| Jhajjar, Haryana, India | Supriya Mallick |

# Contents

# Introduction to Paediatric Oncology

# 1

Renu Madan, Shikha Goyal, and Supriya Mallick

## 1.1 Introduction

Paediatric oncology has witnessed substantial progress over the last few decades. Over the last 50–60 years, childhood cancer has shown a tremendous improvement in the treatment and the survival rate in the developed countries through adoption of uniform treatment guidelines and patient enrolment in multi-centric clinical trials. In the 1950s, only less than 10% childhood cancer patients survived beyond 5 years, as compared to 70–80% in the present era [1]. In the united states, the 5-year survival rate in 2011–2017 was 85% for children and adolescents [2]. Paediatric age ranges from birth to adolescent age, incorporating the individuals with different maturity rate and age adjusted care leads to a difference in the incidence and outcome in various study protocols [3].

## 1.2 Paediatric Oncology in Low Middle-Income Countries (LMICs)

Paediatric cancers are less common in LMICs as compared to Western countries since they often remain undiagnosed due to nonspecific symptoms and cancer illiteracy. The outcome of paediatric cancers remains far behind the current international standards in LMICs [4]. This is because of the paucity of real epidemiological data, lack of infrastructure, financial resources, and cancer illiteracy. Another reason

R. Madan (✉) · S. Goyal
Department of Radiotherapy and Oncology, Postgraduate Institute of Medical Education and Research, Chandigarh, India

S. Mallick
Department of Radiation Oncology, National Cancer Institute, Jhajjar, Haryana, India

2nd Campus AIIMS, New Delhi, Delhi, India



R. Madan et al. (eds.), *Evidence Based Practice in Pediatric Radiation Oncology*, https://doi.org/10.1007/978-981-96-4872-6_1

in that only less than 15% children are included in the clinical trials in LMICs as compared to >90% in Western countries [5]. Paucity of dedicated paediatric oncology set-up is one of the biggest hurdle in improving outcome. In India, dedicated paediatric oncology was almost non-existent till early 1980s, and the first paediatric centre was started in Tata Memorial Hospital in 1985 [6]. Even at present, many of the childhood cancers are treated by adult oncologists. In a survey of 275 medical colleges or cancer centres revealed that more than 50% centres did not have facilities for treating childhood cancer, even in the treating centres, the infra-structure and facilities were limited [5].

## 1.3 Management of Childhood Cancers and Differences from Adults

Common treatment modalities include surgery, chemotherapy, radiation therapy, immunotherapy, and stem cell transplant. Children face unique issues at diagnosis and during and after their treatment. Hence as soon as a malignancy is suspected, the child should be referred to a paediatric oncology centre for subsequent diagnostic workup and management. The principal differences in childhood and adult cancers are as follows:

1. Diagnosis: Diagnosis of paediatric cancers requires a high level of suspicion. These are often difficult to detect in early stage due to non-specific signs and symptoms mimicking other more common disorders.
2. Risk factors: Unlike adults, lifestyle-related risk factors such as smoking or alcoholism do not play a role in childhood cancers.
3. Intensity and response to the treatment: Childhood cancers tend to be more aggressive as compared to adult cancers hence require more intense treatment. However, with some exceptions, they respond better to the treatment.
4. Therapeutic consideration and treatment toxicities: Children are more prone to treatment related toxicities particularly cardiovascular, neurocognitive, skeletal, endocrinal, and subsequent malignant neoplasm (SMN). Chemotherapeutic agents and radiation increase the risk of SMN particularly in children. One of the Childhood Cancer Survivor Study of 14359, 5-years survivors showed that 30 years cumulative incidence of SMN was 20.5%, which was six times higher as compared to the general population [7]. Therefore, long-term side effects are more of a concern in paediatric cancer patients.
5. Anaesthesia during radiation: Immobilisation during radiation therapy is a concern in children. Many of these patients require daily anaesthesia for the treatment.

6. Supportive care: Childhood cancer survivors need a lifetime follow-up to monitor the long-term side effects.

## 1.4 Conclusion

The outcome of childhood cancers in LMICs remains poor as compared to the West. To reach the international standards, we need a collaborative and multi-dimensional efforts. Best ways to improve paediatric oncology service are optimal utilisation of existing infrastructure, to determine the burden by strengthening national registry programme and establishing national paediatric oncology research groups for Indian children rather than blindly following Western protocols.

## References


1. Arora B, Sripad B. Pediatric oncology in India: past, present and future. Indian J Med Paediatr Oncol. 2009;30(04):121–3.
2. American Cancer Society. Cancer facts and figures 2022. American Cancer Society; 2022.
3. Thorp N. Basic principles of paediatric radiotherapy. Clin Oncol (R Coll Radiol). 2013;25(1):3–10.
4. Barr R, Riberio R, Agarwal B, Masera G, Hesseling P, Magrath I. Pediatric oncology in countries with limited resources. In: Pizzo PA, Poplack DG, editors. Principles and practice of pediatric oncology. 5th ed. Philadelphia: Lippincott Williams and Wilkins; 2006. p. 1605–17.
5. Advani SH, Agarwal R, Venugopal P, et al. Pediatric oncology in India. Indian J Pediatr. 1987;54:843–5. https://doi.org/10.1007/BF02761007.
6. Arora R, Arora B. Delivering childhood cancer service across India: current provisions and future options. Pediatr Blood Cancer. 2009;53:827.
7. Friedman DL, Whitton J, Leisenring W, et al. Subsequent neoplasms in 5-year survivors of childhood cancer: the childhood Cancer survivor study. J Natl Cancer Inst. 2010;102(14):1083–95.

# 2 Epidemiology of Pediatric Cancer

Subhas Pandit and Simit Sapkota

## 2.1 Global Burden of Disease

- Each year, an estimated 4,00,000 children and adolescents, 0–19 years of age, develop cancer.
- Children between 0 and 14 years or 0 and 19 years of age are most often included in pediatric cancer studies.
- In recent decades, management of childhood cancer has improved greatly in terms of cure rates and reduced treatment-related morbidity and mortality. A majority of this gain is observed in countries with high incomes.
- Over 90% of children at risk for cancer reside in low- and middle-income countries (LMICs). However, the full scale of pediatric cancer is unclear in many LMICs due to the lack of systematic data on cancer incidence [1].
- Low cure rates in LMICs stem from delayed disease detection, barriers to proper treatment, treatment abandonment due to financial burdens, higher mortality from poorly managed complications, and preventable relapses caused by insufficient follow-up care.
- Improving access to childhood cancer care, including essential medicines and technologies, is feasible and highly cost effective strategy to improve cure rate and survival in all settings [2].

## 2.2 Classification of Childhood Cancers

- Compared to adult cancers, childhood cancers have a different spectrum.
- Histo-morphology based classification is used unlike site based as in adults.

S. Pandit (✉) · S. Sapkota
Kathmandu Cancer Center, Kathmandu, Nepal
e-mail: dr.subhas@kccrc.org


R. Madan et al. (eds.), *Evidence Based Practice in Pediatric Radiation Oncology*,
https://doi.org/10.1007/978-981-96-4872-6_2

- International Classification of Childhood Cancer, third edition (ICCC-3), serves as the current global standard for categorizing pediatric cancers in population-based research and cancer registry systems.
- The ICCC-3 classifies tumors into 12 main groups, and 47 subgroups.

### 2.2.1 International Classification of Childhood Cancer, 3rd edition: main groups

1. Leukemias, myeloproliferative, and myelodysplastic diseases.
2. Lymphomas and reticuloendothelial neoplasms.
3. Central nervous system (CNS) and miscellaneous intracranial and intraspinal neoplasms.
4. Neuroblastoma and other peripheral nervous cell tumors.
5. Retinoblastoma.
6. Renal tumors.
7. Hepatic tumors.
8. Malignant bone tumors.
9. Soft tissue and other extra-osseous sarcomas.
10. Germ cell tumors, trophoblastic tumors, and neoplasms of gonads.
11. Other malignant epithelial neoplasms and malignant melanomas.
12. Other and unspecified malignant neoplasms.

## 2.3 Epidemiology of Different Cancers Around the Globe

- Distribution of cancer in pediatric (0–14 years) and adolescent (15–19 years) is significantly different.
- In pediatric age groups, leukemia and CNS tumors constitute more than 50% of cases. In leukemias, acute lymphoblastic leukemia (ALL) is 4–5 times more common than acute myeloid leukemia (AML). Next common pediatric tumors are CNS tumors. Other common tumors in order of frequency are neuroblastoma, Wilms' tumor, and non-Hodgkin lymphoma (NHL).
- In the adolescent group (15–19 years), Hodgkin's lymphoma (HL), germ cell tumor, NHL, melanoma, thyroid cancer, and bone and soft tissue sarcoma are more commonly seen (Fig. 2.1).

### 2.3.1 Leukemia

- The most common cancer in children worldwide, accounting for approximately 40% of all pediatric cancers.
- ALL has a peak incidence from 2–5 years of age.
- ALL is one of the major success stories of cancer treatment. With modern protocols, survival of children exceeds over 80% in developed countries [4].

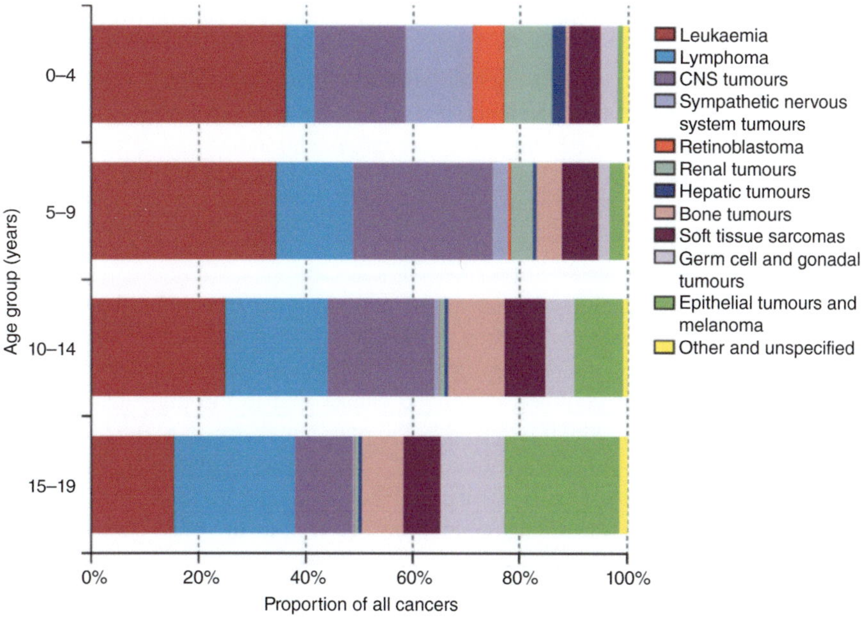


**Fig. 2.1** Proportional distribution of cancer type by age group [3]

- Outcome is better in female compared to male. Other high risk features are diagnosis at age before 1 year or after 10 years, poor socioeconomic and family factors which leads to malnourishment, restricted access to treatment and treatment abandonment.
- Myeloid leukemias are relatively rare in the young population, and constitute around 10% of hematological malignancy in children.

### 2.3.2 Central Nervous System (CNS) Tumor

- In the pediatric population, central nervous system tumors represent both the leading solid tumors and the second most common cancer type, surpassed only by leukemias.
- As the primary cause of cancer-related mortality in children, brain tumors are responsible for over 25% of pediatric cancer deaths.
- Incidence is highest in the younger group, with 75% occurring below 10 years of age.
- Astrocytomas make up roughly half of all pediatric brain tumors, with the low-grade variants, especially pilocytic astrocytoma, being more common than aggressive high-grade forms.
- Astrocytomas and embryonal tumors are the most common entities, followed by ependymomas.

- Medulloblastoma and other embryonal tumors constitute 15–20% of childhood brain tumors.
- In children below 5 years, infratentorial tumors are more common, while supratentorial tumors are more prevalent in the overall pediatric population.
- Unlike adults, metastatic brain tumors are rare in children.

### 2.3.3 Lymphoma

- Lymphoma is the leading cause of cancer among adolescents (15–19 years) and the third most common malignancy in children (0–14 years) in western world.
- However, there is significant geographical variation. In certain regions of Africa, it ranks as the most common childhood cancer due to the high incidence of Burkitt's lymphoma, which is linked to the presence of Epstein–Barr virus and malaria.
- HL accounts for approximately 6–8% of all pediatric neoplasms. This is the most prevalent lymphoma in developed countries, as well as the most common neoplasm in children and young adults aged 10–19 years
- The Epstein–Barr virus (EBV) has been linked to the development of HL. EBV positivity can be observed in approximately 70-80% of mixed-cellularity HL cases, which is the most common histological subvariant of HL in early childhood.
- NHL encompasses a diverse group of tumors, making up around 7% of all pediatric cancers. Like HL, NHL incidence rates vary based on factors such as sex, age, and ethnicity.
- Prior exposure to childhood infections does not influence the incidence of NHL. However, in some areas of Africa, there is a strong link between endemic Burkitt's lymphoma, EBV, and malaria.
- The survival rates of children and adolescents with NHL has risen to over 80% in western world.
- In LMIC, lack of robust national cancer registries make it difficult to accurately estimate incidence and mortality

### 2.3.4 Retinoblastoma

- Though the most common childhood eye cancer, retinoblastoma remains infrequent, with an occurrence rate of approximately one case in every 16,000–18,000 newborns worldwide.
- The incidence of retinoblastoma remains similar across various populations, unaffected by gender, ethnicity, or socioeconomic factors.
- Each year, around 8000 children globally develop retinoblastoma, with the majority being detected in children under 5 years old [5].

### 2.3.5 Renal Tumors

- Malignant renal tumors represent 5% of childhood cancers, the majority of which are Wilms' tumors.
- The age-adjusted occurrence (ASR) of renal tumors in children reached 8.3 per million globally, peaking in North America and Europe (9–10 per million) and showing lowest rates across most Asian regions (4–5 per million)) [6].
- Patient survival rates showed marked economic disparities: 70–97% in wealthy nations, 61–94% in upper-middle-income regions, 0–85% in lower-middle-income areas, and 25–53% in low-income countries.

### 2.3.6 Neuroblastoma

- It is the most frequently occurring tumor in children under the age of one.
- The annual incidence shows a clear economic divide, 1.9 per million children in LMIC, 7.1 per million in upper-middle-income areas, and high-income nations reporting 14.1 per million, with ranges extending to 18.9 per million.
- The annual incidence shows a clear economic divide. In LMIC, the incidence is 1.9 per million children annually. In upper-middle-income countries (UMICs), it increases to 7.1 per million children annually. In high-income countries (HICs), the incidence reaches 14.1 per million children annually.[7].

### 2.3.7 Hepatic Tumors

- Hepatoblastoma is an embryonal tumor and the most common primary liver malignancy in children.
- Estimated incidence is 0.5–1.5 cases per million in children of 0–14 years, with the majority of cases presenting before the age of four.
- Congenital hepatoblastomas are diagnosed either *in utero* or within the first 28 days of life, accounting for less than 10% of all pediatric hepatoblastomas.
- When evaluating intra-abdominal masses in children, renal masses are most frequent, while hepatic masses account for 5–6% of cases. The distribution of liver masses shows a predominance of malignant lesions (66%), with benign tumors making up the remaining 33% [8].

### 2.3.8 Malignant Bone Tumors (MBTs)

- Malignant bone tumors account for 3–5% of cancers in children under 15 years of age.
- This prevalence nearly doubles in adolescents, rising to 7–8% among those aged 15–19 years.
- The peak incidence of malignant bone tumors is in adolescents when the pubertal growth spurt is considered a precipitating factor.

## 2.4 Risk Factors

Risk factors are not known for most pediatric cancers. Genetic factors are more likely to affect childhood cancers than environmental exposure.

- Demographic Risk Factors:
  - Overall incidence is highest in infancy which gradually decreases and reaches nadir at 5–9 years of age and again goes up in the 15–19 years group.
  - Male preponderance is seen in most childhood cancers, mainly in NHL, ALL, CNS tumors, hepatoblastoma, Ewing's sarcoma, and rhabdomyosarcoma. Wilms' tumor however is more common in females.
- Familial Predisposition and Genetic condition:
  - Accounting for an estimated 10% of all cancers occurring in children and adolescents.
  - Several inherited risk factors are linked to ALL, such as trisomy 21 (Down syndrome), which increases the risk by 10–20 times, while genetic conditions like Bloom syndrome, Fanconi anemia, and Nijmegen breakage syndrome also elevate the likelihood of ALL.
  - Children with specific genetic conditions, such as Turcot syndrome, Li-Fraumeni syndrome, neurofibromatosis type 1, and neurofibromatosis type 2, have a higher risk of developing central nervous system (CNS) tumors.
- Immunodeficiency:
  - Congenital immunodeficiency and acquired immunodeficiency are associated with malignancy, particularly with lymphomas.
  - Acquired immune deficiency is mainly associated with HIV infection and post-transplant immune suppression.
- Infection:
  - Infection related cancers are more common in LMIC particularly in sub-Saharan Africa.
  - Endemic Burkitt's lymphoma in Africa is associated with Epstein–Barr Virus (EBV) infection and malaria [9].
  - Children with HIV are at a higher risk of developing Kaposi's sarcoma (KS) and non-Hodgkin lymphoma (NHL) compared to HIV-negative children. Kaposi's sarcoma, which is linked to human herpesvirus 8 (HHV 8), shows a risk increase of up to 30 times among children and adolescents living with HIV [10].
- Ionizing Radiation:
  - Early life exposure to ionizing radiation is linked to an increased risk of leukemia and brain tumors in subsequent years.
  - Medical exposure, X-rays, and CT scans are major sources of ionizing radiation.

- Environment:
  - According to the International Agency for Research on Cancer (IARC), parental smoking is associated with increases in risk of hepatoblastoma with limited evidence suggesting a connection to childhood leukemia, particularly acute lymphoblastic leukemia (ALL) [11].
  - Chemicals like benzene and certain chemotherapy drugs (especially alkylating agents and topoisomerase II inhibitors) are strongly associated with AML.[12]

### 2.4.1 Survival Outcome

- Overall survival in childhood cancer has improved rapidly in the developed world. In high-income countries, approximately 70% of children with cancer survive 5 years after diagnosis.
- Hematological malignancy, such as leukemia and lymphoma, has seen marked improvement in outcome with modern treatment protocols. The survival rate in developed countries is now above 80%.
- Low-income countries, where there are fewer survivors, have not benefited from these improvements. Developing world is still lagging behind in access to treatment and outcome. Over 90% of children at risk for developing cancer reside in LMIC. However, only 40% of these children diagnosed with cancer receive appropriate diagnosis and treatment.

## References


1. Bhakta N, Force LM, Allemani C. Childhood cancer burden: a review of global estimates. Lancet Oncol. 2019;20:e42–53.
2. Lam CG, Howard SC, Bouffet E, Pritchard-Jones K. Science and health for all children with cancer. Science. 2019;363(6432):1182–6. https://doi.org/10.1126/science.aaw4892.
3. Steliarova-Foucher E, Colombet M, Ries LAG, Moreno F, Dolya A, Bray F, Hesseling P, Shin HY, Stiller CA. IICC-3 contributors. International incidence of childhood cancer, 2001–10: a population-based registry study. Lancet Oncol. 2017;18(6):719–31.
4. Pui CH, Yang JJ, Hunger SP, et al. Childhood acute lymphoblastic leukemia: Progress through collaboration. J Clin Oncol. 2015;33:2938–48.
5. Fabian ID, Sagoo MS. Understanding retinoblastoma: epidemiology and genetics. Community Eye Health. 2018;31(101):7.
6. Nakata K, Colombet M, Stiller CA, Pritchard-Jones K. Steliarova-Foucher E; IICC-3 contributors. Incidence of childhood renal tumours: an international population-based study. Int J Cancer. 2020;147(12):3313–27. https://doi.org/10.1002/ijc.33147. Epub 2020 Jul 22.
7. van Heerden J, Abraham N, Schoeman J, Reynders D, Singh E, Kruger M. Reporting incidences of neuroblastoma in various resource settings. JCO Glob Oncol. 2021;7:947–64. https://doi.org/10.1200/GO.21.00054.

8. Lucas B, Ravishankar S, Pateva I. Pediatric primary hepatic tumors: diagnostic considerations. Diagnostics. 2021;11(2):333. https://doi.org/10.3390/diagnostics11020333.
9. van den Bosch CA. Is endemic Burkitt's lymphoma an alliance between three infections and a tumour promoter? Lancet Oncol. 2004;5:738–46.
10. Mbulaiteye SM, Bhatia K, Adebamowo C, Sasco AJ. HIV and cancer in Africa: mutual collaboration between HIV and cancer programs may provide timely research and public health data. Infect Agent Cancer. 2011;6:16.
11. Roman E, Lightfoot T, Smith AG, et al. Childhood acute lymphoblastic leukaemia and birthweight: insights from a pooled analysis of case-control data from Germany, the United Kingdom and the United States. Eur J Cancer. 2013;49:1437–47.
12. Eden T. Aetiology of childhood leukaemia. Cancer Treat Rev. 2010;36(4):286–97. https://doi.org/10.1016/j.ctrv.2010.02.004.

# 3 Evolution of Radiation Therapy Strategies

Sambit Swarup Nanda, Supriya Mallick, and Prashanth Giridhar

## 3.1 Introduction

Radiation therapy in pediatric tumors has undergone a spectral change from conventional two-dimensional radiotherapy to intensity-modulated radiotherapy (IMRT) over last few decades. The complexity of pediatric diseases and its varied presentations have put the focus on the technological advancement to deal with site and disease specific challenges. The radiation therapy strategy has been driven by attempts to improve therapeutic index. This involves improving the disease control by exactly characterizing location and extent of the disease. The integration of technological advancements, such as computed tomography (CT) scans, magnetic resonance imaging (MRI), and positron emission tomography (PET) scans, has enabled radiation oncologists to define the structural and functional aspects of every tumor. The use of these modern imaging techniques and improved pathological classification of pediatric tumors helped oncologists to characterize these tumors according to their nature and predict prognosis. Furthermore, it has helped in predicting the recurrence pattern in various type of tumors. These factors, such as the nature of tumor, its extent, pattern of presentation, and recurrence, have dictated the radiotherapy techniques.

S. S. Nanda · P. Giridhar
Department of Radiation Oncology, Tata Memorial Center, Varanasi, India

S. Mallick (✉)
Department of Radiation Oncology, National Cancer Institute, Jhajjar, Haryana, India

2nd Campus AIIMS, New Delhi, Delhi, India



R. Madan et al. (eds.), *Evidence Based Practice in Pediatric Radiation Oncology*, https://doi.org/10.1007/978-981-96-4872-6_3

## 3.2 Different Forms of RT

The PENTEC data [1] has demonstrated that in pediatric population, each normal tissue has its inherent threshold for radiation, and traditionally it has been shown to have lower than the adult patients. Further, these tolerances are modified by use of concurrent sensitizers, protectors, and chemotherapeutic agents along with RT [2]. This has led to innovation in RT techniques to optimize tumor control while limiting the normal tissue complication probability (NTCP). Numerous RT delivery techniques have been used in pediatric population over time. These include three-dimensional conformal therapy (3DCRT), intensity-modulated radiation therapy (IMRT), intraoperative radiotherapy (IORT), proton therapy, stereotactic radiosurgery, and brachytherapy. Use of radiotherapy to treat malignancy has evolved from use of low-energy orthovoltage photons [3] to high-energy photon or electron. Of late, particle therapy such as proton has taken the center stage, which have a very favorable beam profile that can be of particular significance in pediatric tumors. Unlike photon beam, which has a significant exit dose that contributes to increased integral dose, proton has a sharp Bragg peak followed by rapid dose fall off [4]. This significantly reduces the dose received by OARS [4], which are beyond the tumor along the beam axis. Thus, proton therapy has been hypothesized to reduce the dose received by critical OAR and the region of body receiving lower isodose lines, which are contributory to secondary malignancy.

Prior to 1970, radiation therapy was primarily two–dimensional, using standard opposed field portals guided by surface anatomy as a surrogate marker for target volumes. During 1970 to 1980, with the widespread introduction of cross-sectional imaging, RT techniques evolved to three-dimensional conformal RT techniques. The use of cross-sectional images allowed RT beam placement in different angles than traditional opposed pair techniques. Further couch movement with newer machines allowed the use of non-coplanar beam for the delivery of optimum dose in critical sites, such as pituitary tumors and ethmoid sinus tumors, where vertex beams was used. Introduction of computer-based planning systems allowed beam eye views (BEVs) which allowed better optimization of beam entry angle as per the need of the target volume and adjoining OAR [5]. Further refinement in computer-based planning systems enabled rapid planning, even in complex plans, using both planar and non-co-planar beams and allowed for an appropriate dose distribution, even in complex non-homogenous tissues, with greater degree of accuracy. This approach of defining the target followed by beam placement and optimizing beam angles and weightage to meet the essential planning parameters is known as forward planning [6]. Computer-based planning algorithms enabled quick planning, but they had the inherent limitation of number of beam angles and weightages that can be optimized manually. This led to development of inverse planning system, which forms the basis for IMRT. Here the planning parameters are set and computer-based planning algorithms calculate the optimum angle/arc to meet these parameters. Inverse planning system [7] provided rapid plan generation with higher degree of combination of beam angle/arc, weightage, and beam modulation via multi-leaf collimator movement to attain ideal plan.

## 3.3 IMRT in Pediatric Tumors

- IMRT is the modern radiotherapy technique that uses computer-based reverse optimization to achieve dose intensity modulation in order to deliver the desired dose to the tumor. It has the advantage of optimization, which enables limiting doses to critical adjoining OARS.
- IMRT has been further modified in volumetric modulated arc therapy which uses fixed degree arc in place of static gantry angles, resulting in dynamic beam shaping during continuous gantry rotation.
- VMAT has the potential advantage of reducing on treatment time and providing more degree of freedom for beam optimization than fixed field IMRT. This could be beneficial in very small children requiring daily anesthesia by reducing the treatment time.
- Despite these potential benefits of IMRT, its use in pediatric tumors has been limited. Proponents of IMRT in pediatric malignancy emphasize on the potential benefit of reducing RT-related toxicities in children who have a lesser tolerance level than adult population.
- RT-related acute morbidities, such as mucositis, skin reactions, nausea, and vomiting, may have lasting physical as well as psychological implications in children. Whether, its somnolence syndrome or pituitary and thyroid hypofunctioning, which is a well-documented phenomenon in pediatric patients undergoing cranial RT, can have a long-standing impact on the overall wellbeing of these children.
- Late radiation-related morbidities such as growth retardation or loss of reproductive function may be reduced by use of IMRT.
- The improvement of surgical techniques, RT techniques, and chemotherapeutic agents has resulted in improved survival in many pediatric malignancies. This has put the limelight back on the late toxicities related to RT [8]
- Numerous studies have reported increase in integral dose and low-dose regions in VMAT/IMRT vis-a-vis conventional RT [9, 10]. This has been hypothesized to be contributory to secondary malignancy in long-term survivors.
- The Surveillance, Epidemiology and End Results (SEER) database has reported almost 17–19% patients developing second malignancy after long survival from first malignancy [11].
- Genetic susceptibility, continued exposure to carcinogens, chemotherapy drugs, and RT contribute to it. The exact contribution of RT to the causation of this remains determined. Despite numerous hypothesis, a comparative analysis between conventional RT vis-a-vis IMRT/VMAT with respect to causation of second malignancy is lacking.
- Numerous studies have reported a lower rate of second malignancy with proton therapy compared to photon therapy. Chung et al. reported second malignancy rate 7.5% versus 5.2% for photon therapy and proton therapy, respectively [12]. This has been attributed to the favorable Bragg's peak, which contributes to lower exit dose, thus reducing the integral dose.

## 3.4 Brachytherapy in Pediatric Malignancies

- Children are not small adults. Long-term issues, such as hormone dysfunction, growth abnormalities, and risk of second malignancies, need to be kept in mind while designing protocols for management in children organ preservation being the key target.
- In addition to conservative surgery versus amputation/exenteration, brachytherapy is an option to reduce radiation-related toxicities in certain malignancies of childhood and to achieve local control.
- The section will explain the types of brachytherapy, modifications for pediatric brachytherapy versus adults, common indications and doses, and data on outcomes. The last section will include a description on plaque brachytherapy for ocular tumors.

**Types:** Brachytherapy can be classified as intraoperative HDR brachytherapy (IOHDR), intraoperative electron therapy (IOERT), LDR brachytherapy (LDR), fractionated HDR brachytherapy (f HDR), and temporary plaque brachytherapy (Table 3.1).

**Table 3.1** Types of brachytherapy

| Type | IOHDR | IOERT | LDR | F HDR | Plaque |
|---|---|---|---|---|---|
| Treatment time | Minutes | Minutes | 2–7 days | 6–8 days | 3–7 days |
| Doses | 10–15 Gy | 10–15 Gy | 40–45 Gy | 36–50 Gy in fractions of 3–4 Gy with at least 8 h gap | 40–80 Gy |
| Indication | Sarcoma, lacrimal gland/ orbital tumors as boost to EBRT | Sarcoma, lacrimal gland/ orbital tumors as boost to EBRT | Gynecological, orbital, genito-urinary RMS, < 5 cm sarcoma with negative margins | Gynecological, orbital, genito-urinary RMS, < 5 cm sarcoma with negative margins | Retinoblastoma, melanoma, choroidal metastases |
| Dosimetry | Surface dose: 200% At 2 cm depth: 30% | Surface dose: 80% At 2 cm depth: 90% | NA | NA | NA |
| Re-oxygenation | No role | No role | Yes, involved | Yes, involved | Yes, involved |
| Repair of SLD | No role | No role | Yes, involved | Yes, involved | Yes, involved |
| Re-distribution | No role | No role | Yes, involved | Yes, involved | Yes, involved |

## 3.5 Considerations in Pediatric Patients

The techniques and doses used in pediatric brachytherapy are similar to those in adults with some modifications.

1. Shorter inter-catheter spacing (8 mm–max 1 cm).
2. Reduced margins around clinical target volume.

   *Both the above modifications reduce the total volume receiving the prescribed dose [13].
3. Radiation oncologist should preferably be in the operating theater to note the location of tumor and its relation with growth plate and nerves.
4. A custom-made mold is preferred for vaginal tumors.
5. Mild sedation during brachytherapy treatment should be considered [14].

Common Indications:

1. Soft tissue sarcoma (alone in <5 cm, high grade and negative margins; with EBRT in others)
2. Clear cell adenocarcinoma vagina (alone or with EBRT; custom-made mold or interstitial implant)
3. Lacrimal gland tumors
4. Gynecological/genito-urinary RMS (alone or with EBRT; custom-made mold or interstitial implant)
5. Retinoblastoma (plaque)
6. Ocular melanoma (plaque)

Outcomes (Table 3.2):

**Table 3.2** Disease-specific outcomes [14]

| Disease | Clear cell adenocarcinoma vagina [15] | Ewing sarcoma/ PNET [16] | Neuroblastoma [17] | Retinoblastoma [18] | Rhabdomyosarcoma (vesico-prostatic) [19] | Rhabdomyosarcoma (vulvo-vaginal) [20] | Soft tissue sarcoma [21] |
|---|---|---|---|---|---|---|---|
| Treatment used | Surgery with ovarian transposition f/b EBRT and brachytherapy | IOHDR and EBRT | IOHDR and EBRT | Plaque LDR temporary | LDR brachytherapy +/– EBRT | LDR brachytherapy | LDR brachytherapy +/– EBRT |
| Survival outcome | DFS at 5 years: 78%<br>Organ preservation: 70% | Local control at 2 years: 56–100% | Local control at 2 years: 56% | 4-year local control: 83% | 9-year local control: 56% | 13-year local control: 100% | 5-year local control: 61–68% |
| Toxicity | Grade 2 and 3 late toxicity: 35% | 2-year complication rate: 12% | 2-year complication rate: 12% | 31% cataract<br>25% maculopathy<br>15% proliferative retinopathy<br>11% glaucoma | No grade 2 or higher | 23% risk of stenosis (vaginal/urethral/ ureteral stenosis) | 5-year late toxicity: 23% |

## 3.6 Plaque Brachytherapy

- Malignant tumors of the orbit are usually treated by surgical excision and EBRT. Plaque radiotherapy precisely delivers radiation dose to the tumor apex with minimal dose to the surrounding ocular/orbital tissues.
- It can be done in cases of residual tumor, recurrence of the tumor after prior surgery or EBRT or chemotherapy.
- Common indications for plaque brachytherapy are adenoid cystic carcinoma of the lacrimal gland, orbital invasion of the basal cell and squamous cell carcinoma, orbital melanoma, retinoblastoma, and metastatic tumors.
- Common radiation plaques used are Iodine-125 ($^{125}I$), Palladium-103 ($^{103}Pd$), and Ruthenium ($^{106}Ru$) plaque.
- Plaque brachytherapy involves placing a radioactive implant directly to the target tumor. It is made of a gold-plated dome/shell with appropriately placed radioactive seeds or wires. The eye plaque is 6–22 mm in diameter [15].
- Iodine-125 seeds (model 6711) are available at strength of up to 5 mCi/seed and Palladium-103 seeds (model 200) at strength of 2 mCi/seed [16].
- Duration of the treatment typically varies from 3 to 7 days depending on the thickness and largest basal diameter and type of the tumor.
- The radiation dose varies from 40 to 80 Gy depending on the type of tumor (40 Gy in retinoblastoma; 80 Gy in melanoma) [17].
- *Plaque brachytherapy surgery is* performed under peribulbar or general anesthesia by trained ocular oncologist.
- Depending on the location of the tumor, the area of the tumor is marked, and sutures are preplaced using a dummy plaque. After that, the real gold eye plaque with radioactive seeds is sutured that can cover the target tumor volume.
- Side effects of plaque radiation may include redness, tearing, eyelid swelling, cicatricial scarring leading to ectropion or entropion, acute conjunctivitis, keratitis, dry eyes, iris atrophy, iris neo-vascularization, cataract, secondary glaucoma, sclera thinning and necrosis, radiation maculopathy, radiation retinopathy, vitreous hemorrhage, chorioretinal atrophy, retinal vascular sclerosis (retinal vein/artery occlusions), orbital bone hypoplasia, and orbital bone growth retardation leading to asymmetry and orbital deformities [18]

## 3.7 Role of Image Guidance in Pediatric Malignancies

The children oncology group has recently published practice recommendations for image guidance in pediatric radiotherapy taking into consideration increased radiation dose with more frequent imaging and its possible risks and benefits. The recommendation is summarized below [19].

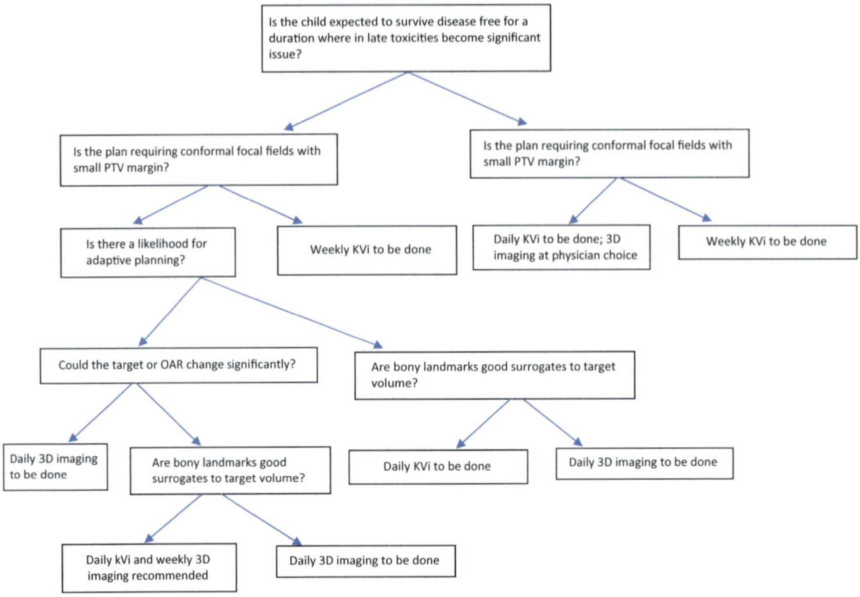


## References


1. Constine LS, Ronckers CM, Hua CH et al. Pediatric Normal Tissue Effects in the Clinic (PENTEC): An International Collaboration to Analyse Normal Tissue Radiation Dose-Volume Response Relationships for Paediatric Cancer Patients. Clin Oncol (R Coll Radiol). 2019;31(3):199–207. https://doi.org/10.1016/j.clon.2019.01.002.
2. Swift P. Novel techniques in the delivery of radiation in pediatric oncology. Pediatr Clin North Am. 2002;49(5):1107–29. https://doi.org/10.1016/s0031-3955(02)00037-8. PMID: 12430628.
3. Tucker MA, D'Angio GJ, Boice JD Jr, Strong LC, Li FP, Stovall M, Stone BJ, Green DM, Lombardi F, Newton W, et al. Bone sarcomas linked to radiotherapy and chemotherapy in children. N Engl J Med. 1987;317(10):588–9 https://doi.org/10.1056/NEJM198709033171002. PMID: 3475572.
4. Steinmeier T, Schulze Schleithoff S, Timmermann B. Evolving radiotherapy techniques in paediatric oncology. Clin Oncol. 2019;31(3):142e150.
5. Purdy JA. 3D treatment planning and intensity-modulated radiation therapy. Oncology (Huntingt). 1999;13:155–68.
6. Verhey LJ. Comparison of three-dimensional conformal radiation therapy and intensity-modulated radiation therapy systems. Semin Radiat Oncol. 1999;9:78–98.
7. Rosenman J. Incorporating functional imaging information into radiation treatment. Semin Radiat Oncol. 2001;11:83–92.
8. Mullenders L, Atkinson M, Paretzke H, Sabatier L, Bouffler S.Assessing cancer risks of low-dose radiation. Nat Rev Cancer 2009;9:596–604.
9. Hall EJ. Intensity-modulated radiation therapy, protons, and the risk of second cancers. Int J Radiat Oncol Biol Phys 2006;65:1–7.
10. Friedman DL, Whitton J, Leisenring W, et al. Subsequent neoplasms in 5-year survivors of childhood cancer: the childhood Cancer survivor study. J Natl Cancer Inst. 2010;102:1083–95.

11. Morton LM, Onel K, Curtis RE, Hungate EA, Armstrong GT. The rising incidence of second cancers: patterns of occurrence and identification of risk factors for children and adults. Am Soc Clin Oncol Educ Book. 2014;2014:e57–67.
12. Chung CS, Yock TI, Nelson K, Xu Y, Keating NL, Tarbell NJ. Incidence of second malignancies among patients treated with proton versus photon radiation. Int J Radiat Oncol Biol Phys. 2013;87:46–52.
13. Martinez-Monge R, Cambeiro M, San-Julián M, Sierrasesúmaga L. Use of brachytherapy in children with cancer: the search for an uncomplicated cure. Lancet Oncol. 2006;7(2):157–66.
14. Nag S, Tippin DB. Brachytherapy for pediatric tumors. Brachytherapy. 2003;2(3):131–8.
15. Shields JA, Shields CL, Freire JE et al (2003 Plaque radiotherapy for selected orbital malignancies: preliminary observations: the Montgomery Lecture, part 2. Ophthalmic Plast Reconstr Surg. 2002;19(2):91–5.
16. Meigooni AS, Sabnis S, Nath R. Dosimetry of palladium-103 brachytherapy sources for permanent implants. Endocuriether Hypertherm Oncol. 1990;6(2):107–117.
17. Stannard C, Sauerwein W, Maree G et al. Radiotherapy for ocular tumours. Eye (Lond) 2013;27(2):119–27.
18. Durkin SR, Roos D, Higgs B et al. Ophthalmic and adnexal complications of radiotherapy. Acta Ophthalmol Scand. 2007;85(3):240–50.
19. Hua CH, Vern-Gross TZ, Hess CB, et al. Practice patterns and recommendations for pediatric image-guided radiotherapy: A Children's Oncology Group report. Pediatr Blood Cancer. 2020 Oct;67(10):e28629.

# Early and Late Effects of Radiotherapy in Children

4

Venkata Krishna Vamsi Gade

## 4.1 Review of Radiobiology

X-rays and gamma rays produce cell kill by indirect free radical damage to DNA. This damage while initially transient and repairable becomes fixed and permanent in the presence of oxygen. This free radical damage leads to various lethal chromosomal aberrations such as dicentric chromosomes, ring chromosomes, and anaphase bridges. The linear quadratic model is best suited and widely used to describe the cell kill after radiation. After an initial straight-line linear component (denoted by $\alpha$), where cell kill is directly proportional to dose and occurs due to single track events, the survival curve bends and becomes curved due to the quadratic component (denoted by $\beta$), where the cell kill is proportional to the square of the dose. In the region of this shoulder, cell kill mainly occurs due to multiple track events [1].

The $\alpha/\beta$ ratio is the ratio at which the linear and quadratic components of cell kill are equal. Different tumors and normal tissues have different $\alpha/\beta$ ratio which are calculated based on clinical isoeffect models. Early reacting tissues are those with high rate of turnover and regenerative capacity. They have a high $\alpha/\beta$ ratio (taken as 10) and are responsible for the acute effects of radiotherapy (skin, mucosal lining, and bone marrow). These effects manifest during or within few weeks of start of radiotherapy and usually subside after a few months. Late-reacting tissues are usually highly differentiated and have a low regenerative capacity. They have a low $\alpha/\beta$ ratio (taken as 3) and are responsible for the late effects of radiotherapy (neural tissue, kidney and heart). These effects manifest 6 months to many years after radiotherapy. Early effects depend on dose per fraction and overall treatment time, whereas late effects depend on dose per fraction alone [2].

V. K. V. Gade (✉)
Department of Radiotherapy and Oncology, PGIMER, Chandigarh, India





R. Madan et al. (eds.), *Evidence Based Practice in Pediatric Radiation Oncology*, https://doi.org/10.1007/978-981-96-4872-6_4

Withers and Taylor introduced the concept of functional subunit (FSU) where all organs were proposed to consist of FSUs. These could be structurally or functionally defined as units capable of being repopulated by a single clonogenic cell. Based on the arrangement of FSUs, various organs are classified into serial or parallel organs. Serial organs (e.g., spinal cord, brainstem, and optic neural structures) have FSUs arranged like links of a chain, where disruption of a single FSU affects the entire organ. High dose at a particular point is relevant in evaluating dose to these organs. In the case of parallel organs (e.g., lung, kidney, and heart), organ function is maintained provided that a limited number of FSUs are functional. Volumetric constraints are relevant in this setting [3, 4].

Radiation-induced side effects can be broadly classified into stochastic or deterministic effects. Stochastic effects occur due to cellular modification and do not have a threshold dose. The probability of occurrence increases with the dose, but the severity is not dose related. Radiation-induced second malignancies and hereditary effects of radiation are classical examples. Deterministic effects are those with a defined threshold dose beyond which the incidence dramatically increases. The severity is dose related. Deterministic effects occur due to cell killing that affects organ function. Radiation-induced cataracts and other dose-related toxicities are deterministic effects [5].

## 4.2 Attempts to Quantify Normal Tissue Toxicity in Adults and Children

Before 1990, dose-related effects of radiotherapy on normal tissues were estimated based on institutional and expert experiences. Rubin first introduced the concept of TD 5/5 and TD 50/5, where TD 5/5 was the tolerance dose for 5% toxicity at 5 years. Pooling the experiences up to that point, various investigators in 1991 published the Emami paper that prescribed TD 5/5 and 50/5 constraints for 26 organs concerning both full volume and partial-volume irradiation. However volumetric information was limited and much of the paper was based on expert opinion [6].

With the advent of 3D treatment planning systems and conformal radiotherapy in the 2000s, it became possible to quantify exact dose-volume characteristics for each organ. In 2007, the ASTRO-AAPM task force was convened to provide a more detailed review of dose-volume characteristics for various organs at risk. In 2010, the QUANTEC (Quantitative Analysis of Normal Tissue Effects in the Clinic) review was published with detailed dose-volume data correlating with clinical endpoints for 16 organs [7]. However, clinicians encountered several uncertainties while applying QUANTEC data to pediatric radiotherapy. This was due to the varied vulnerability of developing tissues and varied sites as compared to adult radiotherapy. Hence, the PENTEC (Paediatric Normal Tissue Effects in the Clinic) group was formed to provide quantitative dose-volume irradiation data for 18 sites in children. The work of the PENTEC group is ongoing and detailed dose-volume data is awaited [8].

## 4.3 Common Early Effects After Radiotherapy

### 4.3.1 Skin Reactions

The skin is composed of the dermis and epidermis. The epidermis consists of stratum corneum, stratum granulosum, stratum spinosum, and stratum basale. The basal layer consists of actively dividing cells that push older layers toward the surface of the skin. It takes approximately 14 days for a cell in the basal layer to reach the stratum corneum. Hence, the first radiation reactions take approximately 2 weeks to manifest since the start of radiotherapy [9].

According to the CTCAE (Common Terminology Criteria for Adverse Events) version 5, Grade 1 changes include follicular or mild generalized erythema and dry desquamation. Grade 2 changes include persistent tender or edematous erythema, which can progress moist desquamation in skin folds with loss of epidermal lining. This usually occurs 4 weeks after radiotherapy and after a dose of 40 Gy. Grade 3 dermatitis includes confluent moist desquamation in areas other than skin folds which usually occurs after a dose of 50 Gy and after 5–6 weeks. Ulceration, necrosis, and hemorrhage suggest Grade 4 dermatitis that can occur with doses over 60 Gy [10–12].

### 4.3.2 Oral Mucositis

Oral mucositis is a consequence of the radiotherapy of the head and neck region. In contrast to the skin, turnover time for mucosal epithelium is faster and hence reactions occur a few weeks earlier. Grade 1 changes include mucosal erythema. Patchy ulceration or pseudomembrane formation signals a Grade 2 change. Grade 3 mucositis includes confluent mucositis or pseudomembrane bleeding with minor trauma. The presence of necrosis, spontaneous bleeding, and life-threatening events suggest Grade 4 mucositis. Maintenance of good oral hygiene, adequate nutritional intake, and hydration can prevent mucositis [13, 14].

### 4.3.3 Esophagitis

Acute esophageal mucosal injury after radiotherapy can present with dysphagia and odynophagia. The patients can have reduced oral intake further worsening their quality of life. Esophageal mucositis is a consequence of thoracic radiotherapy and large field treatments like craniospinal irradiation (CSI) for medulloblastoma. Grade 1 esophagitis is asymptomatic. Patients with Grade 2 esophagitis present with altered swallowing and require a soft solid or semisolid diet. Severely altered swallowing with the requirement of tube feeding and intravenous fluids suggests Grade 3 esophagitis. Grade 4 esophagitis is life-threatening. According to the QUANTEC review, an esophageal mean dose of less than 34 Gy is associated with a 5–20% incidence of Grade 3 or higher esophagitis. Grade 1 and 2 esophagitis can be improved with local anesthetic gels, diet modifications, and antacids to prevent superadded reflux injury. Grade 3 esophagitis may require interruption of radiotherapy [7, 13, 15].

### 4.3.4 Myelosuppression

Dividing bone marrow is extremely sensitive to radiotherapy. From birth to about 1 year of age, hematopoiesis occurs in the red marrow of the bones all through the body. As the child grows older, hematopoiesis becomes restricted to the skull, sternum, ribs, vertebrae, pelvis, and proximal ends of the femur. Yellow marrow, comprised of fat cells with limited potential for division, replaces the red marrow with age [16]. The hematopoietic system is of concern with radiotherapy to the pelvis and large-field radiotherapy such as CSI and total body irradiation (TBI) (Fig. 4.1).

Lymphocytes are the most radiosensitive cells and begin to deplete after a radiation exposure of as little as 0.3 Gy. This is followed by a fall in granulocytes, thrombocytes, and red blood cells in that order in the irradiated marrow. The unirradiated marrow experiences a compensatory hyperplasia. Myelosuppression is more pronounced when chemotherapy is concurrently administered. The bone marrow

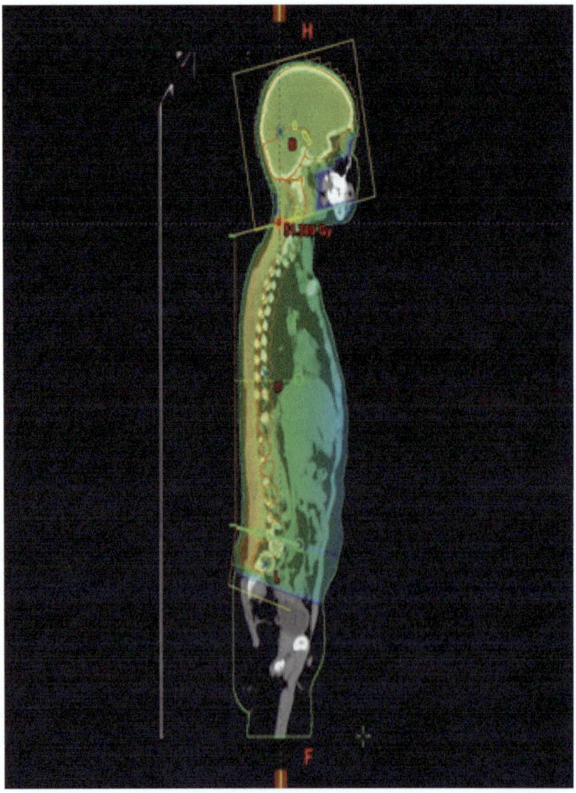


**Fig. 4.1** Large field treatments like craniospinal irradiation in medulloblastoma produce significant myelosuppression due to irradiation of active bone marrow sites

**Table 4.1** CTCAE v5: hematological toxicity

| Blood element | Grade 1 | Grade 2 | Grade 3 | Grade 4 | Grade 5 |
|---|---|---|---|---|---|
| Neutrophils | <LLN to 1500/ microL | 1000 to 1500/ microL | 500 to 1000/ microL | <500/microL | |
| Platelets | <LLN to 75,000/ microL | 50,000 to 75,000/ microL | 25,000 to 50,000/ microL | <25,000/microL | |
| Hemoglobin | <LLN to 10 g/dL | 8.0 to 10.0 g/dL | <8.0 g/dL | Life-threatening consequences; urgent intervention indicated | Death |

stromal cells are relatively resistant to radiotherapy. However, TBI delivered in high-dose rates (>0.5 Gy/min) or high dose per fraction has been found to disrupt the stromal cells preventing transplantation [17–19]. Neutropenia, thrombocytopenia, and anemia are classified separately under CTCAE v5 classification (Table 4.1).

Grade 1 and 2 toxicities are usually managed conservatively. Grade 3 toxicity may require interruption of radiotherapy and growth factors and or blood transfusion.

### 4.3.5 Early Radiation-Induced Brain Injury

The earliest symptom of radiation-induced brain injury is generalized restlessness and somnolence, which is hypothesized to occur due to transient demyelination of neurons in the irradiated field. This can progress to worsening fatigue, headache, projectile vomiting, visual disturbances, and other features of raised intracranial pressure that occurs due to increased edema and disruption of the blood-brain barrier (BBB). Explicit features of raised intracranial pressure with neurological deficits are more likely to be seen on radiotherapy in patients with large disease burden, pre-existing edema, and hypofractionated regimens. Such symptoms may be debilitating and may require interruption of radiotherapy and institution of medical decompressive measures including intravenous glucocorticoids and mannitol [20].

## 4.4 Late Effects of Radiotherapy

### 4.4.1 Effects on the Central Nervous System

#### 4.4.1.1 Radiation Necrosis

Radiation necrosis is the most dreaded endpoint that effects dose-volume prescription in cranial radiotherapy. It may be asymptomatic and detected on imaging alone or may present with focal neurological deficit pertaining to the site of radiation necrosis or with neurocognitive defects. It typically occurs 3 months to several years after radiotherapy. The Emami review mentions a TD5/5 of 60 Gy, 50 Gy, and

45 Gy for 1/third brain, 2/third brain, and whole brain, respectively [6]. According to the QUANTEC review, there is a < 3% risk of radionecrosis for a maximum dose of 60 Gy (conventionally fractionated) which increases to 5% for a dose of 72 Gy and 10% for a dose of 90 Gy. For stereotactic techniques, a V12Gy < 5–10 cc for whole brain is associated with a less than 20% risk of radiation necrosis [7]. The PENTEC group proposed a radiation necrosis model for children that estimates a 5% risk of necrosis for a maximum dose of 59.8 Gy in a primary radiotherapy setting and 63.6 Gy in the reirradiation setting [21].

#### 4.4.1.2 Neurocognitive Dysfunction

Neurocognitive dysfunction following radiotherapy manifests in several months to years after radiotherapy and may take the form of early cognitive decline, impairment of memory, spatial processing, learning, and dementia. The symptoms of cognitive impairment in adults are more apparent if cranial radiotherapy was delivered for childhood cancers. These symptoms may include delayed milestone development, poor academic performance, reduced social interaction, and reduced Intelligence Quotient (IQ) scores [22, 23]. Studies of prophylactic cranial irradiation for acute leukemia in children showed a 13 point IQ reduction at 5 years for a dose of 24 Gy [24]. Studies in medulloblastoma showed that with reduced dose cranial radiotherapy of 23.4 Gy vs. standard dose of 36 Gy, there was 10 to 15 point improvement in IQ scores [25]. The PENTEC group proposed a 5% risk of below average IQ (IQ < 85) when 10%, 20%, 50%, and 100% of the brain received a dose of 35.7, 29.1, 22.2, or 18.1 Gy, respectively. The addition of methotrexate further increased the risk [21]. The use of hippocampal sparing techniques and the use of memantine have shown to improve neurocognitive outcomes after radiotherapy in adults [26, 27]. But data is sparse to support their use in pediatric population.

#### 4.4.1.3 Cerebrovascular Events

Stroke and cerebral ischemia are potentially debilitating events that contribute to significant morbidity and mortality. Radiation-induced damage to the anterior cerebral circulation and circle of Willis is thought to play a major role. A PENTEC modeling study found that the total radiotherapy dose predicted the cerebrovascular event risk and proposed a sigmoidal dose response for cerebrovascular events (CVAs) [28]. Radiotherapy dose exceeding 50 Gy to the temporal or frontal lobes also increased the risk of stroke in childhood survivors of medulloblastoma [29].

#### 4.4.1.4 Effects on the Optic Apparatus

Optic neuropathy is the end point for radiation-induced damage to the optic neural apparatus. The QUANTEC review specifies a 3% risk of optic neuropathy for a maximum dose of 54 Gy that increases to as high as 20% for maximum dose exceeding 60 Gy. For stereotactic radiotherapy, a maximum dose of 12 Gy correlates with a less than 10% risk of optic neuropathy [7]. Radiation-induced cataract is another common late effect of cranial radiotherapy. Posterior subcapsular cataract is characteristically linked with radiation exposure and occurs after a latent period of about 8 years for a dose up to 6.5 Gy. Higher doses are associated with a faster onset. The

International Commission on Radiological Protection (ICRP) classifies cataract as a deterministic effect with a threshold dose of 2 Gy for single acute exposure and 5–8 Gy for prolonged exposure [30].

#### 4.4.1.5 Effects on the Auditory Apparatus

Sensorineural hearing loss (SNHL), tinnitus, and vertigo are consequences of damage to the vestibulo-cochlear apparatus. QUANTEC mentions a cochlear mean dose of 45 Gy to correlate with a less than 30% risk of sensorineural hearing loss, whereas in stereotactic settings a prescription dose of 14 Gy is associated with a 25% risk of of SNHL [7]. In a study of long-term survivors of childhood medulloblastoma, the 30-year risk of tinnitus and hearing loss were 30.1% and 37.4%, respectively, whereas the incidence of problems with balance and coordination was as high as 72% at 30 years. The risks of deafness and hearing loss were also found to be associated with a higher dose received by the temporal or frontal lobe [29]. Acute and chronic serous otitis can occur as a result of radiation exposure to the external and middle ear [31].

#### 4.4.1.6 Effect on the Brainstem and Cranial Nerves

Brainstem necrosis and cranial neuropathy are the endpoints for brainstem and cranial nerve damage. According to the QUANTEC review, a maximum dose of 54 Gy or a maximum volume exceeding 54 Gy of up to 10 cc is associated with a 5% risk of cranial neuropathy. For stereotactic radiosurgery, a maximum dose of 12.5 Gy is associated with a 5% risk of cranial neuropathy. There appears to be a rapid increase in the risk of cranial neuropathy if the maximum dose exceeds 15 Gy per fraction [7, 32].

#### 4.4.1.7 Radiation-Induced Myelopathy

It is a rare but serious late effect of radiotherapy. Radiation-induced endothelial damage of the perineural vessels and damage to the myelin-producing oligodendrocytes are the possible mechanisms [33]. Emami et al. proposed a constraint of TD5/5 of 50 Gy for 5 cm and 10 cm of the cord and a constraint of 47 Gy for 20 cm of the cord. According to the QUANTEC review, a maximum dose of 50 Gy is associated with 0.5% risk of myelopathy which increased to 6% and 50% for a dose of 59 Gy and 69 Gy [6, 7]. Lhermitte's sign is one of the first signs of demyelination which develops several months after radiotherapy. Demyelination and vasculopathy manifest after 6 months to several years after the insult [34].

### 4.4.2 Endocrine Dysfunction

Hypopituitarism is seen in 30–60% of the patients undergoing cranial radiotherapy after a latent period of 5–10 years. Different cells of the pituitary appear to have varying sensitivity to radiotherapy with growth hormone deficiency occurring first at a dose of 18 Gy followed by FSH/LH deficiency at a dose of 30 Gy. This is followed by ACTH and TSH deficiency [35–38]. Growth hormone deficiency can lead to stunting and short stature, whereas FSH/LH deficiency can cause infertility, loss of secondary sexual characteristics, and loss of libido. While TSH deficiency causes secondary hypothyroidism, radiation-induced damage to the thyroid gland causes primary hypothyroidism. According to the PENTEC group, a mean thyroid gland dose of 30 Gy is associated with a 13% risk of clinical hypothyroidism and 44% risk of subclinical hypothyroidism [39].

### 4.4.3 Dysphagia and Aspiration

Dysphagia and aspiration are potentially morbid side effects after radiotherapy to the head and neck region. About 30% of patients with dysphagia develop aspiration. Aspiration after head and neck radiotherapy has a mortality rate as high as 70%. A mean dose to the larynx of 50 Gy is associated with a 30% risk of aspiration. Dysphagia aspiration-related structures (DARS) are said to include the base of tongue, floor of mouth, superior and middle pharyngeal constrictors, cricopharynx, and proximal esophagus. DARS are now being studied together to potentially spare these structures and prevent dysphagia and aspiration [7, 40, 41].

### 4.4.4 Xerostomia

Radiation-induced damage to the major and minor salivary glands leads to xerostomia. The QUANTEC review mentions a bilateral parotid mean dose of 25 Gy to be associated with a 20% risk of long-term salivary dysfunction (<25%) [7]. The PENTEC group mentions that a mean parotid dose of 35–40 Gy in children is associated with a 32% risk of acute xerostomia and 13–32% risk of more than Grade 2 chronic xerostomia [42]. The adoption of IMRT has led to reduced incidences of xerostomia without any differences in clinical outcomes [43].

### 4.4.5 Pulmonary and Cardiac Toxicity

Radiation-induced pneumonitis occurs in two phases. The acute phase occurs 2–6 months following radiotherapy. The chronic fibrotic phase occurs several years after radiotherapy. Vascular endothelial cells and surfactant producing Type 2 pneumocytes are the targets which trigger a complex cytokine-mediated cascade. Acute pneumonitis can be asymptomatic or present with dry cough, dyspnea, and chest pain [44]. Chronic fibrosis is associated with slowly progressing dyspnea on exertion and dry cough. A V20Gy of up to 30% is associated with a 20% risk of symptomatic pneumonitis. Mean lung doses of 7, 13, 20, 24, and 27 Gy are associated with 5%, 10%, 20%, 30%, and 40% risk of pneumonitis, respectively [7]. The PENTEC review suggests that for a mean lung dose of less than 14 Gy and V20Gy < 30%, the risk of symptomatic pneumonitis is very low [45].

The pericardial sac is sensitive to radiotherapy. Pericarditis post radiotherapy usually occurs 12 months to several years after radiotherapy with varying severity. Patients usually complain of dyspnea, low-grade fever, and chest pain. A mean dose of 26 Gy and a V30Gy <46% is associated with a 15% risk of pericarditis [7]. Patients of Hodgkin's lymphoma post thoracic radiotherapy had an up to 85% incidence of coronary artery disease with a twofold increase in risk of death due to myocardial events. Cardiomyopathy post radiotherapy is also described with V25Gy < 10% correlating with a 1% risk of long-term cardiac mortality. The use of drugs such as doxorubicin and trastuzumab along with radiotherapy increases the risk of cardiac toxicity [46–48].

### 4.4.6 Liver and Renal Toxicity

Radiation-induced liver disease (RILD) is of two types. Classic RILD presents in patients with a previously healthy liver with features of anorexia, abdominal pain, and anicteric ascites. It is usually accompanied by alkaline phosphatase (ALP) elevation with normal bilirubin and transaminase. Nonclassic RILD occurs in patients with pre-existing liver disease such as hepatitis or cirrhosis and presents with jaundice and transaminase elevation. A mean dose of 30 Gy to the liver is associated with 5% risk of RILD which rises to 50% with a mean dose of 42 Gy [7, 49].

The FSUs of the kidney are arranged in a unique manner such that the lobules of the kidney are considered to in be parallel arrangement, but nephrons draining into a single collecting tubule have a serial arrangement. Radiation nephropathy typically manifests with arterial hypertension, osteodystrophy, and anemia. A mean dose to bilateral kidneys of 15 Gy is associated with a 5% risk of renal dysfunction which increases to 50% for a dose of 28 Gy [7, 50].

### 4.4.7 Late Bladder and Rectal Toxicity

Radiation cystitis usually manifests several years after radiotherapy. Radiation-induced vascular damage causes obliterative endarteritis that makes the bladder mucosa hypovascular, hypocellular, and hypoxic. Under such circumstances, the bladder mucosa sloughs off causing hematuria. Grade 1 cystitis is usually asymptomatic with microscopic hematuria. Grade 2 cystitis presents with gross hematuria that usually self-subsides. Grade 3 cystitis requires blood transfusions and bladder irrigation, whereas Grade 4 cystitis presents with catastrophic hematuria requiring emergency interventions such as cystoscopic fulguration, ligation of internal iliac arteries, or cystectomy with urinary diversion. With conventional fractionation, it has been seen that V65Gy < 50% is a feasible constraint to prevent Grade 3 cystitis with several other constraints mentioned in the QUANTEC review [7, 51].

Late radiation proctitis presents 6 months to several years after radiotherapy. It occurs due to radiation-induced telangiectasia, submucosal fibrosis, and obliterative endarteritis. Tenesmus, rectal bleeding, and stricture formation are the presenting symptoms. In conventional fractionation, V50Gy <50% and V60Gy < 35% is associated with a < 10% risk of Grade 3 or higher proctitis. Treatment options include oral medication such as 5-aminosalicylic acid derivatives and antibiotics, rectal instillation of steroids, sucralfate, and formalin, and endoscopic therapies such as argon laser photocoagulation [7, 52].

### 4.4.8 Infertility

A dose as less as 0.15 Gy causes a temporary reduction in the number of sperms produced (oligospermia). Doses up to 0.5 Gy cause temporary azoospermia that is reversible in a few months. A dose of 6 Gy delivered in single fraction or 3–4 Gy delivered in fractionated format causes permanent sterility. Male sterility induced due to radiotherapy does not affect libido [53]. In the case of females, during the prepuberal age group, a dose of 12 Gy is required to produce sterility, which reduces to 2 Gy in the premenopausal age group. Radiation-induced sterility in females induces a permanent menopause with reduced libido and changes in bone mineral density [54, 55].

### 4.4.9 Second Malignancies

Radiation-induced second malignancies are becoming more common especially with improved survival outcomes in childhood cancers. A large study of childhood cancer survivors in the UK revealed that the 25-year cumulative risk of second malignancy was 4.2%. A greater risk was seen in individuals who received both radiotherapy and chemotherapy. While leukemias are more often a result of exposure to chemotherapy (especially alkylating agents), sarcomas, meningiomas, and gliomas are more closely related to radiation exposure. Thyroid cancer, especially papillary carcinoma of the thyroid, is well known to occur even after low to moderate doses of ionizing radiation. The median time interval is usually around 10 years and occurs earlier in the case of hematological malignancies [56–58].

## References

1. McMahon SJ. The linear quadratic model: usage, interpretation and challenges. Phys Med Biol. 2018;64(1):01TR01.
2. Barnett GC, West CML, Dunning AM, Elliott RM, Coles CE, Pharoah PDP, et al. Normal tissue reactions to radiotherapy. Nat Rev Cancer. 2009;9(2):134–42.
3. Withers HR, Taylor JM, Maciejewski B. Treatment volume and tissue tolerance. Int J Radiat Oncol Biol Phys. 1988;14(4):751–9.
4. Dale E, Olsen DR. Specification of the dose to organs at risk in external beam radiotherapy. Acta Oncol. 1997;36(2):129–35.
5. Deterministic Effects (Tissue Reactions) and Stochastic Effects [MOE] [Internet]. [cited 2022 Oct 31]. https://www.env.go.jp/en/chemi/rhm/basic-info/1st/03-01-04.html.

6. Emami B, Lyman J, Brown A, Coia L, Goitein M, Munzenrider JE, et al. Tolerance of normal tissue to therapeutic irradiation. Int J Radiat Oncol Biol Phys. 1991;21(1):109–22.
7. Bentzen SM, Constine LS, Deasy JO, Eisbruch A, Jackson A, Marks LB, et al. Quantitative analyses of Normal tissue Effects in the clinic (QUANTEC): an introduction to the scientific issues. Int J Radiat Oncol Biol Phys. 2010;76(3 Suppl):S3–9.
8. Constine LS, Ronckers CM, Hua CH, et al. Pediatric Normal tissue Effects in the clinic (PENTEC): an international collaboration to analyse Normal tissue radiation dose-volume response relationships for Paediatric cancer patients. Clin Oncol. 2019;31(3):199–207.
9. Wysocki AB. Skin anatomy, physiology, and pathophysiology. Nurs Clin North AM. 1999;34(4):777–97.
10. Hymes SR, Strom EA, Fife C. Radiation dermatitis: clinical presentation, pathophysiology, and treatment 2006. J Am Acad Dermatol. 2006;54(1):28–46.
11. Mendelsohn FA, Divino CM, Reis ED, Kerstein MD. Wound care after radiation therapy. Adv Skin Wound Care. 2002;15(5):216–24.
12. Bray FN, Simmons BJ, Wolfson AH, Nouri K. Acute and chronic cutaneous reactions to ionizing radiation therapy. Dermatol Ther (Heidelb). 2016;6(2):185–206.
13. Common Terminology Criteria for Adverse Events (CTCAE)|Protocol Development|CTEP [Internet]. [cited 2022 Oct 25]. https://ctep.cancer.gov/protocoldevelopment/electronic_applications/ctc.htm.
14. Sonis ST. Oral mucositis in head and neck cancer: risk, biology, and management. Am Soc Clin Oncol Educ Book. 2013;33:e236–40.
15. Baker S, Fairchild A. Radiation-induced esophagitis in lung cancer. Lung Cancer (Auckl). 2016;7:119–27.
16. Hematopoiesis KR. In: Enna SJ, Bylund DB, editors. xPharm: The comprehensive pharmacology reference [internet]. New York: Elsevier; 2007. p. 1–5. https://www.sciencedirect.com/science/article/pii/B9780080552323602685.
17. Hoeben BAW, Wong JYC, Fog LS, Losert C, Filippi AR, Bentzen SM, et al. Total body irradiation in haematopoietic Stem cell transplantation for paediatric acute lymphoblastic leukaemia: review of the literature and future directions. Front Pediatr. 2021;9:774348.
18. Croizat H, Frindel E, Tubiana M. Long term radiation Effects on the bone marrow Stem cells of C3H mice. Int J Radiat Biol Relat Stud Phys Chem Med. 1979;36(1):91–9.
19. Croizat H, Frindel E, Tubiana M. The effect of partial body irradiation on Haemopoietic stem cell migration. Cell Prolif. 1980;13:319–25.
20. Yang Z, Bai S, Gu B, Peng S, Liu WL, Yang ZJ, et al. Radiation-induced brain injury after radiotherapy for brain tumor. In: Molecular considerations and evolving surgical management issues in the treatment of patients with a brain tumor. IntechOpen; 2015. https://www.intechopen.com/state.item.id.
21. Mahajan A, Stavinoha PL, Rongthong W, Brodin NP, McGovern SL, Naqa IE, et al. Neurocognitive effects and necrosis in childhood cancer survivors treated with radiation therapy: a PENTEC comprehensive review. Int J Radiat Oncol Biol Phys. 2021;119:401–16. https://www.redjournal.org/article/S0360-3016(21)00127-9/fulltext.
22. Monje M, Dietrich J. Cognitive side effects of cancer therapy demonstrate a functional role for adult neurogenesis. Behav Brain Res. 2012;227(2):376–9.
23. Michaelidesová A, Konířová J, Bartůněk P, Zíková M. Effects of radiation therapy on neural Stem cells. Genes. 2019;10(9):640.
24. Halberg FE, Kramer JH, Moore IM, Wara WM, Matthayi KK, Ablin AR. Prophylactic cranial irradiation dose effects on late cognitive function in children treated for acute lymphoblastic leukemia. Int J Radiat Oncol Biol Phys. 1992;22(1):13–6.
25. Mulhern RK, Kepner JL, Thomas PR, Armstrong FD, Friedman HS, Kun LE. Neuropsychologic functioning of survivors of childhood medulloblastoma randomized to receive conventional or reduced-dose craniospinal irradiation: a pediatric oncology group study. J Clin Oncol. 1998;16(5):1723–8.

26. Gondi V, Pugh SL, Tome WA, Caine C, Corn B, Kanner A, et al. Preservation of memory with conformal avoidance of the hippocampal neural Stem-cell compartment during whole-brain radiotherapy for brain metastases (RTOG 0933): a phase II multi-institutional trial. J Clin Oncol. 2014;32(34):3810–6.
27. Brown PD, Pugh S, Laack NN, Wefel JS, Khuntia D, Meyers C, et al. Memantine for the prevention of cognitive dysfunction in patients receiving whole-brain radiotherapy: a randomized, double-blind, placebo-controlled trial. Neuro-Oncology. 2013;15(10):1429–37.
28. Waxer JF, Wong K, Olch AJ, Modiri A, Charpentier AM, Sprow G, et al. Radiotherapy-induced cerebrovascular events among survivors of childhood and adolescent cancer of the central nervous system: a PENTEC modeling study. Int J Radiat Oncol Biol Phys. 2020;108(3):e241–2.
29. King AA, Seidel K, Di C, Leisenring WM, Perkins SM, Krull KR, et al. Long-term neurologic health and psychosocial function of adult survivors of childhood medulloblastoma/PNET: a report from the childhood cancer survivor study. Neuro-Oncology. 2017;19(5):689–98.
30. The 2007 Recommendations of the International Commission on Radiological Protection. ICRP publication 103. Ann ICRP. 2007;37(2–4):1–332.
31. Christensen JG, Wessel I, Gothelf AB, Homøe P. Otitis media with effusion after radiotherapy of the head and neck: a systematic review. Acta Oncol. 2018;57(8):1011–6.
32. Mayo C, Yorke E, Merchant TE. Radiation associated brainstem injury. Int J Radiat Oncol Biol Phys. 2010;76(3 Suppl):S36–41.
33. Okada S, Okeda R. Pathology of radiation myelopathy. Neuropathology. 2001;21:247–65.
34. Maranzano E, Bellavita R, Floridi P, Celani G, Righetti E, Lupattelli M, et al. Radiation-induced myelopathy in long-term surviving metastatic spinal cord compression patients after hypofractionated radiotherapy: a clinical and magnetic resonance imaging analysis. Radiother Oncol. 2001;60(3):281–8.
35. Appelman-Dijkstra NM, Kokshoorn NE, Dekkers OM, Neelis KJ, Biermasz NR, Romijn JA, et al. Pituitary dysfunction in adult patients after cranial radiotherapy: systematic review and meta-analysis. J Clin Endocrinol Metab. 2011;96(8):2330–40.
36. Chemaitilly W, Cohen LE. Diagnosis of endocrine disease: endocrine late-effects of childhood cancer and its treatments. Eur J Endocrinol. 2017;176(4):R183–203.
37. Darzy KH, Shalet SM. Radiation-induced growth hormone deficiency. Horm Res. 2003;59(Suppl 1):1–11.
38. Darzy KH, Shalet SM. Hypopituitarism following radiotherapy. Pituitary. 2009;12(1):40–50.
39. Milano MT, Vargo JA, Yorke ED, Ronckers CM, Kremer LC, Chafe SMJ, et al. Primary hypothyroidism in childhood cancer survivors treated with radiation therapy: a PENTEC comprehensive review. Int J Radiat Oncol Biol Phys. 2021;S0360–3016(21):00128.
40. Eisbruch A, Schwartz M, Rasch C, Vineberg K, Damen E, Van As CJ, et al. Dysphagia and aspiration after chemoradiotherapy for head-and-neck cancer: which anatomic structures are affected and can they be spared by IMRT? Int J Radiat Oncol Biol Phys. 2004;60(5):1425–39.
41. Pigorsch SU, May C, Kessel KA, Graf S, Bier H, Nüsslin F, et al. MRI-and CT-determined changes of dysphagia / aspiration-related structures (DARS) during and after radiotherapy. PLoS One. 2020;15(9):e0237501.
42. Milgrom SA, van Luijk P, Pino R, Ronckers CM, Kremer LC, Gidley PW, et al. Salivary and dental complications in childhood cancer survivors treated with radiation therapy to the head and neck: a pediatric Normal tissue Effects in the clinic (PENTEC) comprehensive review. Int J Radiat Oncol Biol Phys. 2021;S0360–3016(21):00443.
43. de Felice F, Pranno N, Papi P, Brugnoletti O, Tombolini V, Polimeni A. Xerostomia and clinical outcomes in definitive intensity modulated radiotherapy (IMRT) versus three-dimensional conformal radiotherapy (3D-CRT) for head and neck squamous cell carcinoma: a meta-analysis. In Vivo. 2020;34(2):623–9.
44. Jain V, Berman AT. Radiation pneumonitis: old problem, new tricks. Cancers. 2018;10(7):222.
45. Briere TM, Agrusa JE, Martel MK, Jackson A, Olch AJ, Ronckers CM, et al. Acute and late pulmonary Effects after radiation therapy in childhood cancer survivors: a PENTEC comprehensive review. Int J Radiat Oncol Biol Phys. 2022;S0360–3016(22):00132–8.

46. Heidenreich PA, Hancock SL, Vagelos RH, Lee BK, Schnittger I. Diastolic dysfunction after mediastinal irradiation. Am Heart J. 2005;150(5):977–82.
47. Veinot JP, Edwards WD. Pathology of radiation-induced heart disease: a surgical and autopsy study of 27 cases. Hum Pathol. 1996;27(8):766–73.
48. Yeh ETH, Tong AT, Lenihan DJ, Yusuf SW, Swafford J, Champion C, et al. Cardiovascular complications of cancer therapy. Circulation. 2004;109(25):3122–31.
49. Kim J, Jung Y. Radiation-induced liver disease: current understanding and future perspectives. Exp Mol Med. 2017;49(7):e359.
50. Klaus R, Niyazi M, Lange-Sperandio B. Radiation-induced kidney toxicity: molecular and cellular pathogenesis. Radiat Oncol. 2021;16(1):43.
51. Smit SG, Heyns CF. Management of radiation cystitis. Nat Rev Urol. 2010;7(4):206–14.
52. Leiper K, Morris AI. Treatment of radiation Proctitis. Clin Oncol. 2007;19(9):724–9.
53. De Felice F, Marchetti C, Marampon F, Cascialli G, Muzii L, Tombolini V. Radiation effects on male fertility. Andrology. 2019;7(1):2–7.
54. Biedka M, Kuźba-Kryszak T, Nowikiewicz T, Żyromska A. Fertility impairment in radiotherapy. Contemp Oncol (Pozn). 2016;20(3):199–204.
55. Stroud JS, Mutch D, Rader J, Powell M, Thaker PH, Grigsby PW. Effects of cancer treatment on ovarian function. Fertil Steril. 2009;92(2):417–27.
56. Smith MB, Xue H, Strong L, Takahashi H, Jaffe N, Ried H, et al. Forty-year experience with second malignancies after treatment of childhood cancer: analysis of outcome following the development of the second malignancy. J Paed Surg. 1993;28(10):1342–9.
57. Jenkinson HC, Hawkins MM, Stiller CA, Winter DL, Marsden HB, Stevens MCG. Long-term population-based risks of second malignant neoplasms after childhood cancer in Britain. Br J Cancer. 2004 Nov;91(11):1905–10.
58. Tran TV, Kitahara CM, de Vathaire F, Boutron-Ruault MC, Journy N. Thyroid dysfunction and cancer incidence: a systematic review and meta-analysis. Endocr Relat Cancer. 2020;27(4):245–59.

# Pediatric Radiation Therapy: Preplanning Aspects

5

Ajeet Kumar Gandhi and Jaspreet Kaur

## 5.1 Introduction

The reported incidence of childhood cancer has increased in India over the last 25 years [1]. The five top childhood cancer sites are leukemia, lymphoma, central nervous system (CNS), bone, and retinoblastoma [2]. Radiotherapy has an important role to play in all these malignancies. Planning and treating children with radiotherapy requires an understanding of the differences between adult and pediatric cancers and the consequences of the treatment. Radiation therapy treatment planning is more challenging for children than for adults for many reasons. First, most of the childhood cancers are being treated curatively, while 30–50% of the adults are treated with palliative intent. Second, many tissues in children have a lower tolerance to radiation than adults. Modern radiation therapy practices are precise and require strict immobilization for accurate delivery, and this poses a unique challenge for the pediatric population vis-à-vis adults.

Preplanning preparation of the patient as well as the caregiver is a very important step which is often neglected in our country. Once the patient is selected for treatment by radiation, attempts should be made to reduce the need for anesthesia or sedation by various psychological and behavioral techniques. Preschool-age children and older children with special needs, planned for radiation treatment, often require daily sedation or general anesthesia to ensure adequate motion control [3]. There are very few centers in India equipped to render comprehensive pediatric oncologic care to the afflicted patients. Pediatric radiation therapy in low- and

A. K. Gandhi (✉)
Department of Radiation Oncology, Dr Ram Manohar Lohia Institute of Medical Sciences, Lucknow, India

J. Kaur
Department of Radiation Oncology, Vardhman Mahavir Medical College and Safdarjung Hospital, New Delhi, India


R. Madan et al. (eds.), *Evidence Based Practice in Pediatric Radiation Oncology*, https://doi.org/10.1007/978-981-96-4872-6_5

middle-income countries faces many challenges due to poor social and economic conditions [4]. The infrastructure, equipment, and staff necessary for optimal radiation treatment of pediatric patients, such as immobilization equipment in pediatric sizes, anesthesia equipment, post-anesthesia recovery rooms, play areas and support staff experienced in childcare (nurses, social workers), are either insufficient or not available in many centers.

## 5.2 Alternative Modalities of Treatment

Radical and extra-radical surgeries done earlier for the pediatric malignancies have been replaced over time by conservative surgeries. This has happened with the use of adjuvant and neoadjuvant chemotherapy and radiation therapy. With the advancements in pediatric anesthetic techniques as well as radiation oncology technology, optimal immobilization can be provided during radiation planning and treatment. Radiotherapy is an indispensable part of multidisciplinary cancer care in pediatric oncology. Owing to the effects of radiation therapy on growing/developing pediatric tissues which sometimes can be very debilitating in the long run, several of the groups have tried to explore non-radiation treatment for certain cancer sites with excellent results like omission of prophylactic cranial radiotherapy for acute leukemias, involved field radiotherapy for Hodgkin lymphoma [5] and in yet other tumors like low-grade gliomas and medulloblastomas, molecular characterization has helped in adapting the treatment and refining protocols [6]. In summary, alternative modalities of treatment like surgery and risk-adapted treatment protocols should be explored in all pediatric patients with a multidisciplinary approach to best optimize the use of radiation therapy.

## 5.3 Patient Selection and Requirement for Anesthesia

Age of the patient is one of the most important decisive factors while assessing the need of anesthesia in a pediatric patient undergoing radiation therapy [7]. Age-appropriate preparation may help guide selection of patients requiring anesthesia [8]. For very young children less than 2 years old (or below the age of comprehension/language development), usually sedation or anesthesia is required. Fortunately, the indications of radiation therapy for the same age groups are fewer. For children aged 2–12 years, it is possible to avoid anesthesia with distractions and counseling [9]. This age group is very well managed by behavioral and psychological intervention. Older children with special needs however may require sedation or general anesthesia.

Nevertheless, despite all the efforts and distraction methods, there would be few patients who would require anesthesia for radiation therapy delivery. One important aspect of decision-making is not to presume that the child, based on their initial first assessment, would require anesthesia. Often with two or three visits to the hospital, the children may become more comfortable and do the treatment sessions without anesthesia. It is important to establish early referral for pre-anesthetic check-up and acquire clearance before initiation of treatment. Sometimes, although the treatment can be started without anesthesia, children would stop co-operating midway and may require it for a part of their treatment.

The type of anesthesia required in the patients should also be discussed between radiation oncologist and anesthesiologist. Position of the patient and use of anesthetic devices like airway may interfere with certain radiotherapy delivery, for example, in head and neck region. Overall, propofol-based total intravenous anesthesia without intubation is preferred worldwide, and deviation from this should be individualized [10, 11]. Prolonged and repetitive delivery of anesthetic agent may be harmful but has been proven to be safe, and if there is dilemma, sedation/anesthesia should be preferred as precise delivery of radiation therapy is very important for an optimal oncologic outcome.

## 5.4 Preplanning Counseling and Preparation

When the child is accepted as a candidate for radiation therapy, the treating team should meet the patient and his family. The team should explain the treatment process and should answer the concerns raised by the caregivers. Families are encouraged to write down their questions before the appointment. The doctor should talk to the parents about the need for sedation or anesthesia during radiation treatment. The treatment team should talk to parents about the goal of radiation treatment and side effects. This process is called informed consent.

A preparatory kit consisting of age-adjusted information on tablets, gift of a stuffed toy or a pair of headphones, a parent booklet, and toy models of the computed tomography and RT machines can be handed over to the parents or the caregivers [12]. This systematic, family-centered strategy contributes to parents' understanding and coping with the child's radiation treatment. The presence of friendly staff, along with making the child and the caregivers familiar with the equipment as well as the entire process, goes a long way in making the radiation treatment experience smooth for the patient. Preparation program for radiation treatment in children has been shown to minimize anxiety and increase satisfaction among children, caregivers, and staff.

## 5.5 Behavioral Techniques to Avoid/Reduce the Need of Anesthesia

It takes a lot of teamwork to plan and administer radiation treatment to children. Administration of sedation or anesthesia routinely to pediatric cancer patients leads to a higher chance of clinical complication, inadequate nutrition, disturbed sleep, and is expensive and time-consuming [13, 14]. In some older children, behavioral techniques may be tried to avoid anesthesia for radiation treatment. These techniques involve various ways to teach children to cooperate with the radiation team.

A dedicated pediatric nurse for procedural preparation, audiovisual distraction (television during RT), and two-way audio communication with caregivers are some strategies to decrease the use of GA [15]. Behavioral techniques are also called desensitization or exposure therapy. These techniques entail using videos, stories, cartoons, or music to create a calm state of mind. When the child tries to cooperate, rewards like toys, stickers, praise, and prizes are given. Videotaped movies and cartoons can be used as distractions, relaxation aids, and to help teach young children to comply with radiation treatment. To play movies or cartoons while the child is in the treatment position during radiation therapy, a small television monitor can be hung close to the linear accelerator couch and hooked up to a VCR. The effectiveness of this method was shown in children ranging in age from 2 1/2 to 7 years by Slifer et al. [16]. All of the radiation planning and treatment sessions for nine out of 11 children were completed successfully and without the need for sedation.

A study by Haeberli et al. (2008) was done to evaluate whether a psychoeducational intervention reduces the need for anesthesia in childhood cancer patients. Using a play program and interactive assistance from a qualified nurse, the psychoeducational intervention helped the patient become acquainted with the personnel, equipment, and radiotherapy process. This study showed that only 8.9% of the patients who received psychoeducational intervention needed anesthesia compared to 21.4% of those who did not receive any intervention needed anesthesia [17].

**Modification of the environment for the patient population:** Although radiation is a painless and non-invasive procedure, most children often experience phobia and distress because of the unfamiliarity with the procedure and the idea of staying alone in the radiation room away from their parents. The child has to stay motionless during radiation for optimal results and safety reasons. Studies have shown that presence of friendly staff who listened and explained to the children and their families helps in reducing their distress and anxiety. Children between the ages of three and half to 6 years were given information and instructions about radiation therapy, visited the radiation unit, and participated in an arts therapy intervention in order to reduce their anxiety. Out of the 55 children treated, only five required anesthesia, according to the results. It emphasized how important it is for employees to be adaptable and cognizant of the unique needs and abilities of every child and family [18].

In order to lessen the need for daily anesthesia, an audiovisual system that is compatible with radiation therapy has been developed that enables children to watch streaming video while undergoing treatment. A digital media player with wireless streaming and projector, along with a radiolucent display screen placed within the child's field of vision, provides enough entertainment and distraction for the duration of serial treatments without the need for daily anesthesia. This system is known as an audiovisual-assisted therapeutic ambience in radiation therapy (AVATAR). Patients' experiences receiving treatment were enhanced by this pilot system [19].

**Immobilization techniques:** Immobilization of children is different as compared to the adult patients requiring radiation therapy. Also, immobilization of the pediatric patients pose challenges as compared to other medical specialties where the adult can accompany the children and be there inside the imaging room with personal radiation protective gears. Some of the immobilization methods described for pediatric patients like distraction technique, verbal technique, and feed and sleep technique may not also be applicable, as radiation therapy delivery requires strict immobilization for accurate delivery of radiation therapy. It is important to understand that a comfortable and calm child is ideal for the treatment delivery, and hence restraint measures like forceful physical and verbal methods should strictly be avoided.

The basic principles of immobilization remain the same: the immobilization devices used should be comfortable for the patients, should be reproducible, and should not interfere with the radiation beam entry path. Common immobilization devices used for pediatric population are thermoplastic immobilization devices, VacLok, and customized sand bags. One important point to be kept in mind is not to use adult-sized thermoplastic devices for pediatric population. Customized thermoplastic devices for age group of 0–5 years and 6–12 years are commercially available.

Helpful tips to allay patient's anxiety and ease the process of immobilization and positioning (Fig. 5.1) are as follows:

(a) Magic string technique: Separation of the parents from the child makes the child anxious. A colorful, long piece of magic string, whose one end is held by the child during treatment and other end is held by the parents outside the treatment room at the console, along with audiovisual cues, makes the child believe that their parents are connected to them.
(b) Painting of the patients masks with their favorite cartoons, superhero, fantasy characters and simulating the painted masks on them makes them comfortable. Often, this can be done few days prior to the actual simulation process. Children are encouraged to play with the painted masks and can also be given painted masks to take home with them to become more comfortable.
(c) Decoration of the masks with stickers: While use of paints may get boring with kids as the treatment span may typically last few weeks, use of sticker decoration gives them the feeling to pick and choose and also change the design in between and make it more fun and beautiful.
(d) Picture books and videos: Children often understand interestingly with pictures and demonstrations. Picture books, depicting the flow of radiation therapy treatment in a lucid way, prepare the child mentally and playfully for the treatment. Older children may understand the treatment process from cartoonist videos, some of which are available online [20, 21].
(e) Pretend play with LINAC models: One of the fascinating aspects of making the child acquainted with the treatment machine is pretend play with LINAC models with dummy patients, akin to the dollhouse play joyfully done by most children. "Little LINAC project" at the Leeds Children's Hospital is an excellent example of the same helping several of the pediatric patients [22].
(f) Departmental tour with visualization of other children undergoing the same treatment: Spending more time with the children and making them visualize the execution of treatment on other children help the children.

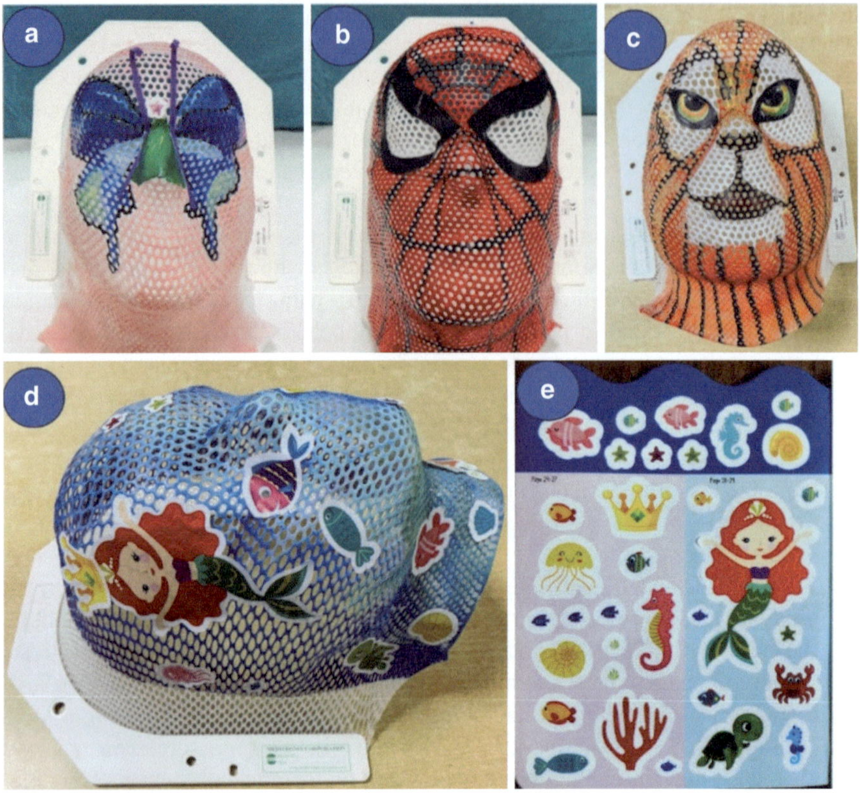


**Fig. 5.1** Painting on thermoplastic cast (author's own images, permission not required). (**a**–**c**)-Painting on thermoplastic casts. (**d**) Decoration of thermoplastic cast with stickers. (**e**) Reusable stickers

**Patient positioning:** Patient positioning must be reproducible, comfortable, and non-interfering with the radiation therapy process. A supine position is preferred for most radiation therapy treatments in children owing to its comfort and ease of administration of anesthesia/sedation. Prone positioning has been used for certain cases like craniospinal irradiation. This position facilitates direct visualization of the cranial and spinal fields and allows matching of the cranial/spinal fields as well. However, prone positioning may lead to difficulty in intubation/anesthetic delivery. Use of total intravenous anesthesia may be preferred if the decision is taken to use prone position and some modifications in techniques may also felicitate radiotherapy process [23]. If the difference between supine and prone positioning does not make a difference in treatment outcome, then a more comfortable supine positioning should be chosen [24]. Different treatment positions like "stool-sitting position," lateral decubitus, and standing may be required for specialized radiotherapy treatment planning such as total body irradiation [25] Other patient positioning methods as mandated by the radiotherapy treatment planning may also be applied on a case-to-case basis like arm akimbo in lymphoma planning and frog leg positioning in inguinal radiotherapy planning. Although less employed, when using palliative radiotherapy in children, it is important not put the child in uncomfortable or painful positions for planning, and this should be optimized on a case-to-case basis.

**Imaging/simulation:** Accurate and adequate simulation is usually the first step toward a successful radiation therapy delivery. Children may be apprehensive about the simulation process. Trained staff members like child life specialists and trained nursing personnel may help prepare them. A preparatory session fitted to child's age before the actual simulation process would help. The children are acquainted with the simulation process, given a tour of the imaging equipment, and walked through the simulation process step by step to ease their apprehension.

The simulation has to be tailored and optimized to the type of radiation therapy modality. A fluoroscopic simulation may be done when X-ray-based two-dimensional radiotherapy is planned. Usually, a non-contrast computed tomographic scan is acquired. Contrast agents should be used very judiciously and should be avoided if possible. Magnetic resonance imaging (MRI) may also be acquired in certain cases like brain tumor to aid in target volume delineation. Positron emission tomography may also be used as an adjunct to simulation scans in certain cases like lymphoma.

Markers are placed on the thermoplastic immobilization devices. In cases where skin markings are to be placed as reference markers, use of permanent paint markers or needle tattoos should be used rather than temporary markers. The use of permanent tattoos if used should be discussed with children and parents beforehand.

## 5.6 Treatment Scheduling Time

Unlike adults, the treatment of pediatric patients may be more time-consuming. Although the exact treatment time may be less, the time required for preparation for the treatment is usually more. The basic principles to be followed in scheduling treatment for the pediatric patients undergoing radiotherapy should be as follows:

(a) Preference to the pediatric patients: Radiation therapy initiation waiting time in busy setups in resource constraint setting may range from few weeks to months in low- and middle-income countries. However, since radiation therapy in children is often done in multimodality setting and owing to certain indications (like Wilms tumor, rhabdomyosarcoma, where early radiotherapy is indicated), it would be prudent not to keep young children waiting for radiotherapy slots. Special efforts should be made in concert with administration to optimize and prioritize pediatric patients on radiotherapy machines.
(b) Grouping treatment of all pediatric patients together at a time: Children often learn by imitating and also do several other things in day-to-day life with imitation and copying. Children often assume the role of treatment as a turn-taking activity in a play, and hence show least resistance and do it playfully when other children are also doing the same. It is important, however, that children of simi-

lar age group or those undergoing similar type of treatment like cancer sites and type of radiation therapy are grouped together, else it may be counterproductive.

(c) Patients requiring anesthesia: Since, children requiring anesthesia/sedation would require them to be nil per oral for 2–4 h, it is always better to schedule the treatment as first few patients on the treatment machines. Scheduling the treatment early in the morning also has other advantages like a relatively less crowded hospital and multidisciplinary scheduling with other departments like anesthesia. Treatment of children also requires a lot of effort, energy, and enthusiasm, and this is easier in the morning than evening times when most of the hospital staffs are worn out with entire days' work.

(d) Adapting the treatment to children's need: For older children, it is important not to interfere with their daily schedule and adapt timings as per their needs. For example, for a child who may be receiving shorter duration of radiotherapy, such as prophylactic cranial irradiation for acute lymphoblastic leukemia, may be continuing with their education and should be scheduled accordingly. Fitting radiotherapy schedules inside the daily routine of children increases the compliance of the treatment.

(e) Flexibility in treatment scheduling time: Children, unlike adults, may not be very conscious and disciplined about their treatment. Attending a sibling's birthday party or get-together may be more important to them than their radiation therapy. On occasion, these situations should be handled with care and compassion, and rescheduling may be allowed on a case-to-case basis to again improve treatment compliance.

(f) Familiar environment: It is important that the children are treated daily on the same treatment machine/unit and if any shift/change in treatment unit is planned, the child should be acclimatized to the new environment beforehand. The duty roster of the radiation therapists should also be designed in a way that same children see the same therapist every day, and this helps in alleviating the anxiety and expediting the treatment process.

## References


1. Arora RS, Eden TO, Kapoor G. Epidemiology of childhood cancer in India. Indian J Cancer. 2009;46(4):264–73.
2. Malhotra RK, Manoharan N, Nair O, Deo SVS, Bakhshi S, Rath GK. Patterns and trends of childhood cancer incidence (0-14 years) in Delhi, India: 1990-2014. Indian Pediatr. 2021;58(5):430–5.
3. Slifer KJ, Bucholtz JD, Cataldo MD. Behavioral training of motion control in young children undergoing radiation treatment without sedation. J Pediatr Oncol Nurs. 1994;11(2):55–63.
4. Anacak Y, Zubizarreta E, Zaghloul M, Laskar S, Alert J, Gondhowiardjo S, et al. The practice of Paediatric radiation oncology in low-and middle-income countries: outcomes of an International Atomic Energy Agency study. Clin Oncol (R Coll Radiol). 2021;33(4):e211–20.

5. Boterberg T, Dunlea C, Harrabi S, Janssens GO, Laprie A, Whitfield G, Gaze MN, SIOP-Europe Radiation Oncology Working Group. European clinical trials in paediatric radiation oncology. Lancet Child Adolesc Health. 2021;5(12):843–5.
6. Shen CJ, Terezakis SA. The evolving role of radiotherapy for pediatric cancers with advancements in molecular tumor characterization and targeted therapies. Front Oncol. 2021;11:679701.
7. Shimazu Y, Otsuki R, Murakami M, Konishi A, Kan K, Seto I, et al. Age as a decisive factor in general anaesthesia use in paediatric proton beam therapy. Sci Rep. 2020;10(1):15096.
8. Gårdling J, Törnqvist E, Månsson ME, Hallström IK. Age-appropriate preparations for children with cancer undergoing radiotherapy: a feasibility study. J Child Health Care. 2017;21(4):370–80.
9. Nagarajan AA, Radhakrishnan V, Ganesharajah S. Radiotherapy in children without anesthesia: a feasibility approach using distraction. Indian J Med Paediatr Oncol. 2019;40:507–9.
10. Owusu-Agyemang P, Tsai JY, Kapoor R, Van Meter A, Tan GM, Peters S, et al. Survey of anesthesia, sedation, and non-sedation practices for children undergoing repetitive cranial or craniospinal radiotherapy. Cureus. 2022;14(4):e24075.
11. Khurmi N, Patel P, Koushik S, Daniels T, Kraus M. Anesthesia practice in pediatric radiation oncology: Mayo Clinic Arizona's experience 2014-2016. Paediatr Drugs. 2018;20(1):89–95.
12. Ångström-Brännström C, Lindh V, Mullaney T, Nilsson K, Wickart-Johansson G, Svärd AM, et al. Parents' experiences and responses to an intervention for psychological preparation of children and families during the child's radiotherapy. J Pediatr Oncol Nurs. 2018;35(2):132–48.
13. Scott MT, Todd KE, Oakley H, Bradley JA, Rotondo RL, Morris CG, et al. Reducing anesthesia and health care cost through utilization of child life specialists in pediatric radiation oncology. Int J Radiat Oncol Biol Phys. 2016;96(2):401–5.
14. Scot L, Langton F, O'Donoghue J. Minimising the use of sedation/anaesthesia in young children receiving radiotherapy through an effective play preparation programme. Eur J Oncol Nurs. 2002;6(1):15–22.
15. Ntoukas SM, Ritchie T, Awrey S, Hodgson DC, Laperriere N, Yee R, et al. Minimizing general anesthetic use in pediatric radiation therapy. PractRadiat. Oncologia. 2020;10(3):e159–65.
16. Slifer KJ. A video system to help children cooperative with motion control for radiation therapy without sedation. J Pediatr Oncol Nurs. 1996;13:91–7.
17. Haeberli S, Grotzer MA, Niggli FK, Landolt MA, Linsenmeier C, Ammann RA, Bodmer N. A psychoeducational intervention reduces the need for anesthesia during radiotherapy for young childhood cancer patients. Radiat Oncol. 2008;3:17.
18. Filin A, Treisman S, Peles BA. Radiation therapy preparation by a multidisciplinary team for childhood cancer patients aged 31/2 to 6 years. J Pediatr Oncol Nurs. 2009;26(2):81–5.
19. Hiniker SM, Bush K, Fowler T, White EC, Rodriguez S, Maxim PG, et al. Initial clinical outcomes of audiovisual-assisted therapeutic ambience in radiation therapy (AVATAR). PractRadiat. Oncologia. 2017;7(5):311–8.
20. https://youtu.be/EA9Al7KeIGs. Accessed 4 Sept 2022.
21. https://youtu.be/8pBjobqdtrc. Accessed 4 Sept 2022.
22. https://stories.swns.com/news/lego-obsessed-seven-year-old-suffering-from-brain-cancer-conquered-fear-of-hospital-machines-by-building-scanner-out-of-toy-bricks-103345/. Accessed 4 Sept 2022.
23. Onal O, Aslanlar E, Ciftci C, Onal M, BengiCelik J. A novel and modified technique in the prone position for radiotherapy processes in children. Anesth Pain Med. 2017;7(4):e57816.
24. Verma J, Mazloom A, Teh BS, South M, Butler EB, Paulino AC. Comparison of supine and prone craniospinal irradiation in children with medulloblastoma. Pract Radiat Oncologia. 2015;5(2):93–8.
25. Hoeben BAW, Pazos M, Seravalli E, Bosman ME, Losert C, Albert MH, et al. ESTRO ACROP and SIOPE recommendations for myeloablative Total body irradiation in children. Radiother Oncol. 2022;173:119–33.

# 6 Anaesthesia in Paediatric Radiation

Shiv Lal Soni and Renu Madan

Paediatric population undergoing any type of medical or surgical procedure under anaesthesia requires constant vigilance and special attention due to various factors such as physiological and anatomical differences between paediatric airway compared to that of adults. These differences are important for the anaesthetist to make a safe and effective anaesthesia plan. Paediatric patients also have anxiety, fear of strangers, aversion towards new environment, fear of syringes, and concerns about procedural pain which makes them more vulnerable for procedural complications [1, 2].

Children with primary brain tumors, Wilms' tumor, Neuroblastoma, Retinoblastoma, Sarcoma etc [3] require anaesthesia assistance in various radiation oncology procedures, including radiation simulation and radiation delivery in external beam radiotherapy and brachytherapy. This helps in making treatment plan and localizing the exact anatomical area to be irradiated [4].

Most of the radiation oncology procedures are OPD procedures and are usually of short duration of approximately 5–25 min. However, as paediatric age group comprises neonates, infants, toddlers, children, and adolescents, management becomes challenging for the team involved which usually consists of an anaesthesiologist, radiation oncologist, anaesthesia technician, and nursing staff.

S. L. Soni (✉)
Department of Anesthesia, PGIMER, Chandigarh, India

R. Madan
Department of Radiotherapy and Oncology, Postgraduate Institute of Medical Education and Research, Chandigarh, India



R. Madan et al. (eds.), *Evidence Based Practice in Pediatric Radiation Oncology*,
https://doi.org/10.1007/978-981-96-4872-6_6

## 6.1 Anaesthesia Concerns and Challenges

The anaesthesia management comprises of pre-procedural preparation of radiation suite, preoperative, intraoperative and postoperative management.

### 6.1.1 Key Points

1. Knowing challenges associated with different paediatric age group.
2. Addressing Non-Operating Room Anaesthesia (NORA) concerns.
3. Ensuring preparedness to handle airway and any emergency scenarios (equipment and drugs should be ready).
4. Maintaining trained staff in Paediatric BLS and Paediatric Advanced Life Support (PALS) (equipment such as defibrillators should be checked and functioning properly).
5. Implementing radiation safety measures.

## 6.2 Pre-Procedural Preparation

1. Develop a procedure plan with the radiation oncologist with a special focus on time required for simulation and radiation exposure time for radiation therapy.
2. Perform a detailed preanaesthetic check as the child can have associated syndromes, CVS, and respiratory diseases.
3. Explain fasting guidelines to concerned team and parents, emphasizing adequate nil per oral that is must needed for the procedure. Minimum fasting period required for clear liquids is 2 h, breast milk is 4 h, infant formula is 6 h, nonhuman milk is 6 h, light meal is 6 h, and for solid heavy oily meal is 8 h.
4. Counsel the parents and child for the procedure planned. Take detailed informed written consent from the parents.
5. Prepare the radiation suite with all required equipment, anaesthesia, and emergency drugs for different paediatric age groups.
6. Develop airway management plan, desired anaesthesia technique, and keep ready difficult airway cart, and check appropriate sizes of facemasks, nasal prongs, nasopharyngeal and oropharyngeal airway, laryngeal mask airways, endotracheal tubes, etc.
7. Check anaesthesia machine.
8. Check for working standard ASA monitors which include NIBP, ECG, $SPO_2$, $ETCO_2$, temperature (as paediatric patients are posted to radiation suite, temperature should be maintained, and all measures to avoid hypothermia should be taken).
9. Check suction pressures, oxygen supply, air supply, etc.
10. Prepare longer tubings needed for the procedure like oxygen tubing, suction, IV lines, and anaesthetic circuits. If TIVA is planned and longer IV line is attached,

special consideration should be taken as per goal-directed fluid management in paediatric and avoiding fluid overload.

11. Check availability of proper lead apron, lead shields, and thyroid shields to protect from radiation exposure.

**Anaesthetic Technique**—Types of anaesthesia that can be used in radiation oncology procedure range from general anaesthesia, monitored anaesthesia care (MAC), and sedation. The most commonly used method in the paediatric age group in sedation with standard ASA monitoring (Table 6.1).

### 6.2.1 Intraprodecureal and Postprocedural Management

1. Prepare necessary drugs and equipment for planned anaesthesia technique.
2. Ensure the airway trolley is ready.

**Table 6.1** Drugs used in sedation [5, 6]

| Drug | Route and dose | Side effects and cautions |
|---|---|---|
| Midazolam | • Oral<br>– Syrup—0.25 mg/kg<br>– Tablet—0.5 mg/kg<br>(onset of action-30 min)<br>• Intramuscular (IM)—0.1–0.01 mg/kg<br>• Intravenous (IV)—0.02–0.05 mg/kg<br>• Intranasal—0.2–0.3 mg/kg (onset of action 5–10 min) | • Precautions to be taken to reduce the risk of respiratory depression and hypotension<br>• May cause nasal irritation |
| Propofol | • IV—2–4 mg/kg<br>• IV infusion—100–200 μg/kg/min | • May cause pain during injection<br>• Watch for apnoea and hypotension |
| Morphine | • IV—0.05–0.1 mg/kg | • May cause respiratory depression<br>• Nausea and vomiting |
| Fentanyl | • IV—1–2μg/kg | • Pruritus<br>• Chest wall rigidity |
| Ketamine | • IV sedation—0.2–2 mg/kg<br>• IV analgesia—0.1 mg/kg<br>• Oral—5–10 mg/kg<br>• IM—3–5 mg/kg | • Hallucination<br>• Increased salivation<br>• Dissociated anaesthesia<br>• Sympathetic stimulation, i.e. hypertension and tachycardia<br>• Nausea and vomiting |
| Dexmedetomidine | • IV infusion—Bolus at 1 μg/kg over 10–15 min<br>• Maintenance dose—0.3–1.5 μg/kg/h | • Hypotension<br>• Bradycardia<br>• Avoid rapid administration to ameliorate transient sudden hypertension |

Table created by the author

3. Prevent hypothermia.
4. Implement goal-directed fluid therapy.
5. Adhere to radiation safety guidelines, maintaining a safe distance from the radiation source as the intensity of the radiation beam is attenuated according to the inverse square law ($1/d^2$).
6. Be aware of potential challenges as the children undergo radiation therapy, as they may experience skin reactions to the moulds used to provide targeted therapy on their face, neck, and shoulders. This may pose challenges such as interference with airway patency, obstruction of the movement of the chest with ventilation, delay in immediate access to the airway in an emergency, and/or result in skin damage or pressure sores.
7. Maintain strict vitals monitoring.
8. Administer PONV prophylaxis.
9. Implement effective pain management.

### 6.2.2 Complications to Be Kept in Mind Throughout Paediatric Radiotherapy

| |
|---|
| 1. Children need multiple sessions in small time interval (days to weeks) for radiation therapy, so take special care to keep intravenous route patent |
| 2. Non-cooperation of children can lead to an inability to provide immobility during the procedure |
| 3. Airway obstruction or comprise can occur due to drug overdose and anatomical variations. Presence of face moulds make airway handling more difficult |
| 4. Airway oedema and swelling |
| 5. Radiation safety concerns |
| 6. Hypothermia |
| 7. Hemodynamic instability in form of hypotension, hypertension, bradycardia, and tachycardia |
| 8. Post-procedure nausea and vomiting. |
| 9. Pain and discomfort |
| 10. Drug reactions or allergies |
| 11. Cardiopulmonary arrest |

## References

1. Singapuri K, Russell GB. Anesthesia and radiotherapy. In: Russell GB, editor. Alternate-site anesthesia: clinical practice outside the operating room. Boston, Mass, USA: Butterworth-Heinemann; 1997.
2. Harris EA. Sedation and anesthesia options for pediatric patients in the radiation oncology suite. Int J Pediatr. 2010;2010:1–9.
3. Halperin EC, Constine LS, Tarbell NJ, et al. Pediatric radiation oncology. 5th ed. New York: Lippincott Williams & Wilkins; 2011.

4. Eric HA. Sedation and anaesthesia options for pediatric patients in radiation oncology suite. Int J Pediatr. 2010;870921:1–9.
5. Theagrajan A, Maddirala S. Non-operating room anaesthesia in children. Indian J Anaesth. 2019;63(9):754.
6. Davis PJ, Cladis FP, Smith RM. Smith's anesthesia for infants and children. Amsterdam: Elsevier; 2022.

# 7 Supportive Care, Quality of Life, and Survivorship Aspects among Pediatrics Cancer Patients

Jaivinder Yadav, Jasbir Singh, and Shikha Goyal

## 7.1 Introduction

The incidence of childhood cancer has risen steadily over the years, and approximately 300000 children younger than 19 years developed cancer in 2020. With improvement in therapeutics, 5-year survival has improved to ~80% in developed world [1]. As a result, more pediatric cancer patients are surviving to adulthood.

During cancer treatments, aggressive tumors like embryonal tumors often require intensive therapy, and ongoing efforts aim to enhance survival rates. Conversely, certain tumors respond well to a combination of treatments, and there is a growing emphasis on reducing treatment intensity to minimize long-term health complications. These treatment approaches encompass various methods such as surgery, chemotherapy, targeted therapy, or radiotherapy.

In some pediatric cancers, like Hodgkin's lymphoma, the use of radiotherapy has decreased due to concerns about potential long-term effects on growth, development, and the risk of second malignancies. Sometimes, decisions regarding treatment modalities, such as surgery or radiotherapy, with similar long-term survival

J. Yadav (✉)
Department of Pediatrics, Post Graduate Institute of Medical Education and Research (PGIMER), Chandigarh, India

J. Singh
Department of Pediatrics, All India Institute of Medical Sciences (AIIMS), Bilaspur, Himachal Pradesh, India

S. Goyal
Department of Radiotherapy and Oncology, Postgraduate Institute of Medical Education and Research, Chandigarh, India



R. Madan et al. (eds.), *Evidence Based Practice in Pediatric Radiation Oncology*,
https://doi.org/10.1007/978-981-96-4872-6_7

probabilities, are made based on expectations of morbidity and disability associated with each option.

Throughout the follow-up period, many complications related to the cancer itself or the treatment interventions become apparent. The improved survival rates bring about increased responsibilities for healthcare providers, leading to the emergence of new areas of research and care. These include supportive care, efforts to enhance the quality of life, and screening for various comorbidities and complications in cancer survivors.

The therapeutic modalities used in cancer care can impact multiple organ systems in the body, necessitating regular assessments to identify and manage abnormalities in these systems.

## 7.2 Endocrine System

The endocrine system is profoundly affected in the therapeutics of pediatric cancer care. Around 40–50% of childhood cancer survivors develop one or more hormonal deficiencies in follow-up. A wide range of endocrinal disturbances can happen due to direct involvement by the tumor or effects of chemotherapy, radiotherapy, and advanced therapies like hematopoietic stem cell transplants. The time duration of onset of endocrinal effects depends on tumor location, chemotherapy agents used, and radiation dose. The delayed onset and late diagnosis of these endocrine complications affect the quality of life.

Different endocrine tissues show differential sensitivity to radiation and chemotherapy. Younger age, brain tumors involving sellar-suprasellar regions, alkylating agents (like busulphan, cyclophosphamide), and high radiation doses (>18 gray) are common risk factors for developing endocrinal complications. Hypothalamic pituitary involvement, thyroid dysfunction, and gonadal toxicity are common endocrine sequelae of cancer treatment.

Hypothalamic pituitary exposure to mean radiotherapy doses of 21–34 Gy leads to ~20% risk of deficiency of pituitary hormones (growth hormone, thyroid-stimulating hormone, adrenocorticotrophic hormone). Many of these toxicities may be difficult to avoid but appropriate counseling and monitoring are important [2]. Irradiation of neck to doses of 10–30 Gy leads to subclinical hypothyroidism risk of 12–44%, the risk being higher for females and exposure after 15 years or age [3].

Different societies have given guidelines for endocrinal evaluation among childhood cancer patients. [4, 5]. The guidelines suggest the frequency of screening of various endocrinal conditions, clinical tools depending on cancer type, impact of chemotherapy, and radiation dose received. The following parameters should be routinely evaluated in the care of childhood cancer patients:

1. Growth monitoring—Height, weight, sitting height, total height to sitting height ratio, body mass index (weight/height$^2$) at baseline, and then at 6 months should be done till growth is completed. Use region, ethnicity, and gender-specific growth charts for growth monitoring (e.g. IAP charts 2015 for India, CDC charts for US population). Any growth faltering should be evaluated for growth hormone - insulin-like growth factor (GH-IGF) axis abnormalities after ruling out

other systemic causes of growth failure. The GH therapy can be administered after 1 year of disease-free status after completion of therapies for cancer. Children with active disease and tyrosine kinase inhibitor (TKI)-based therapy should not be treated with GH therapy.

2. Sexual maturity—All children should be monitored for precocious (onset of secondary sexual characters before 8 years in girls and 9 years in boys) and delayed puberty (absence of secondary sexual characters after 13 years in girls and 14 years in boys).
3. Bone health is assessed with Dual X-ray absorptiometry (DEXA) or quantitative CT-based methods at baseline and then assessed following the clinical indications.
4. Symptoms of lethargy and easy fatiguability are pointers toward secondary adrenal insufficiency.
5. Baseline hormonal evaluation for thyroid function tests (T3, T4, TSH), adrenal hormones (ACTH and cortisol), and IGF-1 should be done in all patients. The hormonal profile is repeated 6 months to yearly in follow-up.
6. Patients developing unusual appetites and rapid weight gain should be evaluated for hypothalamic obesity.
7. Cancers needing head–neck radiation therapy (up to 30 Gy) require surveillance for thyroid cancer. Clinical palpation and ultrasound are usual modalities for screening.
8. Fertility preservation with sperm and oocyte preservation should be offered in adolescents.
9. The children identified through screening tests should be referred to a pediatric endocrinologist for further evaluation and management.

## 7.3 Cardiovascular System

Anthracyclines are one of the most common antineoplastic drugs used in approximately 50% of pediatric cancer patients [6]. While we commonly associate cardiovascular risks with a cumulative anthracycline dose exceeding 300 mg/m$^2$, it is essential to acknowledge that even children receiving less than 100 mg/m$^2$ may exhibit subclinical echocardiographic abnormalities [7]. Anthracycline-mediated cardiovascular complications occur through multiple mechanisms, such as oxidative stress, apoptosis induction, toxic metabolite formation, altered cardiomyocyte gene expression, and impaired adenosine triphosphate (ATP) synthesis. The clinical manifestations of cancer treatment-related cardiotoxicity in childhood cancer survivors can range from subtle cardiovascular impairments, like exercise intolerance or asymptomatic elevations in serum biochemical markers, to more severe abnormalities such as arrhythmias, myocardial ischemia, valvular dysfunction, and congestive heart failure. Several risk factors, such as a young age at the start of therapy, body weight, female gender, concurrent radiotherapy, trisomy 21, and pre-existing cardiomyopathy, should be evaluated before initiating chemotherapy to assess the likelihood of increased cardiac toxicity [8]. It is worth noting that long-term survivors of pediatric cancer are particularly susceptible to these adverse effects, which can manifest either early in therapy or many years later. Genetic factors may also play a role in predisposing patients to cardiac complications. To mitigate the long-term adverse effects of childhood cancer treatment, we can consider modifying therapeutic regimens and employing cardioprotective therapies. Enhanced surveillance and multidisciplinary screening strategies are crucial for reducing the incidence of cardiovascular complications in pediatric cancer patients.

Risk of coronary artery disease is <2% even after 30 years of exposure with mean doses <10 Gy, but doubles with every 10 Gy increase in cardiac radiation dose, while the risk of valvular or other cardiac disease is also high. Increase in cumulative anthracycline dose of 100 mg/m$^2$ is equivalent to 10.5 Gy mean cardiac dose [9].

During follow-up visits, the early detection of heart dysfunction is paramount for implementing preventive measures. The International Late Effects of Childhood Cancer Guideline Harmonisation Group has established guidelines for cardiomyopathy screening, especially for the high-risk group, defined by specific anthracycline and chest radiation exposures. High risk for cardiomyopathy group (defined as those with anthracycline exposure ≥250 mg/m$^2$, or ≥ 35 Gy chest radiation, or a combination of ≥100 mg/m$^2$ of anthracyclines and ≥ 15 Gy chest radiation) will require routine surveillance, depending on the cumulative dose of anthracycline and chest radiation exposure [7]. Although screening might make sense for survivors of lower-dose exposures, there is not enough data to compare various screening methods or schedules against one another. Surveillance echocardiography should commence 2 years after exposure and be repeated at least once every 5 years. While elevated troponin and N-terminal pro-brain natriuretic peptide levels during anthracycline therapy may be associated with subclinical cardiomyopathy, the development of clinically significant disease in the long term remains less certain [10].

## 7.4 Renal System

Nephrotoxic chemotherapy can lead to kidney function deterioration, which can significantly impact morbidity and mortality in these patients. A recent systematic review delved into the early and late nephrotoxic effects of chemotherapy and radiotherapy involving the renal region in pediatric patients. This review revealed a wide prevalence of renal dysfunction, ranging from 0 to 80%. These variations in prevalence could be attributed to differences in how abnormal kidney function is defined, including factors such as inclusion criteria, the type of malignancy, specific antineoplastic drugs used, and radiation therapy [11, 12]. Among the chemotherapy agents, cisplatin, ifosfamide, and high-dose methotrexate are the most commonly associated with nephrotoxicity. Several risk factors have been identified for nephrotoxicity, including the patient's age, the specific chemotherapeutic agent used, the inherent toxicity of the antineoplastic agent, and the pre-treatment status of renal function [13]. Many treatment regimens for commonly prevalent cancer in pediatric age, e.g., leukemia and lymphoma, use high doses of methotrexate. Chemotherapy-related kidney damage can affect several segments of the nephron. Risk of renal toxicity with drugs such as ifosfamide and cisplatin increased even with partial renal exposure to RT [14]. In the pediatric population, traditional indicators of renal dysfunction, such as urine nitrogen or plasma creatinine and proteinuria, may not be sufficiently sensitive. Therefore, it is essential to conduct additional investigations that assess different segments of the nephron. These investigations include estimating the glomerular filtration rate (GFR), measuring serum levels of calcium, magnesium, phosphate, and urate, as well as assessing urine osmolarity [11]. Enzyme markers like N-acetyl-D-glucosaminidase (NAG), alanine aminopeptidase (AAP), lactate dehydrogenase (LDH), as well as smaller protein molecules like cystatin-C and neutrophil gelatinase-associated lipocalin (NGAL), have shown promise as markers of renal injury [15]. Importantly, renal injury can persist even after the cessation of chemotherapeutic agents, underscoring the need for regular and lifelong evaluation of renal function in pediatric cancer patients. The Dutch Childhood Cancer Survivor Study (DCCSS)-LATER 2 kidney analysis has emphasized the importance of lifetime monitoring of glomerular functions in pediatric cancer survivors exposed to high-risk factors [16].

## 7.5 Central Nervous system

Central nervous system (CNS) toxicity manifestations may appear heterogeneously and may be observed early during ongoing treatment or may be seen even after the completion of therapy. Distinguishing between chemotherapy-induced brain injury and recurrent disease is of utmost importance for effective therapeutic planning. Chemotherapeutic agents like methotrexate, cytarabine, vincristine, asparaginase, and corticosteroids are commonly linked to CNS toxicity. Acute encephalopathies and posterior reversible encephalopathies are frequently observed neurotoxic manifestations associated with chemotherapy [17, 18]. Moreover, pediatric patients may experience other CNS dysfunctions such as progressive multifocal leukoencephalopathy, vascular complications like venous sinus thrombosis, ischemic strokes, and hemorrhages, cerebellar dysfunction, spinal cord toxicity with intrathecal chemotherapy, mineralizing microangiopathy, and CNS infections [19]. Chemotherapy can lead to varying degrees of cognitive dysfunction, further complicating the clinical picture. Chemotherapy-induced peripheral neuropathy (CIPN) has also been reported with vincristine and other vinca alkaloids, cisplatin, and carboplatin [19]. It is important to acknowledge that multiple factors contribute to the complex interplay of these issues, including obesity, compromised bone health, and psychosocial factors, all of which can limit physical activity and perpetuate long-term health conditions [20].

Radiotherapy to whole or partial brain or to head and neck region may increase the risk of neurocognitive decline, cataracts, retinopathy, optic neuropathy, and hearing dysfunction. The risk is dose dependent. Intelligence quotient (IQ) decline is progressive with increasing RT dose and increasing RT volume (e.g., 5% risk with 10% volume treated to 35.7 Gy or 100% volume treated to 18.1 Gy). Methotrexate is found to be associated with increased risk for an IQ of $< 85$ to generalised brain to RT dose equivalent of 5.9 Gy [21].

The risk exceeds 5% at doses above 42 Gy for retinopathy, above 57 Gy for optic neuropathy, and 9–12 Gy for cataract [22].

The incidence of CNS toxicity tends to rise with the use of polychemotherapy regimens, particularly in children below the age of 6 years, and it can be associated with a decline in intellectual function. This underscores the need for vigilant monitoring and comprehensive care for pediatric cancer patients to address these multifaceted challenges and mitigate their impact on both short-term and long-term health outcomes [23].

## 7.6 Liver

Chemotherapy drugs are often metabolized by the liver, and some of them can cause variable degree of hepatotoxicity depending on the specific chemotherapy drugs used, the dosages administered, and the individual patient's characteristics. Hepatotoxicity can manifest as elevated liver enzymes, jaundice, or more severe liver dysfunction. Drugs like methotrexate, thioguanine, cisplatin, and asparaginase are known to carry a risk of hepatotoxicity [24]. Agents such as corticosteroids, Actinomycin D, bleomycin, methotrexate, and L-asparaginase can cause steatosis and non-alcoholic fatty liver disease (NAFLD) [25]. Certain chemotherapy drugs used in conditioning regimens for hematopoietic stem cell transplantation (HSCT), such as busulfan and cyclophosphamide, can lead to veno-occlusive disease (VOD), a serious liver condition characterized by hepatic sinusoidal obstruction. VOD can be life-threatening and requires prompt management. Use of high-dose radiotherapy combined with these drugs may enhance the risk of VOD. Most pediatric cancers do not need high-dose radiotherapy to liver (e.g., right flank irradiation for Wilms' tumor) and thus the overall rate of RT-induced VOD is low. With whole liver doses up to 10 Gy, risk of VOD is under 6% [26]. Children on long-term low-dose methotrexate may develop hepatic fibrosis and cirrhosis. Pre-existing liver disease and use of drugs affecting liver enzymes may magnify the toxicity due to antineoplastic therapy. Metabolism of antimetabolites and alkylating agents is compromised in severe liver disease. Although monitoring liver enzymes and bilirubin may help identify and monitor liver injury, effects of drugs such as methotrexate may not always be apparent and patients may need liver biopsy for identification. Other factors such as obesity, hepatic surgery, high alcohol intake, metabolic syndrome, use of statins, and older age at diagnosis may also increase the risk of late effects [27].

## 7.7 Lung

The spectrum of pulmonary complications stemming from anticancer therapy can encompass subclinical changes in pulmonary function tests (PFTs) to severe and potentially life-threatening pulmonary conditions. Bleomycin may cause a range of abnormalities from hypersensitivity pneumonitis to pulmonary fibrosis; the effect is dose-dependent and exceeds 10% for cumulative doses of 400 units. Concurrent or sequential thoracic RT, other drugs (cyclophosphamide, vincristine, doxorubicin, methotrexate), and oxygen therapy may worsen lung injury. High-dose chemotherapy with stem cell transplantation is also associated with pulmonary complications, both infectious and non-infectious, such as obstructive changes following chronic GVHD [28]. Risk of even low-grade RT-related pulmonary toxicity is low with partial thoracic exposure to mean doses <14 Gy and V20 < 30%. Toxicity seems higher with whole lung irradiation, and it is accentuated with use of bleomycin or other antineoplastic agents [29].

Other predisposing factors such as growth defects (kyphoscoliosis, thoracic cage hypoplasia), underlying asthma, infections, cigarette exposure, environmental toxins, and genetic susceptibility may enhance lung effects. Markers predictive of radiation pneumonitis, such as transforming growth factor-β1 and interleukins, may prove useful in initiating early interventions.

## 7.8 Marital Status, Fertility

Alkylating agents are particularly gonadotoxic with Sertoli cells being more sensitive (cyclophosphamide dose >4 $g/m^2$) than Leydig cells (cyclophosphamide dose >20 $g/m^2$); thus, infertility may appear earlier before hypogonadism. Similar effects are also seen in stem cell transplant involving alkylating drugs. Radiation exposure of 2–4 Gy to the testes, even as scatter irradiation, may lead to permanent azoospermia, while doses of 12 Gy can cause testosterone deficiency and delayed puberty. Cranial radiation >30 Gy may produce infertility due to central gonadotropin hormone deficiencies [30].

Only 25–30% of childhood cancer survivors get married, the likelihood lower in males compared to females and in those with CNS tumors probably related to growth deficiency and neurocognitive issues. Marriages are usually in late-twenties and fertility rates were much lower than the general population [31].

Breast hypoplasia is common even with doses <1 Gy if exposure occurs before the age of 4 years. Treated breast was 90% smaller with doses of 10 Gy. With exposure to doses of 42 Gy, nearly 40% are unable to breastfeed [32].

Children exposed to high doses of chemotherapy, total body irradiation, or malignancies requiring radiotherapy to pelvis or testicular region are at risk of gonadal failure and hormonal imbalances leading to infertility. Pre-treatment counseling about fertility-sparing methods, possibility of sperm cryopreservation in adolescent males, oocyte preservation in adolescent females, and possible use of gonadotropin hormone during chemotherapy may help preserve fertility in a segment of patients. Hormone replacement therapy may be warranted in many patients for development and maintenance of secondary sexual characteristics, improved bone and muscle health, and better quality of life (QOL) and sexual function.

## 7.9 Dentition and Oral health

Poor dental health including missing teeth may be a sequel to mucositis, oral infections, and poor nutrition related to anticancer therapy. Nearly one-third experience grade 2 or higher xerostomia with mean parotid doses of 35 Gy. Dentition may be delayed and abnormal both due to oral cavity and dental irradiation and salivary toxicity. RT Doses to teeth is advised to be kept <20 Gy to reduce risk [33].

## 7.10 Second Cancers and Benign Tumors

Childhood cancer survivors have a sixfold higher risk of developing subsequent cancer compared to general population. Certain cancers have higher probability of developing (non-melanoma skin cancers, thyroid, breast, CNS, bone, head and neck), the median interval for development exceeds 15 years. Risk factors may include radiotherapy exposure (linearly increasing risk with dose for breast cancer after thoracic RT, and of meningioma after cranial RT). Exposure to RT doses of 20–29 Gy or to alkylating agents led to higher risk of thyroid cancer. Non-melanoma skin cancers, especially basal cell carcinomas, can occur after skin exposure to >35 Gy. The risk increases with age and interval since first diagnosis. For those surviving second cancer, the risk of subsequent neoplasms also exists (~30% at 10 years) [34].

A Dutch record-linkage study (DCOG-LATER) places the incidence of subsequent benign tumors (leiomyomas, osseous tumors, nerve sheath tumors) over 5–52 years at 9.3%. Many of these were linked to local radiotherapy and dose-dependent [35].

Awareness of the entity of second malignant neoplasmas and appropriate surveillance is recommended. For women with RT >20 Gy, the International Late Effects of Childhood Cancer Guideline Harmonization Group recommends annual mammography and breast MRI starting 8 years after RT or age 25, whichever is later [36]. Children's Oncology Group also gives recommendations to screen for thyroid, skin, GI, and hematological malignancies.

## 7.11 Financial Burden

Cancer treatment cost drains the family members and the caregiver role disrupts employment, leading for further diminution of family resources. Of all malignancies, leukemia therapy is among the most costly. Even in insurance-based societies such as the USA, out-of-pocket medical costs for childhood cancer survivors amount to ~10% of household income [37]. Treatment and monitoring of adverse effects, revision of prosthesis, corrective procedures, etc., lead to additional lifelong financial burden.

Several national and philanthropic agencies attempt to bridge this gap by facilitating cancer treatment, searching employment for parents of these children or for rehabilitation into society for survivors, some even imparting skills and education funding. However, the disability, cognitive impairment, and ongoing financial burdens are difficult hurdles to cross. In developing countries, the availability of these facilities is limited and an even bigger challenge is to maintain compliance to therapy and follow-up for disease control.

## 7.12 Social/Psychosocial Effects

With an improvement in the overall survival rates among pediatric cancer patients, many of them lead to a satisfying life in adulthood. However, psychological stress in patients and among family members is a critical aspect that must be well addressed [38]. These children have faced acute distress and adjustment difficulty during the diagnosis, during prolonged treatment cycles, reduced interaction with peers, and unstable coping with society. They are also at risk for the development of long-term treatment complications and the occurrence of secondary diseases. Because of these incidents, some pediatric cancer survivors may face profound social, impaired social competence and behavioral challenges during adulthood. Although the severity of psychological distress among parents of pediatric cancer patients decrease with time, some parents may continue to experience a high level of psychological distress even after the completion of the child's treatment [39]. Due to the need for repeated hospital admissions for treatment and management of adverse effects, the school education attainment remain low and other important social domains like parents' employment and the socioeconomic state of the family. An increased prevalence of depression and anxiety symptoms has been observed among pediatric cancer survivors [40]. Timely identification and institution of appropriate treatment for psychosocial issues is a critical step to prevent undesirable effects on survivors' quality of life. The psychosocial care of pediatric cancer patients is essential in comprehensive multidisciplinary care.

## 7.13 Quality of Life in Childhood Cancer Survivors

With improvement in survival rates among pediatric cancer patients, there is a growing population of survivors reaching adulthood. This population remains at increased risk of many consequences of treatment and disease that have a long-term impact on the quality of life. Krull et al. reported an incidence of cognitive dysfunction among 29–59% of long-term survivors who have been treated for leukemia, and Brinkman et al. observed approximately 15–85% of adult survivors of childhood brain tumors demonstrate cognitive impairment [41, 42]. So, the primary goal of anticancer treatment should not be limited to curing the disease, it also includes the concept of providing a resilient functioning and favorable health-related quality of life (HRQOL). Diagnosis and treatment cycles of cancer affect all aspects of quality of life for the patient and parents, irrespective of age, gender, and therapeutic regimen used. Still, these issues may disappear during subsequent treatment cycles and improve quality of life (QOL) at the successful completion of treatment. Many patients may report reduced organ function, altered sleep patterns, reduced ability to interact with others, poor psychological status with reduced self-esteem, and may even develop depression, especially during the initial months of treatment. Fatigue is a commonly seen physical symptom among pediatric cancer patients. Because of lower awareness among healthcare workers and children's limited ability to communicate, these symptoms remain unaddressed among pediatric patients. These children may face problems in peer relationships and prosocial behavior, e.g., bullying in schools which may lead to a decline in academic performance and poor self-esteem. The impact of painful, invasive procedures like bone marrow aspiration and intravenous cannulation, tissue biopsy, surgery, intensive chemotherapy, and repeated hospitalization are considered key determinants of quality-of-life deterioration in pediatric cancer patients. The patient's family becomes overprotective toward the child whenever a cancer diagnosis is established. At the same time, the patients may develop their defense mechanisms to adjust to the disease, limiting the overall impact on their QOL [43, 44]. Parental support during the management of cancers has been associated with good quality of life for pediatric patients. Healthcare workers should be made aware and trained to for managing these long-term complications of anticancer treatment.

## 7.14 Status of Childhood Cancer Survivor in developed and LMICs

There is a wide gap in survival rates between developing and developed worlds, varying from 20% in lower-middle-income countries (Sub-Saharan Africa) to more than 80% in high-income nations (the USA, Europe). World Health Organization launched a global collaborative campaign with the theme "Better Survival is achievable #throughyourhand" to achieve at least 60% survival in childhood cancer globally by 2030. Gender, age at diagnosis, type of disease, site, histology grade, and socioeconomic status are significant factors affecting survival in children. Infants and children of more than 10 years have poor survival. Acute lymphoblastic leukemia (ALL) has the best 5-year survival rates (up to 90%), while hepatic and central nervous tumors still have survival rates of 60% even at the best centers. With improvements in the surgical and radiation techniques, chemotherapy agents, more accessibility to quality care and financial support to cancer patients through government and nongovernmental organizations, cancer survival will improve in developing nations as well, and the countries should simultaneously prepare for the long-term care of the survivors [45, 46].

## References

1. Tonorezos ES, Barnea D, Cohn RJ, Cypriano MS, Fresneau BC, Haupt R, et al. Models of Care for Survivors of childhood Cancer from across the globe: advancing survivorship care in the next decade. J Clin Oncol. 2018;36:2223–30.
2. Wheeler G, Grassberger C, Samers J, Dwyer M, Wiltshire K, Daly P, Alvarez B, Campbell BA, Kerr AJ, Kron T, Duane FK, Zacharin M, Downie P, Kyriakou E, Ronckers CM, Constine

LS, Hiniker SM. Central endocrine complications among childhood Cancer survivors treated with radiation therapy: a PENTEC comprehensive review. Int J Radiat Oncol Biol Phys. 2023;S0360–3016(23):00416–9.

3. Milano MT, Vargo JA, Yorke ED, Ronckers CM, Kremer LC, Chafe SMJ, van Santen HM, Marks LB, Bentzen SM, Constine LS, Vogelius IR. Primary hypothyroidism in childhood Cancer survivors treated with radiation therapy: a PENTEC comprehensive review. Int J Radiat Oncol Biol Phys. 2021;S0360–3016(21):00128.
4. Sklar CA, Antal Z, Chemaitilly W, Cohen LE, Follin C, Meacham LR, Murad MH. Hypothalamic-pituitary and growth disorders in survivors of childhood Cancer: an Endocrine Society clinical practice guideline. J Clin Endocrinol Metab. 2018;103(8):2761–84. https://doi.org/10.1210/jc.2018-01175. PMID: 29982476.
5. Dattani MT, Brook CGD. Brook's clinical pediatric endocrinology. 7th ed. Hoboken NJ: Wiley-Blackwell; 2020.
6. Armenian SH, Armstrong GT, Aune G, Chow EJ, Ehrhardt MJ, Ky B, et al. Cardiovascular disease in survivors of childhood Cancer: insights into epidemiology, pathophysiology, and prevention. J Clin Oncol. 2018;36:2135–44.
7. Armenian SH, Hudson MM, Mulder RL, Chen MH, Constine LS, Dwyer M, Levitt G, Kremer LC, et al. International Late Effects of Childhood Cancer Guideline Harmonization Group. Recommendations for cardiomyopathy surveillance for survivors of childhood cancer: a report from the international late effects of childhood Cancer guideline harmonization group. Lancet Oncol. 2015;16:e123–36.
8. Harake D, Franco VI, Henkel JM, Miller TL, Lipshultz SE. Cardiotoxicity in childhood cancer survivors: strategies for prevention and management. Futur Cardiol. 2012;8:647–70.
9. Bates JE, Rancati T, Keshavarz H, Gagliardi G, Aznar MC, Howell RM, Shrestha S, Moiseenko V, Yorke E, Armenian S, Kremer L, Chen MH, van der Pal HJ, Cutter DJ, Constine LS, Hodgson D. Cardiac disease in childhood cancer survivors treated with radiation therapy: a PENTEC comprehensive review. Int J Radiat Oncol Biol Phys. 2023;S0360–3016(23):00285–7.
10. Hutchins KK, Siddeek H, Franco VI, Lipshultz SE. Prevention of cardiotoxicity among survivors of childhood cancer. Br J Clin Pharmacol. 2017;83:455–65.
11. Ruggiero A, Ferrara P, Attinà G, Rizzo D, Riccardi R. Renal toxicity and chemotherapy in children with cancer. Br J Clin Pharmacol. 2017;83:2605–14.
12. Blufpand HN, Hes N, Bökenkamp A, van de Wetering MD, Kaspers GJ. Diversity in renal function monitoring and dose modifications during treatment for childhood cancer: a call for standardization. Pediatr Blood Cancer. 2014;61:337–44.
13. Gatta G, Zigon G, Capocaccia R, Coebergh JW, Desandes E, et al. EUROCARE Working Group. Survival of European children and young adults with cancer diagnosed 1995–2002. Eur J Cancer. 2009;45:992–1005.
14. Poppe MM, Tai A, Li XA, Miften M, Olch A, Marks LB, Qureshi BM, Spunt SL, Shnorhavorian M, Nelson G, Ronckers C, Kalapurakal J, Marples B, Constine LS, Liu AK. Kidney disease in childhood Cancer survivors treated with radiation therapy: a comprehensive PENTEC genitourinary review. Int J Radiat Oncol Biol Phys. 2023;S0360-3016(23):00197–9.
15. Mahmoud AAS, Elsalam HBA, El-Deeb SM, Zanaty FM, Aboelghar HM, Elharoun MS. Evaluation of kidney dysfunction in childhood cancer survivors. Pediatr Res. 2022;92:1689. https://doi.org/10.1038/s41390-022-02015-w.
16. Kooijmans ECM, van der Pal HJH, Pluijm SMF, van der Heiden-van der Loo M, LCM K, Bresters D, et al. Dutch LATER study group. The Dutch childhood Cancer survivor study (DCCSS)-LATER 2 kidney analysis examined long-term glomerular dysfunction in childhood cancer survivors. Kidney Int. 2022;S0085–2538(22):00467.
17. Stone JB, DeAngelis LM. Cancer-treatment-induced neurotoxicity—focus on newer treatments. Nat Rev Clin Oncol. 2016;13:92–105. https://doi.org/10.1038/nrclinonc.2015.152.
18. Abdou MAA, El Kiki HA, Madney Y, et al. Chemotherapy-related neurotoxicity in pediatric cancer patients: magnetic resonance imaging and clinical correlation. Egypt J Radiol Nucl Med. 2021;52:230. https://doi.org/10.1186/s43055-021-00606-x.

19. Moore RJ, Groninger H. Chemotherapy-induced peripheral neuropathy in pediatric Cancer patients. Cureus. 2013;5(6):e124.
20. Kandula T, Farrar MA, Cohn RJ, Mizrahi D, Carey K, Johnston K, Kiernan MC, Krishnan AV, Park SB. Chemotherapy-induced peripheral neuropathy in long-term survivors of childhood Cancer: clinical, neurophysiological, functional, and patient-reported outcomes. JAMA Neurol. 2018;75:980–8.
21. Mahajan A, Stavinoha PL, Rongthong W, Brodin NP, McGovern SL, El Naqa I, Palmer JD, Vennarini S, Indelicato DJ, Aridgides P, Bowers DC, Kremer L, Ronckers C, Constine L, Avanzo M. Neurocognitive effects and necrosis in childhood Cancer survivors treated with radiation therapy: a PENTEC comprehensive review. Int J Radiat Oncol Biol Phys. 2021;S0360–3016(21):00127–9.
22. Shen CJ, Kry SF, Buchsbaum JC, Milano MT, Inskip PD, Ulin K, Francis JH, Wilson MW, Whelan KF, Mayo CS, Olch AJ, Constine LS, Terezakis SA, Vogelius IR. Retinopathy, optic neuropathy, and cataract in childhood Cancer survivors treated with radiation therapy: a PENTEC comprehensive review. Int J Radiat Oncol Biol Phys. 2023;S0360–3016(23):00592–8.
23. Alessi I, Caroleo AM, de Palma L, Mastronuzzi A, Pro S, Colafati GS, et al. Short and long-term toxicity in pediatric Cancer treatment: central nervous system damage. Cancers (Basel). 2022;14(6):1540.
24. Howard SC, McCormick J, Pui CH, et al. Preventing and managing toxicities of high-dose methotrexate. Oncologist. 2016;21(12):1471–82.
25. McDonald GB, Tirumali N. Intestinal and liver toxicity of antineoplastic drugs. West J Med. 1984;140(2):250–9.
26. Hall MD, Howell RM, Jackson A, Owens CA, Hernandez S, Castellino SM, Ronckers CM, Constine LS, Bradley JA. Liver late effects in childhood Cancer survivors treated with radiation therapy: a PENTEC comprehensive review. Int J Radiat Oncol Biol Phys. 2023;S0360-3016(23):00584–9.
27. Mulder RL, Bresters D, Van den Hof M, Koot BG, Castellino SM, YKK L, Post PN, Postma A, Szőnyi LP, Levitt GA, Bardi E, Skinner R, van Dalen EC. Hepatic late adverse effects after antineoplastic treatment for childhood cancer. Cochrane Database Syst Rev. 2019;4(4):CD008205.
28. Huang TT, Hudson MM, Stokes DC, Krasin MJ, Spunt SL, Ness KK. Pulmonary outcomes in survivors of childhood cancer: a systematic review. Chest. 2011;140(4):881–901.
29. Briere TM, Agrusa JE, Martel MK, Jackson A, Olch AJ, Ronckers CM, Kremer LCM, Constine LS, McAleer MF. Acute and late pulmonary effects after radiation therapy in childhood Cancer survivors: a PENTEC comprehensive review. Int J Radiat Oncol Biol Phys. 2022;S0360–3016(22):00132–8.
30. Meacham LR, Burns K, Orwig KE, Levine J. Standardizing risk assessment for treatment-related gonadal insufficiency and infertility in childhood adolescent and young adult Cancer: the pediatric initiative network risk stratification system. J Adolesc Young Adult Oncol. 2020;9(6):662–6.
31. Rauck AM, Green DM, Yasui Y, Mertens A, Robison LL. Marriage in the survivors of childhood cancer: a preliminary description from the childhood Cancer survivor study. Med Pediatr Oncol. 1999;33(1):60–3.
32. Lo AC, Ronckers C, Aznar MC, Avanzo M, van Dijk I, Kremer LCM, Gagliardi G, Howell RM, Rancati T, Constine LS, Marcus KJ. Breast hypoplasia and decreased lactation from radiation therapy in survivors of pediatric malignancy: a PENTEC comprehensive review. Int J Radiat Oncol Biol Phys. 2021;S0360–3016(21):02725.
33. Milgrom SA, van Luijk P, Pino R, Ronckers CM, Kremer LC, Gidley PW, Grosshans DR, Laskar S, Okcu MF, Constine LS, Paulino AC. Salivary and dental complications in childhood Cancer survivors treated with radiation therapy to the head and neck: a pediatric Normal tissue effects in the clinic (PENTEC) comprehensive review. Int J Radiat Oncol Biol Phys. 2021;S0360–3016(21):00443.
34. Morton LM, Onel K, Curtis RE, Hungate EA, Armstrong GT. The rising incidence of second cancers: patterns of occurrence and identification of risk factors for children and adults. Am Soc Clin Oncol Educ Book. 2014;2014:e57–67.

35. Kok JL, Teepen JC, van der Pal HJ, van Leeuwen FE, WJE T, SJCMM N, Loonen JJ, Louwerens M, Versluys B, van den Heuvel-Eibrink MM, van Dulmen-den Broeder E, MMW J, van Santen HM, van der Heiden-van der Loo M, Janssens GO, Maduro JH, Bruggink AH, Jongmans MC, LCM K, Ronckers CM, DCOG-LATER Study Group. Incidence of and risk factors for histologically confirmed solid benign tumors among long-term survivors of childhood Cancer. JAMA Oncol. 2019;5(5):671–80.
36. Mulder RL, Kremer LC, Hudson MM, et al. Recommendations for breast cancer surveillance for female survivors of childhood, adolescent, and young adult cancer given chest radiation: a report from the international late effects of childhood Cancer guideline harmonization group. Lancet Oncol. 2013;14:e621–9.
37. Nipp RD, Kirchhoff AC, Fair D, Rabin J, Hyland KA, Kuhlthau K, Perez GK, Robison LL, Armstrong GT, Nathan PC, Oeffinger KC, Leisenring WM, Park ER. Financial burden in survivors of childhood Cancer: a report from the childhood Cancer survivor study. J Clin Oncol. 2017;35(30):3474–81.
38. Lewandowska A. The needs of parents of children suffering from Cancer-continuation of research. Children (Basel). 2022;9(2):144.
39. Ljungman L, Cernvall M, Grönqvist H, Ljótsson B, Ljungman G, von Essen L. Long-term positive and negative psychological late effects for parents of childhood cancer survivors: a systematic review. PLoS One. 2014;9:e103340.
40. Stuber ML, Meeske KA, Krull KR, Leisenring W, Stratton K, Kazak AE, Huber M, Zebrack B, Uijtdehaage SH, Mertens AC, Robison LL, Zeltzer LK. Prevalence and predictors of posttraumatic stress disorder in adult survivors of childhood cancer. Pediatrics. 2010;125(5):e1124–34.
41. Krull KR, Brinkman TM, Li C, Armstrong GT, Ness KK, Srivastava DK, Gurney JG, Kimberg C, Krasin MJ, Pui CH, Robison LL, Hudson MM. Neurocognitive outcomes decades after treatment for childhood acute lymphoblastic leukemia: a report from the St Jude lifetime cohort study. J Clin Oncol. 2013;3:4407–15.
42. Brinkman TM, Krasin MJ, Liu W, Armstrong GT, Ojha RP, Sadighi ZS, et al. Long-term neurocognitive functioning and social attainment in adult survivors of pediatric CNS tumors: results from the St Jude lifetime cohort study. J Clin Oncol. 2016;34:1358–67.
43. Vlachioti E, Matziou V, Perdikaris P, Mitsiou M, Stylianou C, Tsoumakas K, et al. Assessment of quality of life of children and adolescents with cancer during their treatment. Jpn J Clin Oncol. 2016;46:453–61.
44. Matziou V, Perdikaris P, Galanis P, Dousis E, Tzoumakas K. Evaluating depression in a sample of children and adolescents with cancer in Greece. Int Nurs Rev. 2008;55:314–9.
45. The Lancet Diabetes Endocrinology. Childhood cancer survival: a gap in need of closing. Lancet Diabetes Endocrinol. 2022;10(3):149. https://doi.org/10.1016/S2213-8587(22)00050-X. Epub 2022 Feb 11. PMID: 35157836.
46. Erdmann F, Frederiksen LE, Bonaventure A, Mader L, Hasle H, Robison LL, Winther JF. Childhood cancer: Survival, treatment modalities, late effects and improvements over time. Cancer Epidemiol. 2021;71(Pt B):101733. https://doi.org/10.1016/j.canep.2020.101733. Epub 2020 May 24. PMID: 32461035.

# Challenges in Paediatric Oncology in Low Middle Income Countries (LMICs)

8

Treshita Dey and Renu Madan

## 8.1 Introduction

Children and adolescents make up a modest but crucially essential portion of cancer patients globally (14.1million newly diagnosed adults vs. 160,000 children annually). In the majority of high-income countries (HICs), a kid with cancer is spared roughly 71 life years as opposed to 15 years for an adult. The substantial increase in paediatric cancer survival rates from a dismal 10% to 80–90% has been one of science's biggest successes in the previous 50 years. However, only 20% of children with cancer, residing in the developed countries, have experienced this modern success story. The remaining 80% of cancer-stricken children who reside in developing nations have yet to fully benefit from this achievement. Only 15–37% of children and adolescents in these low-resource environments receive cancer treatment, and the majority of cases are discovered at an advanced stage, making recovery unlikely. The World Health Organization, the United Nations, and other international organizations have pushed for the treatment of cancer to be considered a human right and have started to draw attention to it as a noncommunicable illness that is spreading and endangers public health in LMICs. This chapter discusses the challenges in paediatric cancers in LMICs and provides a possible strategy for resolution of the same.

T. Dey (✉)
Department of Radiotherapy, SGPGIMS, Lucknow, India

R. Madan
Department of Radiotherapy and Oncology, Postgraduate Institute of Medical Education and Research, Chandigarh, India





R. Madan et al. (eds.), *Evidence Based Practice in Pediatric Radiation Oncology*,
https://doi.org/10.1007/978-981-96-4872-6_8

## 8.2 Burden of Paediatric Cancer

Data on adult malignancies demonstrate regional and worldwide variations in incidence rates and distribution, frequently indicating distinct interactions between ethnic background, environment, socioeconomic status, and biology. Although disparities in disease incidence between developed and LMICs have been reported, the same paradigm for paediatric cancer is unknown due to the inadequate cancer registry systems [1]. In 2015, an estimated 397,000 childhood cancer cases occurred globally, but only 224,000 (43%) were diagnosed. Regional disparities were notable, with undiagnosed rates of 3% in western Europe and North America, and 57% in western Africa. In South Asia, 49% of cases were estimated to be undiagnosed. Based on population projections by Ward et al., 6.7 million childhood cancer cases are expected between 2015 and 2030. Without improvements in health system performance, approximately 2.9 million cases are projected to be missed during this period [2]. It is challenging to determine the real burden of paediatric malignancies in LMICs due to the dearth of paediatric cancer registries and the lack of trustworthy data. When compared to developed countries, leukaemia incidence reported as mean annual incidence per million children in LMICs is much lower (16.4 vs. 40.9, respectively) [3]. Given that acute leukaemia presents similarly to an acute infection and that early mortality may occur before malignancy is identified or diagnosed, these disparities may be a sign of underreporting. In reality, LMICs with lowest reported prevalence and incidence of leukaemia also have very high rates of malaria, which in endemic regions can be up to 10,000 times more prevalent than leukaemia [12]. However, the discovery that children between 2 and 5 years of age have a much higher incidence rate of ALL in developed nations, lack of such an age peak in LMICs, and sporadic clustering of childhood ALL cases have prompted infection-based hypotheses of leukemogenesis.

## 8.3 Reasons for Lagging behind in Paediatric Cancer Care

Contrary to common infectious illnesses, paediatric malignancies require multidisciplinary care, higher financial resource allocation, strong infrastructure, and diagnostic facilities. They account for less than 1% of the under-5 mortality rate (U5MR) [4]. As a result, governments and non-governmental organizations (NGOs) in LMICs have not paid much attention to paediatric malignancies since they were not seen worthwhile of the time and effort [5].

In 2000, the United Nations set eight millennium development goals (MDGs), the point 4 (1990–2015) of which was to reduce U5MR by two-thirds. The main causes of U5MR in LMICs have been infections and infant mortality. Therefore, throughout the past three decades, efforts by the government and NGOs have been concentrated on combating illnesses including malaria, malnutrition, diarrhoea, pneumonia, and human immunodeficiency virus (HIV). These measures have paid off, as seen by reduction in U5MR from 10.8 million deaths annually (2000) to 5.6 million deaths (2016), mostly secondary to early diagnosis and reporting [6–8]. However, whilst U5MR has decreased in the majority of countries, childhood cancer incidence and death are rising [9].

## 8.4 Need to Focus on Paediatric Cancer Care

It is a myth that treating paediatric malignancies is expensive and that expenditure incurred on them does not yield a return on investment [10]. According to studies, treating paediatric cancer meets the cost-effectiveness standard set out by World Health Organization (WHO). According to recent study by Force et al., paediatric tumours are linked to the largest proportion of disability-associated life years (DALYs) among all malignancies, LMICs generated majority of the DALYs, while early deaths were responsible for 99% of DALYs [11]. Due to lack of information, the contribution of long-term disabilities brought on by cancer therapy in developing nations is still grossly underestimated. When all prevalent paediatric illnesses were taken into account, paediatric cancers ranked sixth for DALYs.

## 8.5 Risk Factors for Poor Outcomes in LMIC

Most paediatric cancers have no established risk factors, in contrast to adults where 70% cancers are related to underlying risk factors (cigarettes, alcohol, lifestyle, food, etc.). Therefore, early diagnosis and treatment rather than screening and prevention must be primary goals in paediatric oncology. Paediatric cancer outcomes in LMICs are at risk due to social, economic, and political issues in addition to clinical ones, which are elaborated as follows:

| Risk factor | Evaluation | Recommendation |
|---|---|---|
| Late presentation, advanced stage at diagnosis | Data from cancer registries | 1. Expand diagnostic facilities and infrastructure supporting healthcare<br>2. Add paediatric oncology to medical curriculum<br>3. Frequent CME for general practitioners<br>4. Raise awareness among general population via print and social media<br>5. Create registries using international classification of childhood Cancer-3<br>6. Declare cancer a notifiable illness |
| Treatment dropouts | Hospital database to track patients | 1. Utilize technology to monitor your patients<br>2. Provide free universal healthcare to lessen financial load |
| Malnutrition | National survey on nutrition<br>Patient records<br>Survival statistics | 1. Hospital supplemental nutrition<br>2. Severe malnutrition: Ready-to-use meals and tube feeding<br>3. Discharge with dry ration packs |
| Lacking supportive care | Deaths due to toxicity<br>Dose reduction | 1. Create protocols appropriate for local resources<br>2. Enhance nursing and critical care services |

(continued)

| Risk factor | Evaluation | Recommendation |
|---|---|---|
| Limited healthcare professionals | Medical and nursing council recruitments | 1. Adequately trained nurses and doctors<br>2. Increase fellowships and employment in paediatric oncology<br>3. Develop specialized paediatric oncology nurse cadre |
| Access to quality medicines | Frequent random inspections undertaken by government to check drug quality<br>Evaluating ease of access of medications | 1. Construct testing facilities and regulatory frameworks to guarantee drug quality<br>2. Maintain proper cold chain<br>3. Ensure that necessary medicines for treating paediatric malignancies are accessible |

## 8.6 Increase Early Diagnosis and Community Health Worker Engagement

In reality, effective treatment of various paediatric malignancies in LMICs has shown that early detection is essential to guarantee that children and adolescents with cancer have the possibility to be treated. Wilms tumour and Burkitt's lymphoma are two instances of diseases that, when detected early and treated adequately taking into account the regional comorbidities and resource constraints of LMICs, can be cured. In most LMICs, community health workers (CHWs) are on the front lines of the healthcare delivery system, and by utilizing their ties to the local population, it is possible to enhance timely diagnosis and referral. Although CHWs may get brief training, this training frequently omits instruction on the signs and symptoms of paediatric cancer.

## 8.7 Need for Palliative Care and Psycho-Oncology Services

When children with cancer are evaluated, the WHO advocates integrating palliative care. Only 54.5% of children with cancer received any palliative treatment before passing away, according to a comprehensive evaluation of paediatric palliative care programmes in HICs [12]. In the majority of LMICs, there are no services for paediatric oncology palliative care [4]. In LMICs, palliative care services are essential since the majority of children with cancer have advanced illness and a sizeable part of them will have disease-related deaths. The perception that palliative care is expensive, that there is not enough time, that trained professionals are not available, that providers find talking about it uncomfortable, and the idea that palliative care is only useful when other treatments are no longer working are all obstacles to its implementation [13]. Access to opioids, particularly morphine, for treatment of cancer-related pain in children should be top priority. By 2030, LMICs should provide palliative care to 80% of children with cancer and pain management to all children with cancer, according to Lancet Oncology commission on sustainable care of children with cancer [4]. During treatment and follow-up, both children with cancer and their caregivers face considerable physical and psychological symptoms, notable being stress, anxiety, and depression [14]. Thus, it is crucial to manage them by including psycho-oncology services within regular paediatric cancer care. At Tata Memorial Hospital in Mumbai, the provision of psychological counselling for parents of children with cancer has assisted in lowering treatment dropouts and consequently improving results [4].

## 8.8 Future Directions

The important stakeholders have been treating cancer patients unfairly for many years [3]. However, during the past 2 years, things have altered drastically. The WHO started the Global Initiative for Childhood Cancer in September 2018 with the goal of curing at least 60% of paediatric cancer cases worldwide by 2030. Given that we only have 10 years to improve the survival rate of children malignancies, this burden is overwhelming. One million lives will be saved if this goal is met. By collaborating with WHO, St Jude Hospital is playing a crucial part in this initiative.

## 8.9 Conclusion

Progress made mostly in developed world is frequently used to assess improvements in cancer prevention and treatment. However, until we devote resources and intellectual capacity to address the burden of cancer in LMICs and build global efforts, a meaningful influence on cancer outcomes will not happen. It has been shown successful to adopt intensity-graduated therapies and integrate epidemiology and health services research through international collaborations that facilitate the procedures that create capacity. Major academic institutions with a focus on cancer care should adopt leadership responsibilities and be convinced that substantial worldwide initiatives will lead to significant advancements in cancer treatment and control over the course of the next century. The institution's purpose should include a worldwide cancer agenda, which should be shared by all cancer programmes and included into their strategy implementation.

## References

1. Bhakta N, Force LM, Allemani C, Atun R, Bray F, Coleman MP, et al. Childhood cancer burden: a review of global estimates. Lancet Oncol. 2019;20(1):e42–53. https://doi.org/10.1016/S1470-2045(18)30761-7.
2. Ward ZJ, Yeh JM, Bhakta N, Frazier AL, Atun R. Estimating the total incidence of global childhood cancer: a simulation-based analysis. Lancet Oncol. 2019;20(4):483–93. https://doi.org/10.1016/S1470-2045(18)30909-4.
3. Howard SC, Metzger ML, Wilimas JA, Quintana Y, Pui CH, Robison LL, et al. Childhood cancer epidemiology in low-income countries. Cancer. 2008;112(3):461–72.
4. Atun R, Bhakta N, Denburg A, Frazier AL, Friedrich P, Gupta S, et al. Sustainable care for children with cancer: a lancet oncology commission. Lancet Oncol. 2020;21(4):e185–224.

5. Rodriguez-Galindo C, Friedrich P, Morrissey L, Frazier L. Global challenges in pediatric oncology. Curr Opin Pediatr. 2013;25(1):3–15.
6. UNICEF, WHO, The World Bank Group, UN Population Division. Levels and trends in child mortality: report 2017 [Internet]. United Nations Inter-Group for Child Mortality Estimation; 2017. p. 40. https://childmortality.org/wp-content/uploads/2018/10/UN-IGME-Child-Mortality-Report-2017.pdf.
7. Bryce J, Victora CG, Black RE. The unfinished agenda in child survival. Lancet. 2013;382(9897):1049–59.
8. Black RE, Morris SS, Bryce J. Where and why are 10 million children dying every year? Lancet. 2003;361:2226–34.
9. Rodriguez-Galindo C, Friedrich P, Alcasabas P, Antillon F, Banavali S, Castillo L, et al. Toward the cure of all children with cancer through collaborative efforts: pediatric oncology as a global challenge. J Clin Oncol. 2015;33(27):3065–73.
10. Bhakta N. Building the financial case for treating childhood cancer in resource-limited settings. Cancer. 2019;125:1774–6.
11. Force LM, Abdollahpour I, Advani SM, Agius D, Ahmadian E, Alahdab F, et al. The global burden of childhood and adolescent cancer in 2017: an analysis of the global burden of disease study 2017. Lancet Oncol. 2019;20(9):1211–25.
12. Cheng BT, Rost M, De Clercq E, Arnold L, Elger BS, Wangmo T. Palliative care initiation in pediatric oncology patients: a systematic review. Cancer Med. 2019;8(1):3–12.
13. Weaver MS, Heinze KE, Kelly KP, Wiener L, Casey RL, Bell CJ, et al. Palliative care as a standard of Care in Pediatric Oncology. Pediatr Blood Cancer. 2015;62:S829–33.
14. Marcus J. Psychosocial issues in pediatric oncology. Ochsner J. 2012;12(3):211–5.

# Imaging Perspective in Paediatric Tumours

# 9

Anmol Bhatia, Pratibha Bhatia, and Kushaljit Singh Sodhi

## 9.1 Introduction

Radiological imaging is the most important diagnostic tool in the contemporary world. In the field of oncology, imaging is the cornerstone of patient management and care. It plays an important diagnostic role and helps to stage the disease, know the tumour extent, prognosticate the disease, gauge the therapeutic response, and assess for any recurrence during follow-ups [1]. However, radiological imaging has unique challenges, especially in the paediatric population. Children are more susceptible to the risks of ionizing radiations given the higher radiosensitivity of growing organs and their longer expected life spans, thus emphasizing the need for ALARA (As low as reasonably achievable) [2]. The other primary concern in the paediatric population is the need for immobilization and sedation, mainly for prolonged procedures, magnetic resonance imaging (MRI), or interventions. The lack of dedicated paediatric imaging centres and trained paediatric radiologists further aggravates the problem.

## 9.2 Technical Considerations in Paediatric Imaging

Children are not the same as miniature adults, and the major considerations in paediatric imaging, as aforementioned, are radiation safety and sedation. The use of radiography, fluoroscopy, and computed tomography (CT) should be minimized, and ultrasound (US) and MRI should be the preferred modalities wherever possible. Ultrasound is the safest imaging modality in children and, therefore, the initial modality of choice in most paediatric tumours. MRI enables better evaluation of

A. Bhatia (✉) · P. Bhatia · K. S. Sodhi
Department of Radiodiagnosis and Imaging, Postgraduate Institute of Medical Education and Research, Chandigarh, India


R. Madan et al. (eds.), *Evidence Based Practice in Pediatric Radiation Oncology*, https://doi.org/10.1007/978-981-96-4872-6_9

soft tissue tumours of the extremities and trunk as well as tumours in the head and neck [1, 3]. Also, MRI is now gaining ground for the assessment of tumours in the abdomen, retroperitoneum, and pelvis [1].

Radiography and fluoroscopy are less commonly employed in onco-imaging. Radiation exposure can be reduced by appropriate collimation and source-to-image distance, accurate focal spot size, proper positioning to avoid re-exposures, minimizing fluoroscopy time, and utilizing pulsed fluoroscopy and last image hold-up system [4, 5]. Anti-scatter grids can be avoided in children, and added filtration can be used to reduce entrance surface dose [4, 5].

If CT is absolutely necessary, the scanning area should be limited to the area of concern, multiphasic protocols should be minimized, scanning parameters should be adjusted by tube current modulation and low kV techniques, and the use of dual-energy CT [6]. Modern scanners with ultrahigh pitch, wide area detectors, and rapid rotation times have reduced radiation exposure and the need for sedation [6].

MRI, despite being radiation-free, requires longer imaging times and is thus accompanied by risks of sedation and anaesthesia in younger children, which may also have neuro-cognitive sequelae later in life. Faster imaging techniques like parallel imaging, compressed sensing, radial k space-filling techniques, and automated protocol selection techniques have reduced the dependence on anaesthesia [7]. Nuclear medicine imaging is also increasingly being used in onco-imaging, especially for metastatic workup and follow-up scans to detect recurrence; however, it incurs very high radiation doses [1].

There is a need for more standardized prospective studies to define evidence-based guidelines for interval and follow-up imaging in various paediatric malignancies so as to avoid unnecessary repeat imaging and thus reduce cost and radiation exposure. Also, the risk of secondary malignant neoplasms is rising due to high exposure to ionizing radiation in cancer patients from radiotherapy or diagnostic imaging [1, 3].

## 9.3 Imaging in Common Solid Paediatric Tumours

Paediatric solid tumours are a group of non-haematological, extracranial neoplasms that comprise roughly 40% of all childhood malignancies, the common ones being neuroblastoma, Wilms tumour, malignant bone tumours, soft tissue sarcomas, retinoblastoma, and hepatoblastoma [8].

### 9.3.1 Wilms Tumour

Wilms tumour is the most common abdominal malignancy in children, typically occurring between 1 and 5 years of age, with a peak at around 3 years of age [9]. Wilms tumour may occur sporadically or in association with predisposing genetic syndromes, including Beckwith-Wiedemann syndrome, Denys-Drash syndrome, and Sotos. Two loci on chromosome 11—locus 11p13 (WT1 gene) and locus 11p15 (WT2 gene)—are implicated in the pathogenesis of Wilms tumour [9, 10].

Bilateral tumours are seen in 4–13% of children, which may be synchronous or metachronous and are typically associated with nephroblastomatosis [11]. Classic Wilms tumour is triphasic, consisting of epithelial, blastemal, and stromal cells [9]. The teratoid variant consists of tissue of non-renal origin like bone, cartilage, or muscle.

Radiological evaluation of Wilms tumour focuses on identifying the extent of involvement, looking for metastasis, and assessing response to therapy.

On sonography, Wilms tumour is identified as a predominantly solid renal mass causing renal enlargement. It is heterogeneous in echotexture with areas of cystic, necrotic, and haemorrhagic degeneration. There may be underlying hydronephrosis with entrapment of the obstructed pelvicalyceal systems within the malignant mass. A pseudocapsule is typically seen around the mass. The tumour may invade the renal vein and extend through the IVC into the right atrium, which is better assessed on the Doppler. Ultrasound is an excellent modality for the primary tumour evaluation and vascular extension of tumours; however, it is limited in its ability to detect small contralateral tumours, extracapsular growth or metastasis, and lymph node involvement [9].

Computed tomography better delineates the tumour extent and overcomes the shortcomings seen with sonography. The tumour appears as a well-defined, large renal mass forming a positive beak sign with the kidneys signifying its renal origin. It displaces the adjacent structures rather than uplifting or encasing them. Areas of fat attenuation or calcification may be seen. The extracapsular extension is suggested by contour irregularity and exophytic growth pattern. On contrast-enhanced scans, the tumour is hypoenhancing relative to the normal renal parenchyma (Fig. 9.1). Tumour rupture is a dreaded complication and can increase the risk of

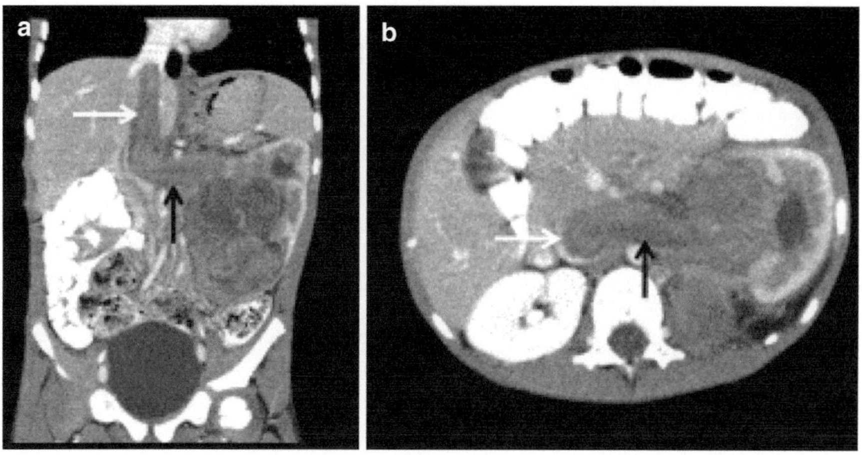


**Fig. 9.1** Wilms tumour. Contrast-enhanced computed tomography images in the coronal (**a**) and axial (**b**) planes are showing a heterogeneous mass arising from the left kidney causing its expansion. There is tumour thrombus involving the left renal vein (black arrow in **a** and **b**) and the inferior vena cava (white arrow in **a**, **b**) causing their expansion

post-operative recurrence in patients. The radiological signs of rupture include ill-defined margins, peritumoral fat stranding, ascites beyond cul-de-sac, extracapsular retroperitoneal fluid, and ipsilateral pleural effusion. Peritoneal, omental, or mesenteric spread can also be well assessed on CT scans, along with detecting spread to the liver or lungs. Lymphadenopathy can help in prognostication; however, differentiating malignant from reactive lymphadenopathy is best done histologically [9, 12].

On MRI, the tumour is heterogeneous and appears predominantly iso-to hypointense than normal renal parenchyma on T1 WI, iso-to hyperintense on T2-weighted imaging, and is relatively hypoenhancing to normal renal parenchyma on post-contrast scans. The pseudocapsule is seen as a hypointense rim on all sequences [9]. The tumour's solid component restricts on diffusion-weighted imaging and can be targeted for tumour biopsies. DWI can also be used to predict response after chemotherapy with the reduction in tumour size and increase in ADC implying a positive response. DWI can also help pick small synchronous tumours in the same or contralateral kidney [13].

Wilms tumour is FDG avid; however, the role of FDG PET is still not clearly defined for its evaluation. Predicting response to therapy or tumour recurrence and detection of metastatic lung nodules can be some of its potential benefits.

Staging in Wilms tumour is directed by the American COG (Children's Oncology Group) and the European SIOP (International Society of Paediatric Oncology) systems. Although both the systems are primarily post-operative staging systems, the SIOP follows initial neoadjuvant chemotherapy followed by surgery, while the COG recommends upfront surgery followed by adjuvant chemotherapy [14].

### 9.3.2 Neuroblastoma

Neuroblastoma is the third most common paediatric malignancy after leukaemia and CNS tumours. Neuroblastomas arise from the primordial neural crest cells, and two-thirds of neuroblastomas are seen in the abdomen, out of which two-thirds originate from the adrenal medulla and the rest from the extra-adrenal sympathetic chain in the retroperitoneum or posterior mediastinum; 90% of the tumours are seen in less than 5 years, with the median age being 2 years. Tumours of neural crest origin comprise neuroblastoma, ganglioneuroblastoma, and ganglioneuroma in increasing order of cellular maturation, differentiation, and positive outcomes. Metastasis to lymph nodes, bone marrow, bone, liver, and skin is common. The biopsy is the diagnostic gold standard; however, combinations of bone marrow aspirate, imaging, and urinary catecholamine levels (vanillylmandelic acid and homovanillic acid) may suffice [15, 16].

Ultrasound shows an ill-defined, heterogeneous, echogenic mass with or without posterior acoustic shadowing. Mass tends to displace and encase the adjacent vasculature rather than invading them and displaces adjacent organs. The mass may rarely infiltrate the adjoining kidney, thus making it difficult to differentiate from Wilms tumour on imaging alone [15, 17].

Computed tomography shows a lobulated, ill-defined soft tissue mass with heterogeneous enhancement in the post-contrast scan. Calcifications are seen in >90% of abdominal and 50% of thoracic neuroblastomas, which may display a fine stippled, curvilinear, or coarse pattern (Fig. 9.2). Areas of low attenuation depicting cystic/necrotic or haemorrhagic degeneration may be seen. Tumour is more likely to displace the adjacent structures with typical inferior displacement of kidneys and anterior displacement and encasement of aorta and IVC [17, 18].

MRI shows a mass with a low signal on T1 and a high signal on T2 with a variable enhancement pattern. Solid areas of tumour typically restrict on DWI. Involvement of the spinal canal and marrow is best appreciated on MRI [15, 17, 18].

Metastasis to the liver may be seen as multiple nodules or diffuse infiltration (typically in neonates). Metastasis to the marrow may be seen as diffuse or focal altered signal intensity with MDG/MIBG uptake on scintigraphy scans. MIBG (Metaiodobenzylguanidine) scans are more sensitive and specific for detecting primary tumours and metastasis to organs other than bone, in which case MDP (Tc-99 m Methylene diphosphonate) scans are more specific [19, 20]. Metastasis to the bone may be seen as geographic lucent area, permeative pattern, or metaphyseal lucency with or without periosteal reaction and soft tissue deposit. Metastasis to the head is commonly seen with involvement of the skull, dura, and orbit.

International Neuroblastoma Risk Group Staging System (INRGSS) system utilizes the role of pre-operative imaging evaluation vis-a-vis the International Neuroblastoma Staging System (INSS), which is a post-operative staging system; however, both are being used and complement each other in the management of neuroblastoma. Image-derived risk factors have been stated under INRG, wherein the risk of surgical resection is envisaged based on the number of body compartments involved, relationship to adjacent vasculature, infiltration of adjacent organs, and spinal extension [16].

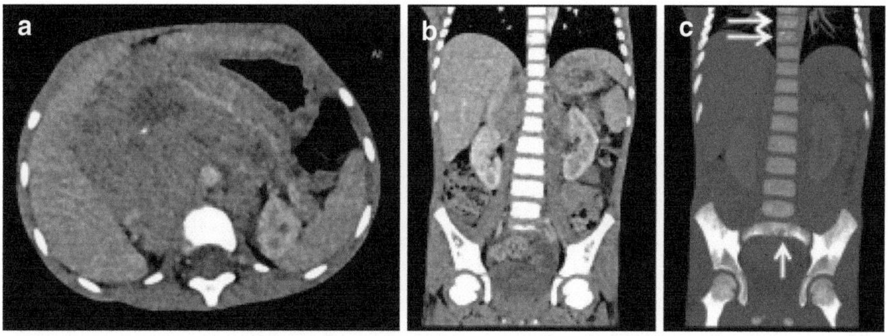


**Fig. 9.2** Neuroblastoma. Axial (**a**) and coronal (**b**) contrast-enhanced computed tomography images are showing a mass in the right suprarenal location which is extending across the midline with encasement of aorta and reaching on to the left side. Bilateral kidneys are seen normal. Bone window image (**c**) is showing lytic lesions in sacrum and dorsal vertebrae (arrows in **c**) suggestive of metastases

### 9.3.3 Hepatoblastoma

Hepatoblastoma is the most common primary malignancy of the liver in children, with the highest incidence in children under 5 years. Association with hemihypertrophy, Beckwith-Wiedemann syndrome, familial adenomatous polyposis, Gardner syndrome, and Wilms tumour is seen. Also, some studies have recorded an increased incidence in pre-term or low birth weight babies. AFP levels are raised in up to 90% of patients and can be used as a tumour marker to monitor treatment and recurrence [21, 22]. Metastasis to the lungs is most common, followed by lymph nodes. There are two pathological variants: epithelial and mixed type [22].

On sonography, the tumour is usually seen as a well-defined, inhomogeneous, predominantly hyperechoic mass in the liver. It commonly presents as a solitary mass in the right lobe of the liver; however, infrequently, it may be multifocal or even diffusely infiltrate the liver. A rare cystic variant of hepatoblastoma is also known [23, 24]. The mixed histopathological variant is more likely to present as heterogeneous mass with anechoic areas of cystic/necrotic or haemorrhagic degeneration and hyperechoic foci with posterior acoustic shadowing suggestive of calcifications. Vascular invasion into the portal or hepatic veins and IVC is known to occur. Demonstration of flow within the thrombus on Doppler evaluation suggests tumour thrombus [19, 22].

Computed tomography of the abdomen reveals a well-circumscribed, heterogeneous mass showing low attenuation compared to the normal liver parenchyma. Amorphous or speckled calcifications are seen in more than 50% of patients. On contrast-enhanced CT, the mass may show peripheral enhancement in the early phase, becoming iso-to hypodense in delayed phases [19, 22, 25] (Fig. 9.3).

On MRI, hepatoblastoma is seen as a predominantly hypointense mass on T1 WI, becoming hyperintense on T2-weighted sequences relative to normal liver parenchyma. T1–T2 hypointense fibrous bands are seen traversing the tumour.

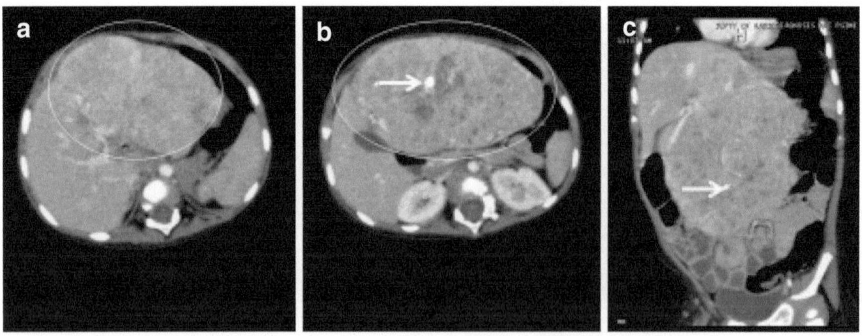


**Fig. 9.3** Hepatoblastoma. Contrast-enhanced computed tomography images in axial plane (**a**, **b**) and coronal plane (**b**) are showing a heterogeneously enhancing mass lesion in the left lobe of the liver (circled in **a**, **b**) and causing its expansion with exophytic component along the inferior aspect. A few small foci of calcification are also seen in it (arrows in **b**, **c**)

Heterogeneous enhancement is seen on post-contrast scans. Vascular invasion is seen as the loss of normal flow voids [19, 25].

Surgical resection is the treatment for hepatoblastoma. PRETEXT (PRE-Treatment EXTent of tumour) system is used for risk stratification. It comprises two subgroups—i) PRETEXT, which stages patients into groups I–IV based on the number of adjoining liver sections that are involved or free of tumour, and ii) the annotation factors, which are denoted by V (hepatic venous/IVC involvement), P (portal venous involvement), E (extrahepatic disease contiguous with the main liver tumour), F (multifocality), R (tumour rupture), C (caudate lobe involvement), N (lymph node involvement), and M (distant metastasis). Imaging plays a crucial role in assessing the resectability of hepatoblastomas before and after chemotherapy [26].

## References

1. Weiser DA, Kaste SC, Siegel MJ, Adamson PC. Imaging in childhood cancer: a society for pediatric radiology and children's oncology group joint task force report. Pediatr Blood Cancer. 2013;60(8):1253–60.
2. Hall EJ. Radiation biology for pediatric radiologists. Pediatr Radiol. 2008;39(1):57.
3. Kaste SC. Imaging challenges: a US perspective on controlling exposure to ionizing radiation in children with cancer. Pediatr Radiol. 2009;39(Suppl 1(Suppl 1)):S74–9.
4. Uffmann M, Schaefer-Prokop C. Digital radiography: the balance between image quality and required radiation dose. Eur J Radiol. 2009;72(2):202–8.
5. Willis CE. Optimizing digital radiography of children. Digit Radiogr. 2009;72(2):266–73.
6. Zacharias C, Alessio AM, Otto RK, Iyer RS, Philips GS, Swanson JO, et al. Pediatric CT: strategies to lower radiation dose. AJR Am J Roentgenol. 2013;200(5):950–6.
7. Kozak BM, Jaimes C, Kirsch J, Gee MS. MRI techniques to decrease imaging times in children. Radiographics. 2020;40(2):485–502.
8. Allen-Rhoades W, Whittle SB, Rainusso N. Pediatric solid tumors of infancy: an overview. Pediatr Rev. 2018;39(2):57–67.
9. Lowe LH, Isuani BH, Heller RM, Stein SM, Johnson JE, Navarro OM, et al. Pediatric renal masses: Wilms tumor and beyond. Radiographics. 2000;20(6):1585–603.
10. Geller E, Smergel EM, Lowry PA. Renal neoplasms of childhood. Radiol Clin North Am. 1997;35(6):1391–413.
11. Lonergan GJ, Martínez-León MI, Agrons GA, Montemarano H, Suarez ES. Nephrogenic rests, nephroblastomatosis, and associated lesions of the kidney. Radiographics. 1998;18(4):947–68.
12. Bates G, Feinsein K. Renal neoplasms. In: Caffeys pediatric diagnostic imaging. 12th ed. Elsevier Saunders; 2013.
13. Gawande RS, Gonzalez G, Messing S, Khurana A, Daldrup-Link HE. Role of diffusion-weighted imaging in differentiating benign and malignant pediatric abdominal tumors. Pediatr Radiol. 2013;43(7):836–45.
14. Brillantino C, Rossi E, Minelli R, Bignardi E, Coppola M, Zeccolini R, et al. Current role of imaging in the management of children with Wilms tumor according to the new UMBRELLA protocol. Transl Med. 2020;8:206.
15. Papaioannou G, McHugh K. Neuroblastoma in childhood: review and radiological findings. Cancer Imaging. 2005;5:116–27.
16. Brisse HJ, McCarville MB, Granata C, Krug KB, Wootton-Gorges SL, Kanegawa K, et al. Guidelines for imaging and staging of Neuroblastic tumors: consensus report from the international neuroblastoma risk group project. Radiology. 2011;261(1):243–57.

17. McHugh K. Renal and adrenal tumours in children. Cancer Imaging. 2007;7(1):41–51.
18. Navarro OM, Daneman A. Acquired conditions. In: Caffey's pediatric diagnostic imaging. 12th ed. Elsevier Saunders; 2013.
19. Chung EM, Lattin GE, Cube R, Lewis RB, Marichal-Hernández C, Shawhan R, et al. From the archives of the AFIP: pediatric liver masses: radiologic-pathologic correlation part 2. Malignant tumors. RadioGraphics. 2011;31(2):483–507.
20. Lonergan GJ, Schwab CM, Suarez ES, Carlson CL. From the archives of the AFIP. Radiographics. 2002;22(4):911–34.
21. Miller JH, Greenspan BS. Integrated imaging of hepatic tumors in childhood. Part I: malignant lesions (primary and metastatic). Radiology. 1985;154(1):83–90.
22. Dubois J, Lowe LH. Neoplasia. In: Caffey's pediatric diagnostic imaging. 12th ed. Elsevier Saunders; 2013.
23. Men S, Hekimoğlu B, Tüzün M, Arda İS, Pinar A. Unusual US and CT findings in hepatoblastoma: a case report. Pediatr Radiol. 1995;25(7):507–8.
24. Dachman AH, Pakter RL, Ros PR, Fishman EK, Goodman ZD, Lichtenstein JE. Hepatoblastoma: radiologic-pathologic correlation in 50 cases. Radiology. 1987;164(1):15–9.
25. Helmberger TK, Ros PR, Mergo PJ, Tomczak R, Reiser MF. Pediatric liver neoplasms: a radiologic–pathologic correlation. Eur Radiol. 1999;9(7):1339–47.
26. Towbin AJ, Meyers RL, Woodley H, Miyazaki O, Weldon CB, Morland B, et al. 2017 PRETEXT: radiologic staging system for primary hepatic malignancies of childhood revised for the Paediatric hepatic international tumour trial (PHITT). Pediatr Radiol. 2018;48(4):536–54.

# Imaging Perspective in Pediatric Tumors: CNS Tumors

# 10

Vikas Bhatia and Bharat Hosur

## 10.1 Background

Pediatric brain tumors are the commonest of solid tumors and overall, the second most common malignancy in children. Neuroimaging is an integral part of the initial assessment, diagnosis, treatment guidance and titration, focused interventions, surgical and combined therapies in real time as well as their short- and long-term follow-up. Imaging forms the sine qua non in complete understanding of the anatomical localization, pathophysiology, histology, and to an extent the molecular genotype of a tumor in the central nervous system (CNS). With the advancing technology and research in the imaging sciences, pre-clinical diagnosis of brain tumors incidentally or with correlative subtle inputs is increasingly becoming the new norm. A precise and detailed understanding of the imaging nuances related to the pediatric tumors of the CNS is helpful in optimizing the apt, effective, and timely management. In this chapter, we are deliberating on the supratentorial pediatric tumors except for the diffuse midline gliomas.

## 10.2 Imaging Approach

Non-contrast CT (NCCT) scan, which is a workhorse for the clinical setting of focal seizures in adults, is not always the best choice in children due to radiation concerns. The limitations include truncated lesion detection, characterization, and suboptimal soft tissue resolution including gray-white differentiation. However, CT is

V. Bhatia (✉)
Department of Radiodiagnosis and Imaging, PGIMER, Chandigarh, India

B. Hosur
Department of Radiodiagnosis, AFMC, Pune, India





R. Madan et al. (eds.), *Evidence Based Practice in Pediatric Radiation Oncology*,
https://doi.org/10.1007/978-981-96-4872-6_10

a fast, cheap, easily acquired, and widely available imaging modality, effective for timely decision-making at the time of initial presentation, surgical planning, and follow-up in some settings. Hyperdense tumors like lymphoma, calcified metastases, and medulloblastoma can be readily diagnosed on NCCT. Calcifications, blood degradation products, cystic components, ventricular dilatation, intracranial mass effects, and bony landmarks related to the tumors can be precisely picked up on the CT images. Also, many a time, it may be the only feasible imaging modality, especially in low- and middle-income countries, for symptomatic children with brain tumors. Transcranial ultrasound is another excellent bedside modality for neonates and small children till the open fontanels provide an acoustic window. Although the diffuse and small focal tumors may be missed, tumoral bleed, hydrocephalus, and calcifications can be picked up without the requirement of significant patient preparation or sedation. Transcranial and abdomino-thoracic ultrasound in combination sometimes readily aids in the complete syndromic diagnosis in a single sitting, especially in phacomatoses.

Magnetic resonance imaging (MRI) is the modality of choice in the diagnosis of all CNS tumors, once the child is clinically apt to undergo the same. The inherent soft tissue contrast, gray-white matter differentiation, cytotoxic edema, tumoral vascularity, the spectroscopic composition of the molecules, and radiation-free screening of the entire neuraxis are some of the points that make it indispensable. However, it should be used with clear clinical reasoning and treating team consensus, because the children may require anesthesia support, be susceptible to gadolinium contrast deposition-related health hazards, and in developing nations, may have to travel long distances and suffer long waiting periods, apart from the higher cost. Optimal clinical stabilization of the child including anti-seizure medications, pain relief, reassurance, and pre-scan rehearsals can yield better image quality.

## 10.3 Classification

The recent fifth edition, 2021-World Health Organization (WHO) Classification of CNS Tumors after consolidating all the updates of The Consortium to Inform Molecular and Practical Approaches to CNS Tumor Taxonomy – Not Official WHO (cIMPACT-NOW), has categorized the pediatric tumors separately for the first time [1]. It is increasingly clearer that pediatric brain tumors are distinct in many more ways than hitherto known, even among the histologically identical adult counterparts. Keeping with the diagnostic approach toward molecular targeted therapies, a four-layered diagnosis is prescribed. Integrated diagnosis (combined histological and molecular), histopathological diagnosis, CNS WHO grade, and molecular information, respectively, are the components of the diagnostic layers [2]. The imaging correlates aid in the prediction of each layer in a non-invasive and reproducible manner.

## 10.4 Tumor Types

### 10.4.1 Sellar and Suprasellar Tumors

The sellar and suprasellar region, a compact cross-road for the cranial nerves (II to VI), arteries leading to circle of Willis, and venous channels of cavernous sinuses harbor approximately 10% of the intracranial tumors in children [3]. Identification of the normal pituitary gland with T1-hyperintense posterior pituitary bright spot, distinctly from a mass lesion, forms an initial step in tumor diagnosis. The smoothly tapering infundibulum inserting at the center of the pituitary may become a subtle marker of a focal lesion when effacement, nodularity, and abrupt change in dimensions are present. Craniopharyngioma is by far the commonest tumor in this location, found in up to 90% of the sellar and parasellar lesions of children. Adamantinomatous type with variable-sized cysts with mucinous contents is common in children, compared to the relatively solid papillary type of adults. The rule of 90% seems to apply for its calcification, enhancement, suprasellar location, and mixed solid-cystic contents. Pituitary adenomas form the least common subset of these tumors with ≤3% incidence. Also, they are almost always functioning tumors in children, prolactinoma being the commonest histological type. The non-functioning pituitary adenomas are extremely rare in children, so much as to incite a detailed review and work-up before labeling them so. Germ cell tumors are intensely enhancing lesions arising from the infundibular recess that may cause thickening and nodularity of the pituitary stalk. Langerhans cell histiocytosis, sarcoidosis, and tuberculosis may be other causes of the thickened stalk. Hypothalamic hamartomas that appear as ill-defined non-enhancing expansile lesions in relation to the tuber cinereum may be associated with the "molar tooth syndrome."

### 10.4.2 Pineal Region Tumors

Germ cell tumors, constituting up to 8% of the brain tumors, are the commonest masses in the pineal region. They seem to "engulf" the pineal physiological calcification, in contradistinction with the pineoblastomas that "blast" the calcific foci toward the periphery. Multifocality is also common with bifocal germinomas occurring concerning both the pineal and pituitary glands, similar to the trilateral retinoblastomas occurring in conjunction with the pineoblastomas. Pineal parenchymal tumors are rare in pediatric age, with benign pineal cyst being the commonest. The vein of Galen on both sides should be looked into carefully on post-contrast T1 images and/or CT/MR venograms to confirm the tumoral infiltration or mass effects.

### 10.4.3 Hemispheric Tumors

Pediatric gliomas are by far the commonest tumors of the cerebral hemispheres, especially in children of less than two and more than 10 years of age. Although most of the diffuse gliomas are distributed primarily in the white matter, some oligodendrogliomas, pleomorphic xanthoastrocytoma (PXA), or gangliogliomas can be cortical based and present with focal seizures. Glioneural tumors like dysembryoplastic neuroepithelial tumor (DNET) and gangliogliomas can involve both gray and white matter ab initio. Meticulous look out for the subtle syndromic markers within and outside the neuroparenchyma aids in superior diagnosis as well as management decisions; for example, recognizing the subtle abnormal focal areas of signal intensities (FASI) in a patient with cortical-based tumor suggests a high-grade glioma as an association with the neurofibromatosis type-1 (Fig. 10.1). The presence of subependymal nodules in conjunction with a cortical lesion is suggestive of a tuber in a case of tuberous sclerosis. As per the fifth edition of WHO-classification, pediatric gliomas are grouped into diffuse and circumscribed based on the topography; high-grade and low-grade based upon genetic and histological markers that have imaging pointers (Table 10.1). The newly recognized pediatric-type diffuse gliomas in the 2021-WHO Classification consist of four low-grade and four high-grade tumors [4]. The diffuse astrocytoma MYB or MYBL1-altered, angiocentric glioma, diffuse low-grade glioma, mitogen-activated protein kinase (MAPK)-altered, and polymorphous low-grade neuroepithelial tumor of the young (PLNTY) are the low-grade gliomas. Diffuse midline glioma, H3K27-altered, diffuse hemispheric glioma, H3

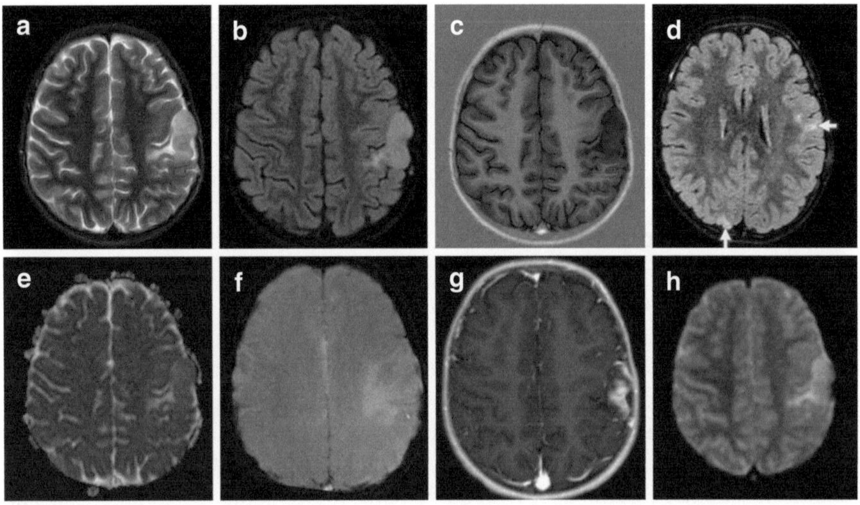


**Fig. 10.1** Contrast-enhanced MRI brain of a 5-year-old-boy with right-sided focal seizures. Axial images at the supratentorial levels with T2 (**a**), FLAIR (**b**), T1-inversion recovery (**c**), apparent diffusion coefficient (**e**), susceptibility-weighted imaging (**f**), post-contrast T1 (**g**), and source image of dynamic susceptibility contrast-based perfusion-weighted imaging show focal peri-Rolandic focal gyral thickening with mild perilesional edema and intense heterogeneous enhancement within the non-restricting, non-blooming cortical-based tumor. The abnormal subcortical focal areas of signal intensity (FASI) in the right occipital and left frontal regions (arrows in **d**), unrelated to the tumor and the cutaneous cafe au lait spots helped in the diagnosis of the high-grade glioma in the child with neurofibromatosis type-1 which was confirmed on histopathology

**Table 10.1** Common supratentorial tumors and their key imaging features

| Tumor groups based on the location | Common tumors | Imaging features |
|---|---|---|
| Sellar and suprasellar tumors | Craniopharyngioma | Adamantinomatous type: Commonly in 5–15 years<br>Cystic components with "machinery oil" like cholesterol-rich T1-hyperintense contents<br>90%-cystic components, 90%-calcify, 90%-enhance |
| | Germ cell tumor | Intense contrast enhancement<br>Thickening of the infundibulum<br>Early CSF seeding/drop metastasis |
| | Pituitary adenoma | Macroadenoma when size >10 mm<br>Snowman sign—Figure of 8 appearances of the tumor on both sides of diaphragma sellae<br>Intra-tumoral hemorrhage—when adenoma overgrows its own circulation<br>PPBS displaced and usually intact |
| | Meningioma | Identified separate from the pituitary gland<br>Dural tail—enhancing dural outline adjacent to the tumor margins<br>May be associated with NF-2 |
| Pineal region tumors | Pineoblastoma | Heterogeneously hyperdense with peripheral (exploded) calcifications<br>Necrotic and hemorrhagic contents with strong enhancement of the rest of the tumor<br>Diffusion restriction of enhancing part |
| | Germ cell tumor | Eccentric (engulfed) calcification<br>Homogeneous intense enhancement<br>Associated with retinoblastomas<br>Early CSF spread |
| | Pineocytoma | Iso-hypodense lesions with discrete margins<br>Peripheral calcific foci with variable rim or nodular enhancement |
| Hemispheric tumors | Ganglioglioma | Usually a cystic temporal lesion with an eccentric enhancing mural nodule<br>Variable rim enhancement; rare patchy enhancement associated with sinister prognosis |

(continued)

**Table 10.1** (continued)

| Tumor groups based on the location | Common tumors | Imaging features |
|---|---|---|
| | Dysembryoplastic neuroepithelial tumor (DNET) | Multinodular, multicystic "bubbly" lesion, pointing toward the ventricle<br>Lack of enhancement and mass effect<br>FLAIR hyperintense rim<br>Associated with focal cortical dysplasias |
| | Pediatric-type low-grade gliomas | T2-hyperintense, T1-hypointense lesions with indistinct margins<br>Lack of enhancement, diffusion restriction, and intra-tumoral susceptibility changes<br>Chunky calcification in PLNTY |
| | Pediatric-type high-grade gliomas | Necrotic, hemorrhagic contents with variable heterogeneous enhancement<br>Foci of restricted diffusion, susceptibility changes, high fractional anisotropy, raised rCBV and high choline:Creatinine ratio |
| Ventricular and periventricular tumors | Supratentorial ependymoma | Subventricular frontoparietal parenchyma<br>"Periwinkle sign" on an NCCT with centripetal calcification and peripheral cysts<br>Diffusion restriction in up to two thirds |
| | Subependymal giant cell astrocytoma | Usually in the vicinity of foramen of Monro<br>Associated with tuberous sclerosis<br>Peripheral calcification, avid enhancement |
| | Choroid plexus papilloma | Trigones of lateral ventricles<br>Lobulated margins, T2-hypointensity, hydrocephalus<br>Intense enhancement |
| | Choroid plexus carcinoma | Heterogeneous enhancement<br>Parenchymal infiltration with perilesional edema<br>Early CSF dissemination |

G34-mutant, diffuse high-grade glioma, H3 and IDH-wild-type and infant-type hemispheric glioma are the high-grade masses. Although routine MRI and CT images remain incapable of specifically diagnosing individual tumors, grade segregation and tumor characterization provide valuable diagnostic pointers. Thus, the hemispheric pediatric tumors are way different from their adult counterparts and have better prognoses with lesser mutation burden.

### 10.4.4 Ventricular and Periventricular Tumors

Approximately 10% of supratentorial tumors occur within or in the vicinity of the ventricles. The lateral ventricle, especially around the trigones is the commonest location that harbor about half of the lesions. Most of the intraventricular lesions are indolent with delayed presentation, especially in a non-verbal child. The subependymal giant cell astrocytomas (SEGA), which are seen in patients with tuberous sclerosis are found in the vicinity of the foramen of Monro and show intense contrast enhancement. The CSF-flow-related artifacts around the ventricular outlets may interfere with the optimal delineation of the small tumors. Choroid plexus papillomas (CPP), the commonest lateral ventricular tumor in children, usually occupy the trigones of the choroid plexus in toddlers and the fourth ventricle in adolescents [5]. They cause ventriculomegaly due to CSF overproduction, malabsorption, as well as ventricular outflow obstructions, hence presenting sometimes with catastrophic acute hydrocephalus. Although avid enhancement is common to both CPP and choroid plexus carcinoma (CPC), the periventricular parenchymal invasion, heterogeneity in enhancement, perilesional edema, and craniospinal CSF seeding point to the latter. Supratentorial ependymomas unlike the infratentorial counterparts are largely parenchymal lesions adjacent to the lateral ventricles. The typical calcification, variable-sized cysts, and minimal enhancement optimally establish the diagnosis. The central neurocytomas, although rarer in children are found usually around the septum pellucidum and the frontal horns, with typical microcysts that are best delineated on the high resolution heavily T2-weighted sequences.

## 10.5 Imaging Patterns

On conventional sequences, most of the neuroparenchymal tumors in children appear hyperintense on T2 and Flair images, and hypointense on T1-weighted images, usually with indistinct margins. Although the eccentric or peripheral diffusion restriction may be present in high-grade tumors, central restriction of diffusion suggests an abscess or tuberculoma. The calcification and hemorrhage related to the tumor are promptly picked up by susceptibility-weighted imaging (SWI). The foci of intra-tumoral susceptibility signal (ITSS) also signify the neovascularity in high-grade tumors [6]. Contrast enhancement on T1-weighted images simply indicates the breach of blood-brain barrier in relation to the mass lesion and is not an indicator of tumor histology or grade.

Although not always does the conventional MRI suffice for a pinpoint diagnosis of brain tumors, some imaging phenotypes are characteristic of the individual lesions. Bubbly cystic tumor with a Flair hyperintense rim is classically seen in DNET. Lobulated periventricular tumor with chunky calcifications showing the "Periwinkle sign" is consistent with the supratentorial ependymoma [7]. The increasing T2-hyperintensity toward the subependymal aspect termed the "Transmantle-like sign" in a tumor showing focal calcification and cystic changes is considered diagnostic of the PLNTY [4]. Suprasellar loculated cystic lesion with T1-hyperintense machine-oil-like contents and enhancing eccentric solid components is typical of adamantinomatous craniopharyngioma. "T2-Flair mismatch sign," which is otherwise validated as an imaging marker of IDH-mutation and 1p19q co-deletion in adult gliomas, has not been found useful in pediatric age group even in the tumors with IDH genotypes [8, 9]. However, it is found commonly in pediatric mixed glioneural tumors with central suppression of signal intensity on Flair images [10].

## 10.6 Advanced Imaging and Their Applications

Compressed Sensitivity Encoding (C-SENSE) is a newer technology, used in conjunction with the parallel imaging techniques of MRI. Superior image quality (especially the tumoral and peritumoral interface regions) with a reduction in acquisition times (by around 21%) and lower energy deposition are possible with C-SENSE-based pediatric tumor MRI protocols [11]. Faster acquisition of MR-spectroscopy without significant loss of information is also possible in C-SENSE [12]. This reduces the time required for the acquisition of the diagnostically optimal images and also higher resolution for the given scan time. It further implies a reduction in sedative or anesthetic drug requirements for toddlers and infants. The newer gradient sequences with variable flip angles with faster k-space-filling protocols further lower the movement-related artifacts, commonly encountered in children. The non-contrast perfusion techniques like arterial spin Labeling (ASL) and intravoxel incoherent motion (IVIM) based on utilizing the flow-dependent proton spins and the differentiation of diffusivity from perfusion fraction are of immense use when repeated scans are needed for follow-up [13]. An exponentially increasing application of Artificial Intelligence (AI) in imaging has facilitated efficient and standardized data management, tumor detection, lesion segmentation, and texture analysis that may be par excellence [14]. The advances in the understanding of tumorigenesis pathways and the feasibility to link them to the imaging phenotypes have led to the evolution of "Radiogenomics," which aligns well with molecular diagnosis and targeted therapy [15]. Transcranial Magnetic Resonance-Guided High-Intensity Focused Ultrasound (MRg-HIFU) is a promising newer minimally invasive therapeutic advancement, which uses the HIFU beams to open up the blood-brain barriers to the chemotherapeutic as well as non-invasive ablation of the tumors [16].

## 10.7 Summary

Neuroimaging is an integral part of pediatric brain tumor diagnosis as well as management. It forms the vital link between the clinical presentation and the treatment decisions at various stages of the management. Commensurate with the principle of a child being not just a small adult, the supratentorial neuroparenchymal tumors vary significantly in terms of imaging phenotype and genotypes, compared to the adult brain tumors. A clear understanding of the pediatric neuroimaging nuances, challenges, and possible artifacts aids in optimal imaging and corroborative clinical benefit. Knowledge about the latest WHO CNS classification and advanced imaging techniques enable reproducible, reliable, treatment-oriented reporting that can save lives, time, and cost.

## References

1. Louis DN, Perry A, Wesseling P, et al. The 2021 WHO classification of tumors of the central nervous system: a summary. Neuro-Oncology. 2021;23:1231–51.
2. Johnson DR, Guerin JB, Giannini C, Morris JM, Eckel LJ, Kaufmann TJ. 2016 updates to the WHO brain tumor classification system: what the radiologist needs to know. Radiographics. 2017;37:2164–80.
3. Harrington MH, Casella SJ. Pituitary tumors in childhood. Curr Opin Endocrinol Diabetes Obes. 2012;19:63–7.
4. Kurokawa R, Kurokawa M, Baba A, Ota Y, Pinarbasi E, Camelo-Piragua S, Capizzano AA, Liao E, Srinivasan A, Moritani T. Major changes in 2021 World Health Organization classification of central nervous system tumors. Radiographics. 2022;42:1474.
5. Suh DY, Mapstone T. Pediatric supratentorial intraventricular tumors. Neurosurg Focus. 2001;10:E4.
6. Gaudino S, Marziali G, Pezzullo G, et al. Role of susceptibility-weighted imaging and intratumoral susceptibility signals in grading and differentiating pediatric brain tumors at 1.5 T: a preliminary study. Neuroradiology. 2020;62:705–13.
7. Mangalore S, Aryan S, Prasad C, Santosh V. Imaging characteristics of supratentorial ependymomas: study on a large single institutional cohort with histopathological correlation. Asian J Neurosurg. 2015;10:276–81.
8. Broen MPG, Smits M, Wijnenga MMJ, Dubbink HJ, Anten MHME, Schijns OEMG, Beckervordersandforth J, Postma AA, van den Bent MJ. The T2-FLAIR mismatch sign as an imaging marker for non-enhancing IDH-mutant, 1p/19q-intact lower-grade glioma: a validation study. Neuro-Oncology. 2018;20:1393–9.
9. Pinto C, Noronha C, Taipa R, Ramos C. T2-FLAIR mismatch sign: a roadmap of pearls and pitfalls. Br J Radiol. 2022;95:20210825.
10. de Narvaez EO, Inada BSY, de Almeida PRSF, et al. Myxoid glioneuronal tumour—report of three cases of a new tumour in a typical location and review of literature. BJR Case Rep. 2021;7:20200139.
11. Meister RL, Groth M, Jürgens JHW, Zhang S, Buhk JH, Herrmann J. Compressed SENSE in pediatric brain tumor MR imaging : assessment of image quality, vol. 32. Examination Time and Energy Release: Clin Neuroradiol; 2022. p. 725. https://doi.org/10.1007/s00062-021-01112-3.
12. Vidya Shankar R, Hu HH, Bikkamane Jayadev N, Chang JC, Kodibagkar VD. 2-D magnetic resonance spectroscopic imaging of the pediatric brain using compressed sensing. Pediatr Radiol. 2019;49:1798–808.
13. Wang DJJ, Le Bihan D, Krishnamurthy R, Smith M, Ho M-L. Noncontrast pediatric brain perfusion: arterial spin labeling and Intravoxel incoherent motion. Magn Reson Imaging Clin N Am. 2021;29:493–513.
14. Huang J, Shlobin NA, Lam SK, DeCuypere M. Artificial intelligence applications in pediatric brain tumor imaging: a systematic review. World Neurosurg. 2022;157:99–105.
15. AlRayahi J, Zapotocky M, Ramaswamy V, Hanagandi P, Branson H, Mubarak W, Raybaud C, Laughlin S. Pediatric brain tumor genetics: what radiologists need to know. Radiographics. 2018;38:2102–22.
16. Grasso G, Midiri M, Catalano C, Gagliardo C. Transcranial magnetic resonance-guided focused ultrasound surgery for brain tumor ablation: are we ready for this challenging treatment? World Neurosurg. 2018;119:438–40.

# Imaging Perspective in Pediatric Tumors: Role of PET Scan

11

Rajender Kumar, Kritin Shankar, and Bhagwant Rai Mittal

## 11.1 Introduction

The origins of the first PET (positron emission tomography) scanner used for human studies can be traced back to the early 1970s when it was unveiled at Washington University in St. Louis, USA [1]. Various changes in design, instrumentation, and technology have advanced the functional imaging modality. The combination of PET with morphological imaging modalities such as CT (computed tomography) and MRI (magnetic resonance imaging) has given rise to superior hybrid imaging modalities capable of simultaneously providing functional and anatomical information. With the limited availability of PET/MRI, especially in low-middle-income countries, PET/CT stands at the forefront of oncology and various other clinical specialities such as neurology and cardiology. Specific challenges in the pediatric population include minimizing radiation burden, using oral or intravenous contrast agents, and the need for sedation or anesthesia for the procedure. Here we will focus on commonly used radiopharmaceuticals, acquisition protocols, physiologic distribution (along with normal variants), and the utility in commonly encountered pediatric malignancies.

## 11.2 Radiopharmaceuticals

Although numerous radiopharmaceuticals with different uptake mechanisms have been developed and displayed promising results in early-phase clinical studies [2], $^{18}$F-fluorodeoxyglucose (FDG) continues to be the workhorse of oncological PET

Rajender Kumar and Kritin Shankar both contributed equally as first author.

R. Kumar (✉) · K. Shankar · B. R. Mittal
Department of Nuclear Medicine, PGIMER, Chandigarh, India





R. Madan et al. (eds.), *Evidence Based Practice in Pediatric Radiation Oncology*, https://doi.org/10.1007/978-981-96-4872-6_11

imaging. FDG is a glucose analog that can be a surrogate marker for evaluating tissue metabolism. Most cancer cells demonstrate continuous glycolytic activity due to the "Warburg effect" and an increase in glucose metabolism [3, 4]. The transportation of FDG into the cell, similar to glucose, is through glucose transporters (GLUT). Hexokinase then phosphorylates glucose and FDG into Glucose-6-phosphate and FDG-6-phosphate, respectively. FDG-6-phosphate cannot enter the glycolytic pathway and remains metabolically "trapped" within the cell. FDG accumulation is also largely dependent on the upregulation of GLUT and increased level of Hexokinase, which occurs in many cancers [5–8].

One major limitation, however, is the non-specific uptake of FDG in inflammatory cells by a similar mechanism. Although an easily obtained semi-quantitative parameter exists to express FDG accumulation, the standard uptake value (SUV), no absolute threshold can be determined to differentiate malignancy from inflammatory uptake [9, 10].

The other commonly used PET radiopharmaceuticals include $^{68}$Ga-DOTA-conjugated somatostatin receptor analogs and $^{18}$F-DOPA. $^{68}$Ga-DOTA-conjugated peptides such as DOTANOC/DOTATOC/DOTATATE can be used to evaluate conditions with high expression of somatostatin receptors (SSTRs) such as neuroblastoma and other neuroendocrine tumors (NETs) [11–13]. $^{18}$F-DOPA is an amino acid analog and has provided utility in tumors with enhanced intracellular amino acid transportation and decarboxylation, such as brain tumors and NETs with low/variable SSTR expression [14].

## 11.3 Patient Preparation

The SNMMI (Society of Nuclear Medicine and Molecular Imaging) Procedure Standard/EANM (European Association of Nuclear Medicine) Practice Guideline on Paediatric $^{18}$F-FDG PET/CT for Oncology comprehensively elaborates on the required preparation and acquisition protocols [15]. After the details of the procedure have been explained to the patient and their parents/caregivers, the child should be instructed to fast for a minimum period of 4–6 h before the scheduled appointment. Fasting is required to decrease blood glucose levels (<200 mg/dL; ideally <140 mg/dL) and maintain a low endogenous insulin level. Elevated blood glucose or insulin level can result in non-specific accumulation of FDG in the normal tissues, particularly increasing muscular uptake [16, 17]. If the child is not required to be NPO (nil per oral) for anesthesia/sedation, they can drink plain, unflavored water. Optimal hydration is encouraged to ensure adequate clearance of the radiotracer. Cold exposure and warm clothing or blankets should be used to minimize the physiological uptake of FDG in the brown adipose tissue (more common in children and adolescents). Premedication with oral propranolol (1 mg/kg, usually 20–40 mg, maximum 40 mg), intravenous fentanyl (0.75–1.0 μg/kg, maximum 50 μg; under the supervision of a trained physician), or oral diazepam (0.080–0.096 mg/kg, maximum 7.5 mg) has also shown to be effective in reducing brown fat uptake [18–21]. The child should avoid talking, playing, or exercising before and after FDG is administered and stay in a quiet, dimly lit room during the uptake phase. To reduce radiation dose and image artifacts, the child should urinate or change their diapers just before image acquisition.

## 11.4 Imaging Protocols and Acquisition

Protocols usually vary depending on PET/CT instrumentation, indication for the study, and other variables. It is advisable to develop and follow institutional protocols. The administered activity of $^{18}$F-FDG should be 3.7–5.2 MBq/kg (0.10–0.14 mCi/kg) with a minimum of 26 MBq (0.7 mCi) [22]. The effective radiation dose can range from 0.02 to 0.2 mSv/MBq [15, 23]. CT acquisition can vary depending on the indication and institutional protocols while adhering to the ALARA (as low as reasonably achievable) principles. Low-dose non-contrast CT can be acquired for attenuation correction or anatomical localization. Diagnostic quality CT with or without intravenous or oral contrast can also be performed depending on the requirement.

## 11.5 Normal Physiologic Variants

In addition to sites of high physiologic FDG uptake (brain, myocardium, liver, kidneys, and sites of urinary excretion), there are numerous physiologic variants that one should be aware of to avoid misinterpretation of normal findings. FDG uptake in the lymphoid tissue of the Waldeyer's ring (adenoids, palatine, and lingual tonsils), terminal ileum, and reactive avidity in cervical lymph nodes are commonly encountered in the pediatric age group. Uptake in the laryngeal muscles and the vocal cord can occur due to talking, while crying can increase activity in the diaphragm and intercostal muscles. Recent use of a specific muscle or muscle spasm can increase FDG uptake. Homogeneous uptake can be noted in the thymus, which decreases with age as the thymus undergoes fatty infiltration. Thymic rebound resulting in increased size and uptake can also be seen after chemotherapy. Using hematopoietic agents (such as G-CSF), anemia and fever can lead to diffuse and homogeneously increased uptake in the bone marrow and spleen. Brown adipose tissue is commonly seen to show bilateral, symmetrical uptake in the cervical, supraclavicular, axillary, mediastinal, paravertebral, and perinephric regions [15, 24].

## 11.6 PET in Specific Malignancies

PET imaging serves a vital purpose in various stages of patient management, including initial diagnosis, disease staging, treatment planning, response assessment, and follow-up. In this section, we shall briefly discuss the role of PET in a few of the most common pediatric malignancies encountered (kindly note that lymphoma shall be discussed separately).

## 11.7 Sarcomas

### 11.7.1 Osteosarcoma

Osteosarcoma (OS) originates from primitive mesenchymal stem cells that improperly form osteoblasts that deposit malignant osteoid [25]. OS is the most common primary bone malignancy, with the peak incidence in children and adolescents with a second peak after 60 years of age [26]. The combination of high-dose chemotherapy and limb-salvage surgery has been shown to prolong the overall survival of localized osteosarcoma; however, a large majority of patients present with occult metastases in the lung, bone, and lymph nodes [26, 27]. Therefore, it is imperative to detect metastatic disease for risk stratification and treatment. As approximately 13% of patients develop local recurrence after limb salvage surgery, it is also crucial to detect recurrence early [28]. FDG PET has been seen to have 100% sensitivity for detecting the primary tumor. The sensitivity of FDG PET for lung, bone, and other distant metastasis has been estimated to be approximately 81%, 93%, and 90%, respectively, while its specificity for the same is 94%, 97%, and 96%. FDG PET also serves an important role in detecting recurrent disease with sensitivity and specificity of 91% and 93%, respectively [29]. FDG PET can also be used as a prognostic indicator, with higher SUVmax (standard uptake value) correlating with shorter progression-free survival and overall survival [30, 31].

### 11.7.2 Ewing Sarcoma

The Ewing sarcoma family of tumors (ESFT) consists of a group of tumors characterized by morphologically similar round-cell neoplasm and by the presence of a common chromosomal translocation, i.e., t(11;22)(q24;q12) in 85–90% of the cases [32]. Ewing sarcoma (ES) is the third most common primary malignant bone tumor. It is seen more frequently in children and adolescents but can also occur in adults. They may arise from bone, soft tissues, or visceral sites. The median age at diagnosis is 15 years, with a male predominance (1.5:1) [33–36]. Approximately 25% of patients with ES have detectable metastases at diagnosis, most commonly in lung and bone [lung (10%); bone/bone marrow (10%); combinations or others (5%)] [37–40]. Metastatic evaluation is usually done using a CT chest for pulmonary metastasis, bone marrow aspiration, biopsy for bone marrow involvement, $^{99m}$Tc-MDP skeletal scintigraphy (SSC) for osseous metastasis, and $^{18}$F-FDG PET/CT. FDG PET can visualize abnormal glucose metabolism by malignant cells before osteoblastic reactions or structural changes occur in the bone. Meta-analyses have determined $^{18}$F-FDG PET/CT to have high specificity (86–96%) and sensitivity (80–92%) to detect bone metastases (especially bone marrow metastasis) in ESFT [41, 42]. Multiple studies have also shown FDG PET is superior to bone marrow biopsy for detecting marrow involvement [43–46]. FDG PET can also serve an important role in prognostication and response assessment [47, 48] (Fig. 11.1).

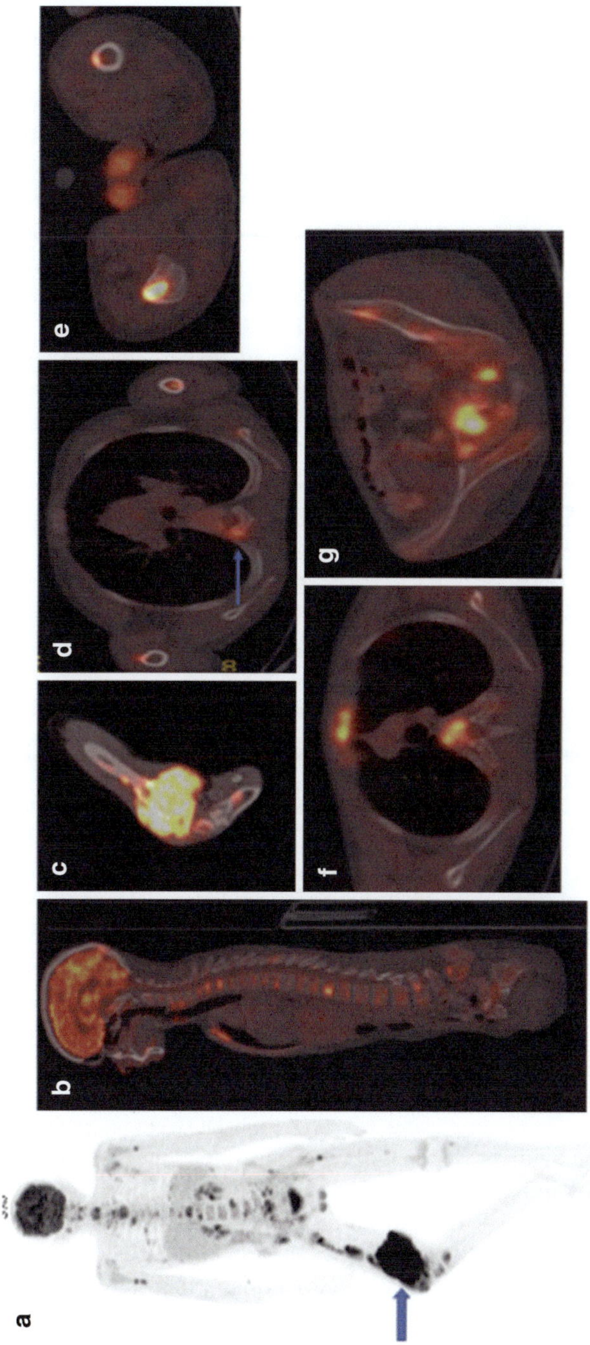


**Fig. 11.1** A 15-year-old male patient with biopsy-proven Ewing sarcoma of the right femur. FDG PET/CT images demonstrating the primary lesion (**a**-arrow, **c**) and multiple lytic and marrow-based metastatic skeletal lesions (**b**, **d-g**) and a metastatic paraspinal lesion in the right neural foramina (**d**-arrow) at the D5 vertebral level

### 11.7.3 Rhabdomyosarcoma

Rhabdomyosarcoma (RMS) is the most common soft tissue sarcoma in children and young adults, accounting for 4–5% of all childhood malignancies [49]. RMS is a highly aggressive tumor originating from primitive cells demonstrating myogenic differentiation. The most important prognostic factor is the presence of metastasis at the time of diagnosis, which occurs in approximately 20% of patients (most frequently involving lungs, bone and bone marrow, and distant nodes). A prospective, international, multi-institutional trial performed by the European Pediatric Soft Tissue sarcoma Study Group (EPSSG) dedicated to metastatic RMS was retrospectively reviewed to determine the impact of FDG PET/CT in staging the disease. Compared to the standard radiology workup, PET/CT was superior in detecting loco-regional (96.2% v/s 78.5%, $p = 0.0013$) and distant (94.8% v/s 79.3%, $p = 0.0242$) lymph nodes. PET/CT was more sensitive than bone scintigraphy (96.4% v/s 67.9%, $p = 0.0116$) for bone metastasis and could detect marrow involvement with sensitivity and specificity of 91.8% and 93.8%, respectively. PET/CT was, however, lower in sensitivity for lung metastasis compared to CT chest (79.6% v/s 100%, $p = 0.0025$) [50, 51]. FDG PET can also serve a prognostic role with higher SUVmax, indicating an unfavorable prognosis [52, 53].

## 11.8 Neuroblastoma

Neuroblastoma is an embryonic tumor derived from the sympathoadrenal lineage of neural crest cells. The primary lesion can originate from the adrenal medulla or anywhere along the sympathetic trunk but is most commonly seen in the abdomen (70%). About 50% of patients present with distant metastasis, which most commonly involves the bone marrow, bone, and lymph nodes and less frequently involves the liver and skin [54, 55]. It is the most common extracranial solid malignancy in children, and more than 95% of patients are below 10 years of age [56]. Various modalities have been used to image and treat patients with neuroblastoma. $^{123}I$ and $^{131}I$ labeled with the norepinephrine analog metaiodobenzylguanidine (mIBG) have several limitations, such as limited sensitivity for smaller lesions, limited spatial resolution, longer uptake period and acquisition time, and need for thyroid blockade. Despite these limitations, mIBG is recommended as the first-line modality for radionuclide imaging [57]. However, the limited availability of mIBG has led to increased PET imaging using $^{18}F$-FDG, $^{68}Ga$-DOTA-conjugated peptides, or $^{18}F$-DOPA. PET imaging provides utility in evaluating clinically suspected neuroblastoma, disease staging, treatment planning, response assessment, follow-up, and before planning radionuclide therapy. PET imaging can also play a crucial role in evaluating mIBG-negative disease. A meta-analysis comparing PET/CT (using various radiopharmaceuticals) and mIBG showed higher per-lesion accuracy and sensitivity of PET/CT (89% vs. 79%) with mIBG showing a comparable diagnostic performance in per-patient analysis and higher specificity (84% vs. 71%) [58] (Fig. 11.2).

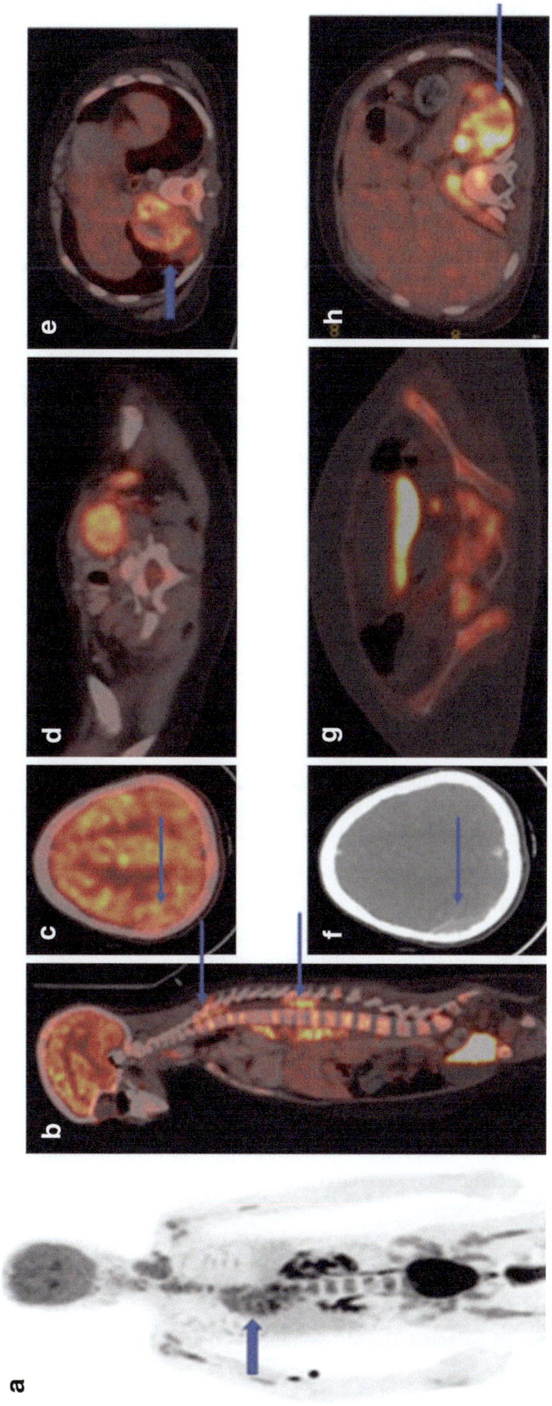


**Fig. 11.2** A 6-year-old female patient presenting with acute onset paraparesis. MRI revealed a paraspinal mass in relation to the dorsal vertebrae. Biopsy from the mass was reported as neuroblastoma. FDG PET/CT images demonstrate the primary lesion (**a**, **e**- arrow), multiple meningeal lesions in the dorsal spinal cord (**b**- arrow) & right parietal cortex (**c**, **f**- arrow), left cervical, supraclavicular (**d**) and retrocrural lymph nodes (**h**), skeletal lesions (**g**), and lesion in the left kidney (**h**)

## 11.9 Other Malignancies

Emerging evidence highlights the utility of PET/CT in various other pediatric malignancies. CNS malignancies represent the most common pediatric solid tumors. Due to the high physiological uptake of FDG in the brain cortex, it is not frequently used to evaluate these neoplasms, especially low-grade gliomas. FDG PET can, however, show increased tracer uptake in high-grade gliomas compared to the surrounding brain parenchyma. Other tracers, such as $^{18}$F-DOPA, $^{11}$C-methylmethionine ($^{11}$C-MET), and $^{18}$F-fluoro-ethyl-tyrosine ($^{18}$F-FET), have also been studied for the evaluation of brain tumors. However, the limited availability of these radiopharmaceuticals and the limited evidence base prevent their incorporation into routine clinical practice.

Langerhans cell histiocytosis (LCH) is an inflammatory myeloid neoplasm characterized by clonal proliferation of Langerhans cells in various organs, including skin, bones, lymph nodes, soft tissue, lung, and liver. Few studies have shown the usefulness of FDG PET/CT in evaluating patients with LCH. It can identify metabolically active disease sites not picked up on conventional imaging and differentiate between metabolically active disease and inactive lesions with residual morphological changes to prevent unnecessary therapy [59, 60].

## 11.10 Conclusion

Hybrid imaging techniques combining PET with CT or MRI have revolutionized imaging by simultaneously providing functional and anatomical information. With advances in imaging technology, the development of newer radiopharmaceuticals for molecular imaging and clinical research to promote evidence-based practice, we can further improve the scope of PET imaging. The development of standardized protocols will help promote uniformity in multi-institutional data. Feature extraction from a high volume of data and its incorporation using radiomics will pave the way for developing surrogate imaging biomarkers that can significantly impact patient management.

## References

1. Portnow LH, Vaillancourt DE, Okun MS. The history of cerebral PET scanning: from physiology to cutting-edge technology. Neurology. 2013;80(10):952–6. https://doi.org/10.1212/WNL.0b013e318285c135.
2. Giammarile F, Castellucci P, Dierckx R, et al. Non-FDG PET/CT in diagnostic oncology: a pictorial review. Eur J Hybrid Imaging. 2019;3(1):20. https://doi.org/10.1186/s41824-019-0066-2.
3. Warburg O. On the origin of cancer cells. Science. 1956;123(3191):309–14. https://doi.org/10.1126/science.123.3191.309.
4. Koppenol WH, Bounds PL, Dang CV. Otto Warburg's contributions to current concepts of cancer metabolism. Nat Rev Cancer. 2011;11(5):325–37. https://doi.org/10.1038/nrc3038.

5. Smith TA. Facilitative glucose transporter expression in human cancer tissue. Br J Biomed Sci. 1999;56(4):285–92.
6. Medina RA, Owen GI. Glucose transporters: expression, regulation and cancer. Biol Res. 2002;35(1):9–26. https://doi.org/10.4067/s0716-97602002000100004.
7. Smith TA. Mammalian hexokinases and their abnormal expression in cancer. Br J Biomed Sci. 2000;57(2):170–8.
8. Mathupala SP, Ko YH, Pedersen PL. Hexokinase II: cancer's double-edged sword acting as both facilitator and gatekeeper of malignancy when bound to mitochondria. Oncogene. 2006;25(34):4777–86. https://doi.org/10.1038/sj.onc.1209603.
9. Keyes JW. SUV: standard uptake or silly useless value? J Nucl Med. 1995;36(10):1836–9.
10. Rahman WT, Wale DJ, Viglianti BL, et al. The impact of infection and inflammation in oncologic 18F-FDG PET/CT imaging. Biomed Pharmacother. 2019;117:109168. https://doi.org/10.1016/j.biopha.2019.109168.
11. Moertel CL, Reubi JC, Scheithauer BS, Schaid DJ, Kvols LK. Expression of somatostatin receptors in childhood neuroblastoma. Am J Clin Pathol. 1994;102(6):752–6. https://doi.org/10.1093/ajcp/102.6.752.
12. Zhang L, Vines DC, Scollard DA, et al. Correlation of somatostatin Receptor-2 expression with Gallium-68-DOTA-TATE uptake in neuroblastoma Xenograft models. Contrast Media Mol Imaging. 2017;2017:9481276. https://doi.org/10.1155/2017/9481276.
13. Tirosh A, Kebebew E. The utility of 68Ga-DOTATATE positron-emission tomography/computed tomography in the diagnosis, management, follow-up and prognosis of neuroendocrine tumors. Future Oncol. 2018;14(2):111–22. https://doi.org/10.2217/fon-2017-0393.
14. Masselli G, Casciani E, De Angelis C, Sollaku S, Gualdi G. Clinical application of 18F-DOPA PET/TC in pediatric patients. Am J Nucl Med Mol Imaging. 2021;11(2):64–76.
15. Vali R, Alessio A, Balza R, et al. SNMMI procedure standard/EANM practice guideline on pediatric $^{18}$F-FDG PET/CT for oncology 1.0. J Nucl Med. 2021;62(1):99–110. https://doi.org/10.2967/jnumed.120.254110.
16. Surasi DS, Bhambhvani P, Baldwin JA, Almodovar SE, O'Malley JP. $^{18}$F-FDG PET and PET/CT patient preparation: a review of the literature. J Nucl Med Technol 2014;42(1):5–13. https://doi.org/10.2967/jnmt.113.132621.
17. Lindholm H, Brolin F, Jonsson C, Jacobsson H. The relation between the blood glucose level and the FDG uptake of tissues at normal PET examinations. EJNMMI Res. 2013;3(1):50. https://doi.org/10.1186/2191-219X-3-50.
18. Gelfand MJ, O'Hara SM, Curtwright LA, MacLean JR. Pre-medication to block [18F]FDG uptake in the brown adipose tissue of pediatric and adolescent patients. Pediatr Radiol. 2005;35(10):984–90. https://doi.org/10.1007/s00247-005-1505-8.
19. Söderlund V, Larsson SA, Jacobsson H. Reduction of FDG uptake in brown adipose tissue in clinical patients by a single dose of propranolol. Eur J Nucl Med Mol Imaging. 2007;34(7):1018–22. https://doi.org/10.1007/s00259-006-0318-9.
20. George A, Sinha P, Conrad G, Memon AA, Dressler EV, Wagner LM. Pilot study of propranolol premedication to reduce FDG uptake in brown adipose tissue on PET scans of adolescent and young adult oncology patients. Pediatr Hematol Oncol. 2017;34(3):149–56. https://doi.org/10.1080/08880018.2017.1338806.
21. Cousins J, Czachowski M, Muthukrishnan A, Currie G. Pediatric brown adipose tissue on 18F-FDG PET: diazepam intervention. J Nucl Med Technol. 2017;45(2):82–6. https://doi.org/10.2967/jnmt.116.187385.
22. Treves ST, Gelfand MJ, Fahey FH, Parisi MT. 2016 update of the North American consensus guidelines for pediatric administered radiopharmaceutical activities. J Nucl Med. 2016;57(12):15N–8N.
23. Stabin MG, Siegel JA. RADAR dose estimate report: a compendium of radiopharmaceutical dose estimates based on OLINDA/EXM version 2.0. J Nucl Med. 2018;59(1):154–60. https://doi.org/10.2967/jnumed.117.196261.

24. Shammas A, Lim R, Charron M. Pediatric FDG PET/CT: physiologic uptake, normal variants, and benign conditions. Radiographics. 2009;29(5):1467–86. https://doi.org/10.1148/rg.295085247.
25. Biermann JS, Adkins DR, Agulnik M, et al. Bone cancer. J Natl Compr Cancer Netw. 2013;11(6):688–723. https://doi.org/10.6004/jnccn.2013.0088.
26. Mirabello L, Troisi RJ, Savage SA. Osteosarcoma incidence and survival rates from 1973 to 2004: data from the Surveillance, Epidemiology, and End Results Program. Cancer. 2009;115(7):1531–43. https://doi.org/10.1002/cncr.24121.
27. Su W, Lai Z, Wu F, et al. Clinical efficacy of preoperative chemotherapy with or without ifosfamide in patients with osteosarcoma of the extremity: meta-analysis of randomized controlled trials. Med Oncol. 2015;32(2):19. https://doi.org/10.1007/s12032-014-0481-y.
28. Yin K, Liao Q, Zhong D, et al. Meta-analysis of limb salvage versus amputation for treating high-grade and localized osteosarcoma in patients with pathological fracture. Exp Ther Med. 2012;4(5):889–94. https://doi.org/10.3892/etm.2012.685.
29. Liu F, Zhang Q, Zhou D, Dong J. Effectiveness of 18F-FDG PET/CT in the diagnosis and staging of osteosarcoma: a meta-analysis of 26 studies. BMC Cancer. 2019;19(1):323. https://doi.org/10.1186/s12885-019-5488-5.
30. Costelloe CM, Macapinlac HA, Madewell JE, et al. $^{18}$F-FDG PET/CT as an indicator of progression-free and overall survival in osteosarcoma. J Nucl Med. 2009;50(3):340–7. https://doi.org/10.2967/jnumed.108.058461
31. Hack RI, Becker AS, Bode-Lesniewska B, et al. When SUV matters: FDG PET/CT at baseline correlates with survival in soft tissue and Ewing sarcoma. Life (Basel). 2021;11(9):869. https://doi.org/10.3390/life11090869.
32. Burchill SA. Ewing's sarcoma: diagnostic, prognostic, and therapeutic implications of molecular abnormalities. J Clin Pathol. 2003;56(2):96–102. https://doi.org/10.1136/jcp.56.2.96.
33. Stiller CA, Trama A, Serraino D, et al. Descriptive epidemiology of sarcomas in Europe: report from the RARECARE project. Eur J Cancer. 2013;49(3):684–95. https://doi.org/10.1016/j.ejca.2012.09.011.
34. Whelan J, McTiernan A, Cooper N, et al. Incidence and survival of malignant bone sarcomas in England 1979-2007. Int J Cancer. 2012;131(4):E508–17. https://doi.org/10.1002/ijc.26426.
35. Valery PC, Laversanne M, Bray F. Bone cancer incidence by morphological subtype: a global assessment. Cancer Causes Control. 2015;26(8):1127–39. https://doi.org/10.1007/s10552-015-0607-3.
36. van den Berg H, Kroon HM, Slaar A, Hogendoorn P. Incidence of biopsy-proven bone tumors in children: a report based on the Dutch pathology registration "PALGA.". J Pediatr Orthop. 2008;28(1):29–35. https://doi.org/10.1097/BPO.0b013e3181558cb5.
37. Potratz J, Dirksen U, Jürgens H, Craft A. Ewing sarcoma: clinical state-of-the-art. Pediatr Hematol Oncol. 2012;29(1):1–11. https://doi.org/10.3109/08880018.2011.622034.
38. Grier HE. The Ewing family of tumors. Ewing's sarcoma and primitive neuroectodermal tumors. Pediatr Clin N Am. 1997;44(4):991–1004. https://doi.org/10.1016/s0031-3955(05)70541-1.
39. Paulussen M, Ahrens S, Burdach S, et al. Primary metastatic (stage IV) Ewing tumor: survival analysis of 171 patients from the EICESS studies. European Intergroup Cooperative Ewing Sarcoma Studies. Ann Oncol. 1998;9(3):275–81. https://doi.org/10.1023/a:1008208511815.
40. Bernstein ML, Devidas M, Lafreniere D, et al. Intensive therapy with growth factor support for patients with Ewing tumor metastatic at diagnosis: Pediatric Oncology Group/Children's Cancer Group Phase II Study 9457--a report from the Children's Oncology Group. J Clin Oncol. 2006;24(1):152–9. https://doi.org/10.1200/JCO.2005.02.1717.
41. Huang T, Li F, Yan Z, et al. Effectiveness of 18F-FDG PET/CT in the diagnosis, staging and recurrence monitoring of Ewing sarcoma family of tumors: a meta-analysis of 23 studies. Medicine (Baltimore). 2018;97(48):e13457. https://doi.org/10.1097/MD.0000000000013457.
42. Treglia G, Salsano M, Stefanelli A, Mattoli MV, Giordano A, Bonomo L. Diagnostic accuracy of $^{18}$F-FDG-PET and PET/CT in patients with Ewing sarcoma family tumours: a systematic review and a meta-analysis. Skeletal Radiol. 2012;41(3):249–56. https://doi.org/10.1007/s00256-011-1298-9.

43. Kopp LM, Hu C, Rozo B, et al. Utility of bone marrow aspiration and biopsy in initial staging of Ewing sarcoma. Pediatr Blood Cancer. 2015;62(1):12–5. https://doi.org/10.1002/pbc.25212.
44. Newman EN, Jones RL, Hawkins DS. An evaluation of [F-18]-fluorodeoxy- D -glucose positron emission tomography, bone scan, and bone marrow aspiration/biopsy as staging investigations in Ewing Sarcoma. Pediatr Blood Cancer. 2013;60(7):1113–7. https://doi.org/10.1002/pbc.24406.
45. Yağci-Küpeli B, Koçyiğit-Deveci E, Adamhasan F, Küpeli S. The value of 18F-FDG PET/CT in detecting bone marrow involvement in childhood cancers. J Pediatr Hematol Oncol. 2019;41(6):438–41. https://doi.org/10.1097/MPH.0000000000001499.
46. Kasalak Ö, Glaudemans AWJM, Overbosch J, Jutte PC, Kwee TC. Can FDG-PET/CT replace blind bone marrow biopsy of the posterior iliac crest in Ewing sarcoma? Skeletal Radiol. 2018;47(3):363–7. https://doi.org/10.1007/s00256-017-2807-2.
47. Albano D, Dondi F, Schumacher RF, et al. Clinical and prognostic role of 18F-FDG PET/CT in pediatric Ewing sarcoma. J Pediatr Hematol Oncol. 2020;42(2):e79–86. https://doi.org/10.1097/MPH.0000000000001518.
48. Bestic JM, Peterson JJ, Bancroft LW. Use of FDG PET in staging, restaging, and assessment of therapy response in Ewing sarcoma. Radiographics. 2009;29(5):1487–500. https://doi.org/10.1148/rg.295095024.
49. Rhee DS, Rodeberg DA, Baertschiger RM, et al. Update on pediatric rhabdomyosarcoma: a report from the APSA Cancer Committee. J Pediatr Surg. 2020;55(10):1987–95. https://doi.org/10.1016/j.jpedsurg.2020.06.015.
50. Bisogno G, Jenney M, Bergeron C, et al. Addition of dose-intensified doxorubicin to standard chemotherapy for rhabdomyosarcoma (EpSSG RMS 2005): a multicentre, open-label, randomised controlled, phase 3 trial. Lancet Oncol. 2018;19(8):1061–71. https://doi.org/10.1016/S1470-2045(18)30337-1.
51. Mercolini F, Zucchetta P, Jehanno N, et al. Role of 18F-FDG-PET/CT in the staging of metastatic rhabdomyosarcoma: a report from the European paediatric Soft tissue sarcoma Study Group. Eur J Cancer. 2021;155:155–62. https://doi.org/10.1016/j.ejca.2021.07.006.
52. Dong Y, Zhang X, Wang S, Chen S, Ma C. 18F-FDG PET/CT is useful in initial staging, restaging for pediatric rhabdomyosarcoma. Q J Nucl Med Mol Imaging. 2017;61(4):438–46. https://doi.org/10.23736/S1824-4785.17.02792-3.
53. El-Kholy E, El Nadi E, Hafez H, et al. Added predictive value of 18F-FDG PET/CT for pediatric rhabdomyosarcoma. Nucl Med Commun. 2019;40(9):898–904. https://doi.org/10.1097/MNM.0000000000001040.
54. Tas ML, Reedijk AMJ, Karim-Kos HE, et al. Neuroblastoma between 1990 and 2014 in The Netherlands: increased incidence and improved survival of high-risk neuroblastoma. Eur J Cancer. 2020;124:47–55. https://doi.org/10.1016/j.ejca.2019.09.025.
55. Morgenstern DA, London WB, Stephens D, et al. Prognostic significance of pattern and burden of metastatic disease in patients with stage 4 neuroblastoma: a study from the International Neuroblastoma Risk Group database. Eur J Cancer. 2016;65:1–10. https://doi.org/10.1016/j.ejca.2016.06.005.
56. Irwin MS, Park JR. Neuroblastoma. Pediatr Clin N Am. 2015;62(1):225–56. https://doi.org/10.1016/j.pcl.2014.09.015.
57. Bar-Sever Z, Biassoni L, Shulkin B, et al. Guidelines on nuclear medicine imaging in neuroblastoma. Eur J Nucl Med Mol Imaging. 2018;45(11):2009–24. https://doi.org/10.1007/s00259-018-4070-8.
58. Xia J, Zhang H, Hu Q, et al. Comparison of diagnosing and staging accuracy of PET (CT) and MIBG on patients with neuroblastoma: systemic review and meta-analysis. Curr Med Sci. 2017;37(5):649–60. https://doi.org/10.1007/s11596-017-1785-x.
59. Jessop S, Crudgington D, London K, Kellie S, Howman-Giles R. FDG PET-CT in pediatric Langerhans cell histiocytosis. Pediatr Blood Cancer. 2020;67(1):e28034. https://doi.org/10.1002/pbc.28034.
60. Ferrell J, Sharp S, Kumar A, Jordan M, Picarsic J, Nelson A. Discrepancies between F-18-FDG PET/CT findings and conventional imaging in Langerhans cell histiocytosis. Pediatr Blood Cancer. 2021;68(4):e28891. https://doi.org/10.1002/pbc.28891.

# Pathological Aspects and Recent Advances in Pathology

# 12

Aanchal Kakkar, Shilpi Thakur, Adarsh Barwad, and Asit Ranjan Mridha

## 12.1 Pediatric Sarcoma

Among pediatric sarcomas, rhabdomyosarcoma and Ewing sarcoma are unique in their exquisite response to radiotherapy and therefore will be the focus of this chapter.

## 12.2 Rhabdomyosarcoma

Rhabdomyosarcoma (RMS) is a family of malignant soft tissue neoplasms with evidence of myogenic differentiation. It is the most common soft tissue sarcoma in children and adolescents. It is comprised of embryonal rhabdomyosarcoma (ERMS), alveolar rhabdomyosarcoma (ARMS), spindle cell/sclerosing rhabdomyosarcoma (SSRMS), and pleomorphic rhabdomyosarcoma (PRMS). Each of these subtypes is a unique disease with distinct presentation. Intraosseous spindle cell rhabdomyosarcoma is a recently described distinct entity with characteristic *NCOA2* or *TFCP2* gene rearrangements [1].

### 12.2.1 Epidemiology

ERMS accounts for nearly three-fourths of pediatric RMS and is usually seen in the first decade of life, while ARMS accounts for 20–25% and usually occurs in the second decade [2]. SSRMS is rare, accounting for less than 10% of all RMS, and is seen across all ages; it is often seen in infancy, being designated congenital/infantile

A. Kakkar (✉) · S. Thakur · A. Barwad · A. R. Mridha
Department of Pathology, All India Institute of Medical Sciences, New Delhi, India





R. Madan et al. (eds.), *Evidence Based Practice in Pediatric Radiation Oncology*,
https://doi.org/10.1007/978-981-96-4872-6_12

SSRMS. PRMS is exceptional in the pediatric age group and will not be discussed further.

### 12.2.2 Location and Clinical Features

The most common anatomical site of RMS is the head and neck (35%), followed by genitourinary system (24%), retroperitoneum (22%) and extremities (19%) [2]. In the head and neck region, parameningeal RMS accounts for 16% of all tumors [2]. All three histological types occur most frequently in the head and neck, with ERMS favoring the orbit and parameningeal region and ARMS favoring the nasal cavity. ERMS is also common in the genitourinary system and retroperitoneum, while ARMS also affects the deep soft tissues of extremities and perineum, and SSRMS is seen in the in the paratesticular region. *TFCP2* rearranged RMS has a striking predilection for craniofacial bones.

The clinical manifestations are site-specific, for example, orbital tumors present with proptosis and loss of vision. In mucosa-lined hollow organs or cavities such as nasal cavity and urinary bladder, RMS may present as a polypoid mass and is known as botryoid RMS (Greek: bunch of grapes).

### 12.2.3 Gross Examination

RMS are grossly infiltrative tumors with poor circumscription. They are fleshy pale tan, may be lobulated, and have a bulging cut surface. Botryoid ERMS are polypoid masses with a glistening surface and gelatinous consistency. ARMS frequently show hemorrhagic and necrotic foci. SSRMS appear firm and may have a whorled appearance.

### 12.2.4 Histopathology

#### 12.2.4.1 Embryonal RMS

ERMS is composed of primitive mesenchymal cells that recapitulate the various stages in myogenesis, displaying variable evidence of rhabdomyoblastic differentiation (Fig. 12.1). Undifferentiated round to ovoid to spindled tumor cells with amphophilic cytoplasm are admixed with a variable number of rhabdomyoblasts having densely eosinophilic cytoplasm and eccentric round nuclei. Tadpole cells, strap cells, and cytoplasmic cross-striations may occasionally be seen. There are alternating hypercellular and hypocellular areas with a loose myxoid stroma. Rhabdomyoblastic differentiation is often prominent following chemotherapy. Botryoid ERMS displays a characteristic subepithelial condensation of tumor cells separated from an intact epithelium by a zone of hypocellular stroma known as cambium layer. Anaplastic ERMS is defined by similar criteria as for Wilms Tumor, that is, markedly enlarged nuclei (at least three times the size of neighboring nuclei) with hyperchromasia and/or atypical mitoses [3]. Anaplasia may be focal or diffuse. Intranuclear cytoplasmic inclusions are frequent. Anaplasia is an indicator of poor prognosis [4]. Heterologous elements like cartilage may be identified in ERMS associated with *DICER1* syndrome. (Fig. 12.1).

#### 12.2.4.2 Alveolar RMS

Classic ARMS are comprised of discohesive islands of oval to round tumor cells with variable amount of cytoplasm that cling to slender fibrovascular septae at the periphery. The central discohesion and peripheral monolayer impart an alveolar appearance. Nuclei are monomorphic as compared to ERMS. ARMS with solid pattern shows similar tumor cells but without the intervening septae. Multinucleated tumor cells, degenerated cells with pyknotic nuclei and cellular debris are frequent in both patterns. Rhabdomyoblasts are infrequent.

#### 12.2.4.3 Spindle Cell/Sclerosing Rhabdomyosarcoma

SSRMS shows elongated spindled cells in fascicles, whorls and storiform pattern. The sclerosing pattern consists of single file arrays of small tumor cells in a collagenized stroma, with a microalveolar or pseudovascular pattern. The stroma appears hyalinized or pseudochondroid, often mimicking osteosarcoma. Infantile RMS may

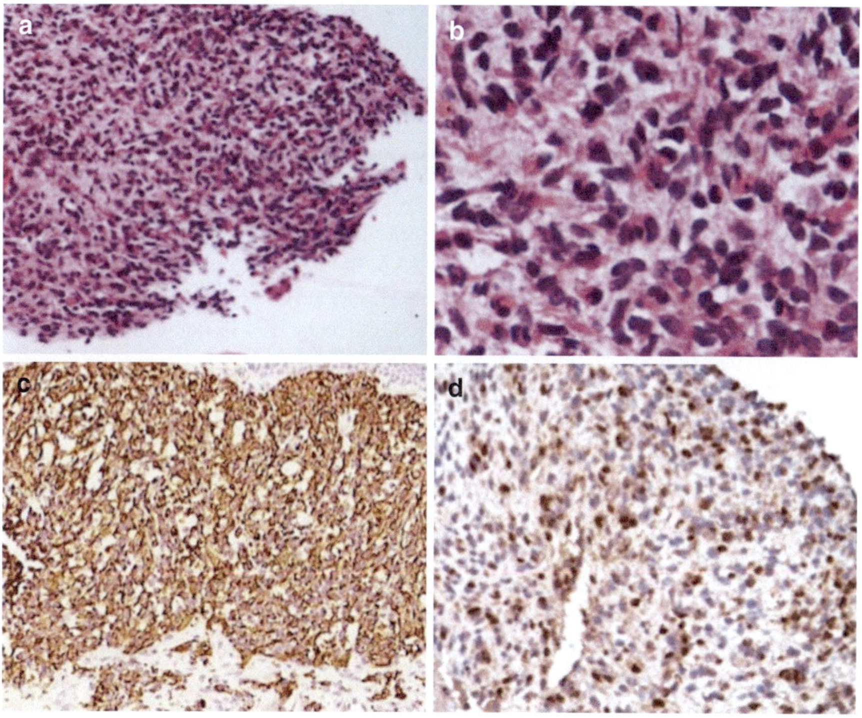


**Fig. 12.1** ERMS composed of primitive ovoid to spindled cells (**a**) with variable amount of amphophilic to eosinophilic cytoplasm (**b**). The tumor cells are immunopositive for desmin (**c**) and myogenin (**d**)

show rhabdomyoblasts admixed with spindled cells. Intraosseous RMS shows spindled and/or epithelioid cells with mild nuclear pleomorphism [5].

### 12.2.5 Histochemistry and Immunohistochemistry

Phosphotungstic acid hematoxylin (PTAH) highlights cytoplasmic cross striations. Cytoplasmic glycogen is not exclusive to Ewing sarcoma and is seen in most RMS, demonstrable with Periodic acid–Schiff reaction (PAS) with and without diastase.

For a diagnosis of RMS, cells must display evidence of skeletal muscle differentiation, as evidenced by immunopositivity with desmin, myogenin (Myf4), and/or MYOD1. Among these, desmin is most sensitive and myogenin is most specific. Muscle-specific actin (HHF-35), sarcomeric actin and myoglobin may also be positive but lack specificity. The extent of immunoexpression of myogenic markers correlates with the degree of skeletal muscle differentiation. Desmin may be completely negative in the most primitive tumor cells. ERMS shows more diffuse positivity for desmin, while myogenin and myoD1 may be patchy. ARMS shows homogeneous strong myogenin positivity. SSRMS shows focal weak desmin and myogenin and diffuse, strong MyoD1 staining.

Approximately 50% of RMS show cytokeratin immunostaining. Variable expression of neuroendocrine markers may be seen. CD99 is positive in a subset of cases. These aberrant immunostaining patterns can cause difficulty in distinguishing from other small round cell tumors.

### 12.2.6 Molecular Pathogenesis and Its Implications

ERMS show consistent losses of chromosome 2, 8, 11, 12, 13 and/or 20. Loss of heterozygosity is seen at chromosome 11p15.5, the locus of multiple genes including *IGF2*. RAS pathway gene mutations are described in 50% of RMS. Anaplasia may be associated with *TP53* mutations. Genitourinary ERMS occur in association with germline *DICER1* mutations [6].

ARMS is characterized by t(2;13)(q35;q14) translocation in 75% and t(1;13)(p36;q14) in 20–25%, with resultant *PAX3::FOXO1* and *PAX7::FOXO1* gene fusions, the latter being associated with amplification of the fusion gene [7]. The *PAX3::FOXO1* fusion gene encodes for a chimeric transcription factor, resulting in excessive activation of *PAX3* binding sites including *MYCN* [8]. Fusion-positive RMS, irrespective of morphology, have inferior outcome as compared to fusion-negative RMS, with *PAX3::FOXO1* fused tumors having worse prognosis than *PAX7::FOXO1* fused RMS. Gene fusions are detected by fluorescence in situ hybridization (FISH) or reverse-transcription PCR, on both frozen as well as paraffin-embedded tissue [9, 10]. However, these are not readily accessible to most labs in LMICs, particularly the latter which requires an expensive fluorescence microscope for visualization of results. Recent studies have implicated fibroblast growth factor receptor genes *FGFR4* and *FGFR1* in the pathogenesis of ARMS, with 11%

fusion-negative ARMS and 6% ERMS showing *FGFR1* amplification [11]. Majority of SSRMS in older children and adults harbor *MYOD1* point mutation, associated with poor prognosis, while a subset of infantile SSRMS display *VGLL2* or *NCOA2* gene rearrangements and have excellent prognosis [12]. Intraosseous RMS harbor either *EWSR1/FUS::TFCP2* or *MEIS1::NCOA2* gene fusions [5].

### 12.2.7 Differential Diagnosis

Differential diagnosis includes all poorly differentiated round cell tumors encountered at a given location (Table 12.1). Cases diagnosed as PRMS in children are likely anaplastic ERMS. Ewing family of tumors, neuroblastoma, synovial sarcoma, malignant lymphoma, granulocytic tumors are the major differential diagnoses for RMS.

## 12.3 Undifferentiated Round Cell Sarcomas

The recent WHO classification of tumors of bone and soft tissue (2020) classifies undifferentiated round cell sarcomas into Ewing sarcoma, round cell sarcoma with *EWSR1*–non-ETS fusions, CIC-rearranged sarcoma, and sarcoma with BCOR genetic alterations, based on their characteristic molecular pathogenesis and clinical attributes [13].

## 12.4 Ewing Sarcoma

Ewing sarcoma is an undifferentiated round cell tumor that primarily affects the bone but can arise in soft tissue. It is a highly aggressive malignant tumor, and the patients often harbor micrometastases. Approximately 20–30% of Ewing sarcoma patients develop metastatic disease at presentation, which is associated with poor survival. Ewing sarcoma is the second most common primary bone malignancy in children and adolescents after osteosarcoma and the fourth most frequent primary malignant bone tumor after multiple myeloma, osteosarcoma and chondrosarcoma. Adamantinoma-like Ewing sarcoma (ALES), a histological subtype first recognized in extremities, is increasingly being described in head and neck locations like sinonasal tract, thyroid and salivary glands [14].

### 12.4.1 Molecular Pathogenesis

Ewing sarcoma is characterized by gene fusions involving a FET family gene encoding for RNA-binding proteins, most frequently *EWSR1*, and a member of the ETS family of transcription factors which share a conserved DNA binding domain (Table 12.2). *EWSR1::FLI1* fusion is seen in 85–95% of cases, followed by

**Table 12.1** Differential diagnosis of common pediatric malignant small round cell tumors

| Diagnosis | Clinical features | Morphology | IHC | Diagnostic genetic alterations |
|---|---|---|---|---|
| ERMS | 1st decade; head and neck, genitourinary | Dispersed cells with anisocytosis, including undifferentiated small round cells, oval, stellate, strap, tadpole cells; myxoid stroma | Desmin; variable myogenin | Nil |
| ARMS | 2nd and 3rd decades; head and neck, extremities | Monomorphic small round cells in alveolar or solid pattern; multinucleated tumor cells, myxoid background | Diffuse strong myogenin; variable desmin | *PAX3::FOXO1; PAX7::FOXO1* fusions |
| Neuroblastoma | Age < 5 years; primary adrenal, mediastinal, paravertebral; metastases to liver, craniofacial bones, marrow | Fibrillary matrix, rosettes, salt and pepper chromatin, nuclear molding; ganglionic differentiation | Synaptophysin, chromogranin, CD56, NB84, PHOX2B; NKX2.2 ± | |
| Ewing sarcoma | Older children, adolescents; bone, soft tissue; thigh, axial skeleton | Primitive small round cells, scant pale cytoplasm, slightly irregular nuclei with inconspicuous nucleoli | CD99, NKX2.2, FLI1, ERG | *EWSR1* gene rearrangements |
| Wilms tumor | Age < 5 years; kidney; lung metastases | Undifferentiated blastemal cells, tubules, abortive glomeruli, mesenchymal cells | WT1, PAX8, cytokeratin | Alterations in *WT1, IGF2, CTNNB1* genes |
| Non-Hodgkin lymphoma | Children and adolescents; mediastinal mass, bone marrow, lymph nodes | Discohesive small to medium sized monomorphic cells with crushing; tingible-body macrophages | CD3/CD79a, Tdt, Cd34; CD99 ± | T-cell receptor gene rearrangement in T-LBL; several genetic alteration in B-LBL subtypes |

**Table 12.2** Chromosomal rearrangements and fusion genes in Ewing sarcoma and other undifferentiated small round cell sarcomas [25, 26]

| FET family | ETS family | Translocation | Fusion gene |
|---|---|---|---|
| *EWSR1* | *FLI1* | t(11;22)(q24;q12) | *EWSR1::FLI1* |
| | *ERG* | t(21;22)(q11;q12) | *EWSR1::ERG* |
| | *ETV1* | t(7;22)(p22;q12) | *EWSR1::ETV1* |
| | *ETV4* | t(17;22)(q21;q12) | *EWSR1::ETV4* |
| | *FEV* | t(2;22)(q33;q12) | *EWSR1::FEV* |
| *FUS* | *ERG* | t(16;21)(p11;q22) | *FUS::ERG* |
| | *FEV* | t(2;16)(q35;p11) | *FUS::FEV* |
| *EWSR1* | **Non-ETS family** | | |
| | *NFATC2* | t(20;22)(q13;q12) | *EWSR1::NFATC2* |
| | *POU5F1* | t(20;22)(p21;q12) | *EWSR1::POU5F1* |
| | *SMARCA5* | t(4;22)(q31;q12) | *EWSR1::SMARCA5* |
| | *PATZ1* | t(1;22)(p36.1;q12)[with inv(22)] | *EWSR1::PATZ1* |
| | *SP3* | t(2;22)(q31;q12) | *EWSR1::SP3* |
| **Non-TET family** | | | |
| *CIC* | *DUX4* | t(4;19)(q35;q13) | *CIC::DUX4* |
| | *FOXO4* | t(X;19)(q13;q13.3) | *CIC::FOXO4* |
| *BCOR* | *CCNB3* | inv(X)(p11.4p11.22) | *BCOR::CCNB3* |
| | *MAML3* | t(x;4)(p11.4;q31.1) | *BCOR-MAML3* |
| | *ZC3H7B* | | *ZC3H7B::BCOR* |
| *CRTC1* | *SS18* | | *CRTC1::SS18* |

*EWSR1::ERG* fusion in 5–10%. Rare fusions account for the rest. Undifferentiated small round cell sarcomas harboring genetic alterations other than these, previously termed “Ewing-like sarcomas” and “Ewing family tumors,” are now recognized as distinct entities, and these terminologies are no longer used in practice (Table 12.2) [15].

### 12.4.2 Gross Appearance

Most Ewing sarcomas occur in the diaphysis and meta-diaphyseal region of long bones; only metaphyseal involvement is seen in 5–15% of cases. Epiphyseal extension is rarely observed. Primary soft tissue involvement accounts for 10–20% of cases. Tumors are soft, grey-white masses with well to poorly-defined margins. Osseous tumors originate in the central medullary cavity, invade cortical bone, and involve soft tissues. Periosteal lifting is common. Soft-tissue masses are often large, circumferential about the affected portion of the bone.

### 12.4.3 Microscopy

Ewing sarcoma is comprised of undifferentiated small round blue cells in sheets or in lobules separated by thin fibrous stroma. Nuclei are round, often with nuclear

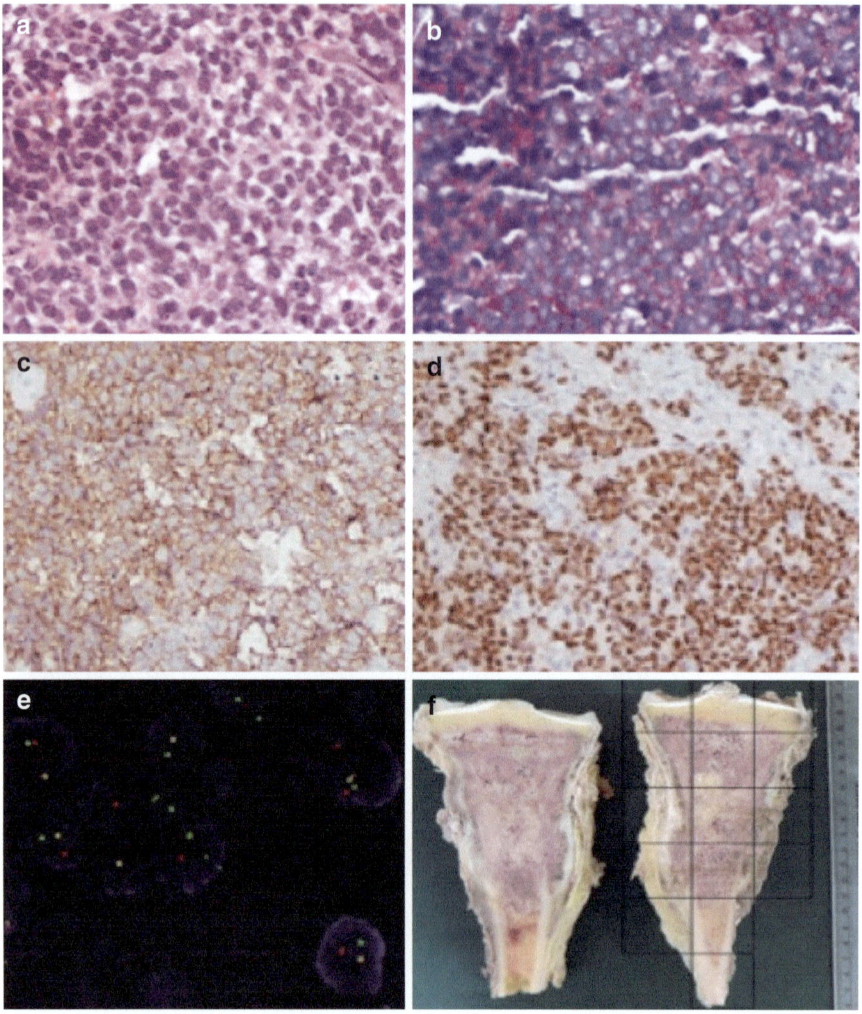

**Fig. 12.2** Undifferentiated small round cells with indentations in the nuclear membrane, inconspicuous nucleoli and clear cytoplasm with indistinct cell membranes (**a**). Periodic acid–Schiff stain demonstrates intracytoplasmic glycogen (**b**). Tumor cells show strong membranous positivity with CD99 (**c**) and diffuse positivity with NKX2.2 (**d**). *EWSR1* break-apart FISH shows *EWSR1* rearrangement (**e**). A large grey tan tumor involving the medullary bone of upper diaphysis and metaphysis of the tibia with cortical destruction, periosteal lifting and soft tissue involvement; the right side shows a grid for microscopic assessment of the percentage of necrosis in the tumor bed (**f**)

membrane indentations, and inconspicuous nucleoli. Cytoplasm is scant or may be clear with an indistinct cell membrane (Fig. 12.2). Homer-Wright and perivascular pseudorosettes may be seen. Foci of hemorrhage and necrosis are frequent. Extensive necrosis is observed after chemotherapy or radiotherapy. Mitoses are present but generally are not numerous. New bone formation occurs in areas of devitalized bone. ALES is composed of nests and lobules of undifferentiated cells with peripheral palisading and foci of squamous differentiation.

### 12.4.4 Histochemistry and Immunohistochemistry

Ewing sarcoma cells contain intracytoplasmic glycogen, which can be demonstrated by PAS positivity and digestion by diastase (Fig. 12.2). Tumor cells are immunoreactive to CD99, FLI1, NKX2.2, neuron-specific enolase, Leu7 (CD57), and vimentin. However, each of these has limited specificity. CD99 positivity is seen in other undifferentiated round cell sarcomas, lymphoblastic lymphoma, synovial sarcoma, etc., while FLI1 stains synovial sarcoma, melanoma, lung adenocarcinoma, Merkel cell carcinoma, etc. NKX2.2 is expressed in mesenchymal chondrosarcoma, poorly differentiated synovial sarcoma, small cell carcinoma, neuroblastoma, desmoplastic round cell tumor, and myoepithelial neoplasms. Adamantinoma-like Ewing sarcoma is positive for pan-cytokeratin, CK5/6, p63, and p40.

### 12.4.5 Differential Diagnosis

Histomorphological differential diagnoses include metastatic neuroblastoma, non-Hodgkin lymphoma, desmoplastic small round cell tumor, rhabdomyosarcoma, small cell osteosarcoma, poorly differentiated synovial sarcoma, etc. The morphology, immunohistochemical profile and molecular genetic testing usually distinguish these tumors.

### 12.4.6 Evaluation of Post-Therapy Resection Specimens

After neoadjuvant chemotherapy (NACT) or radiotherapy, careful mapping should be done to determine the extent of chemotherapy-induced necrosis in the tumor bed, and the percentage of residual tumor should be stated in the report (Fig. 12.2). Residual tumor of <10% indicates a favorable prognosis.

## 12.5 Round Cell Sarcomas with *EWSR1*–non-ETS Fusions

Round cell sarcomas with *EWSR1*–non-ETS fusions are rare and occur in children and adults [13]. *EWSR1-NFATC2* fusion sarcomas occur primarily in the bone, with a ratio of 4:1 over soft tissue, while *FUS-NFATC2* sarcomas are seen primarily in the long bones of the extremities [16]. These sarcomas show small- to medium-sized round and/or spindled cells in cords, trabeculae, small nests and pseudoacinar patterns in a fibrohyaline or myxohyaline stroma. Nuclear pleomorphism, prominent nucleoli and cytoplasmic clearing may be seen. Diffuse CD99 immunopositivity is seen in about half of the cases; nuclear PAX7 and NKX2.2 immunopositivity may be seen. *EWSR1::PATZ1* sarcomas usually occur in the deep soft tissue of the chest wall and abdomen. Tumor cells show mild variation in size and shape, with coarse chromatin [17]. Variable co-expression of myogenic (e.g., desmin, myogenin, MYOD1) and neurogenic (e.g., S100 protein, SOX10, and GFAP) markers is seen. CD99 is consistently negative in this subtype.

## 12.6 *CIC*-Rearranged Sarcomas

*CIC*-rearranged sarcomas often show either t(4;19)(q35;q13) or t(10;19)(q26;q13) translocations resulting in the formation of *CIC::DUX4* fusion gene [13]. It affects patients with a wide age range and occurs in deep soft tissues of the limbs, trunk, head and neck, and retroperitoneum. Primary bone involvement is seen in <5% of cases [18]. About 5% of *CIC*-rearranged sarcomas show fusion with non-*DUX4* gene partners, such as *FOXO4*, *LEUTX*, *NUTM1* and *NUTM2A* [13]. Microscopy shows diffuse sheets of undifferentiated round cells with a lobulated growth pattern. Spindled or epithelioid morphology may be present. Tumor cells usually show mild pleomorphism, with vesicular chromatin, prominent nucleoli and moderate amount of pale eosinophilic or clear cytoplasm. Brisk mitoses and necrosis are usually present. One-third of cases show myxoid appearance of the stroma. Diffuse, strong nuclear DUX4 immunopositivity and usually patchy CD99 staining are present; WT1 and ETV4 are positive in most cases. *CIC::NUTM1* fusion sarcomas express NUT protein [19]. *CIC*-rearranged sarcomas have an aggressive clinical course.

## 12.7 Sarcomas with *BCOR* Genetic Alterations

Sarcomas with *BCOR* genetic alterations include sarcomas with *BCOR* fusions (most frequently *BCOR::CCNB3*) and sarcomas with BCOR internal tandem duplication (ITD). *BCOR::CCNB3* sarcomas usually affect young children with a male predominance and are seen slightly more often in bone than in soft tissue, affecting the pelvis, lower limbs and paraspinal region. Undifferentiated small round to ovoid cells are seen in solid sheets and groups surrounded by a capillary network [20]. Sarcoma with *BCOR* ITDs usually occurs in infancy, primarily in the soft tissues of the trunk, retroperitoneum, and head and neck. Tumors are variably cellular, with primitive round-to-spindled cells in solid sheets or dispersed in a hypocellular myxoid matrix with a network of delicate vessels [21].

Most sarcomas with *BCOR* genetic alterations show BCOR and CCNB3 immunopositivity; however, these stains lack sensitivity and specificity. SATB2, TLE1 and cyclin D1 are often positive. CD99 positivity is seen in approximately 50% of cases.

## References


1. Rudzinski ER, Dry SM, Kohashi K, Bisogno G, Kelsey A. Rhabdomyosarcoma. In: WHO Classification of Tumours Editorial Board. Paediatric tumours. Lyon (France): International Agency for Research on Cancer; 2022. (WHO classification of tumours series, 5th ed.; vol. 7). https://publications.iarc.fr/608.
2. Pappo AS, Shapiro DN, Crist WM, et al. Biology and therapy of pediatric rhabdomyosarcoma. J Clin Oncol. 1995;13(8):2123–39.
3. Kohashi K, Kinoshita I, Oda Y. Soft tissue special issue: skeletal muscle tumors: a clinicopathological review. Head Neck Pathol. 2020;14(1):12–20.
4. Kodet R, Newton WA Jr, Hamoudi AB, et al. Childhood rhabdomyosarcoma with anaplastic (pleomorphic) features. A report of the Intergroup Rhabdomyosarcoma Study. Am J Surg Pathol. 1993;17(5):443–53.
5. Agaram NP, Zhang L, Sung YS, et al. Expanding the spectrum of intraosseous rhabdomyosarcoma: correlation between 2 distinct gene fusions and phenotype. Am J Surg Pathol. 2019;43(5):695–702.
6. Davicioni E, Anderson MJ, Finckenstein FG, et al. Molecular classification of rhabdomyosarcoma--genotypic and phenotypic determinants of diagnosis: a report from the Children's Oncology Group. Am J Pathol. 2009;174(2):550–64.
7. Mercado GE, Barr FG. Fusions involving PAX and FOX genes in the molecular pathogenesis of alveolar rhabdomyosarcoma: recent advances. Curr Mol Med. 2007;7(1):47–61.
8. Mercado GE, Xia SJ, Zhang C, et al. Identification of PAX3-FKHR-regulated genes differentially expressed between alveolar and embryonal rhabdomyosarcoma: focus on MYCN as a biologically relevant target. Genes Chromosomes Cancer. 2008;47(6):510–20.
9. Downs-Kelly E, Shehata BM, Lopez-Terrada D, et al. The utility of FOXO1 fluorescence in situ hybridization (FISH) in formalin-fixed paraffin-embedded specimens in the diagnosis of alveolar rhabdomyosarcoma. Diagn Mol Pathol. 2009;18(3):138–43.
10. Arden KC, Anderson MJ, Finckenstein FG, et al. Detection of the t(2;13) chromosomal translocation in alveolar rhabdomyosarcoma using the reverse transcriptase-polymerase chain reaction. Genes Chromosomes Cancer. 1996;16(4):254–60.
11. Zhu B, Davie JK. New insights into signalling-pathway alterations in rhabdomyosarcoma. Br J Cancer. 2015;112(2):227–31.
12. Alaggio R, Zhang L, Sung YS, et al. A molecular study of pediatric spindle and sclerosing rhabdomyosarcoma: identification of novel and recurrent VGLL2-related fusions in infantile cases. Am J Surg Pathol. 2016;40(2):224–35.
13. Choi JH, Ro JY. The 2020 WHO classification of tumors of soft tissue: selected changes and new entities. Adv Anat Pathol. 2021;28(1):44–58.
14. Kakkar A, Bharati V, Pulimala S, Kumar R, Bhalla AS. Fine-needle aspiration cytology of adamantinoma-like Ewing sarcoma: an unusual parotid tumor [published online ahead of print, 2022 Oct 3]. Diagn Cytopathol. 2022; https://doi.org/10.1002/dc.25061.
15. Sbaraglia M, et al. Ewing sarcoma and Ewing-like tumors. Virchows Arch. 2020;476(1):109–19.
16. Diaz-Perez JA, et al. EWSR1/FUS-NFATc2 rearranged round cell sarcoma: clinicopathological series of 4 cases and literature review. Hum Pathol. 2019;90:45–53.
17. Chougule A, et al. Spindle and round cell sarcoma with EWSR1-PATZ1 gene fusion: a sarcoma with polyphenotypic differentiation. Am J Surg Pathol. 2019;43(2):220.
18. Gambarotti M, et al. CIC–DUX 4 fusion-positive round-cell sarcomas of soft tissue and bone: a single-institution morphological and molecular analysis of seven cases. Histopathology. 2016;69(4):624–34.
19. Le Loarer F, et al. Clinicopathologic features of CIC-NUTM1 sarcomas, a new molecular variant of the family of CIC-fused sarcomas. Am J Surg Pathol. 2019;43(2):268–76.
20. Kao Y-C, et al. BCOR-CCNB3-fusion positive sarcomas: a clinicopathologic and molecular analysis of 36 cases with comparison to morphologic spectrum and clinical behavior of other round cell sarcomas. Am J Surg Pathol. 2018;42(5):604.
21. Antonescu CR, Kao YC, Xu B, et al. Undifferentiated round cell sarcoma with BCOR internal tandem duplications (ITD) or YWHAE fusions: a clinicopathologic and molecular study. Mod Pathol. 2020;33(9):1669–77.

# Pathology of Pediatric Brain Tumors 13

Debajyoti Chatterjee

Although almost all types of tumors that are described in adults can be seen in children, we will discuss mainly those tumors which have a predilection for the pediatric age group. As per the 2021 world health organization (WHO) classification of the central nervous system (CNS) tumors (WHO CNS 5), the tumors have been classified based on their histological and molecular features [1].

The following tumors will be discussed in this section:

- CNS embryonal tumors
- Pediatric gliomas
- Ependymoma
- Choroid plexus tumors
- Germ cell tumors
- Pineal region tumors

## 13.1 CNS Embryonal Tumors

### 13.1.1 Medulloblastoma

Medulloblastoma (MB) is the commonest CNS embryonal tumor that arises in cerebellar parenchyma or grows in the fourth ventricle. It is classified into different histological and molecular subtypes; however, all are considered WHO grade 4 tumors [1].

D. Chatterjee (✉)
Department of Histopathology, Postgraduate Institute of Medical Education and Research, Chandigarh, India



R. Madan et al. (eds.), *Evidence Based Practice in Pediatric Radiation Oncology*, https://doi.org/10.1007/978-981-96-4872-6_13

#### 13.1.1.1 Histopathology of Medulloblastoma

Depending on the architecture and cellular morphology, MB is classified into the following types:

**Medulloblastoma, histologically defined** Four histological subtypes of MBs have been described:

(a) **Classic medulloblastoma:** It comprises 70–80% of all MBs [2, 3]. It is composed of small blue round cells, arranged in diffuse sheets. Homer-wright rosettes are commonly found. Mitotic and apoptotic activities are increased.
(b) **Desmoplastic/Nodular (D/N) medulloblastoma:** It accounts for 15–20% of all medulloblastomas. It is the commonest type of MB under 3 years of age [4]. Histological examination reveals a prominent nodular architecture. The center of the nodules is pale and composed of cells showing variable neurocytic differentiation. The internodular areas are highly cellular and composed of undifferentiated small, blue round cells. The stroma in the internodular areas is compressed and shows an intercellular reticulin-rich framework (Fig. 13.1a and b).
(c) **Medulloblastoma with extensive nodularity (MBEN):** It is a rare variant of MB, comprising 3–4% of all MBs. It is more common under 3 years of age [3–5]. On histological examination, MBEN shows an extensive nodular pattern. These nodules are large and serpentine, compared to D/N type MB. The nod-

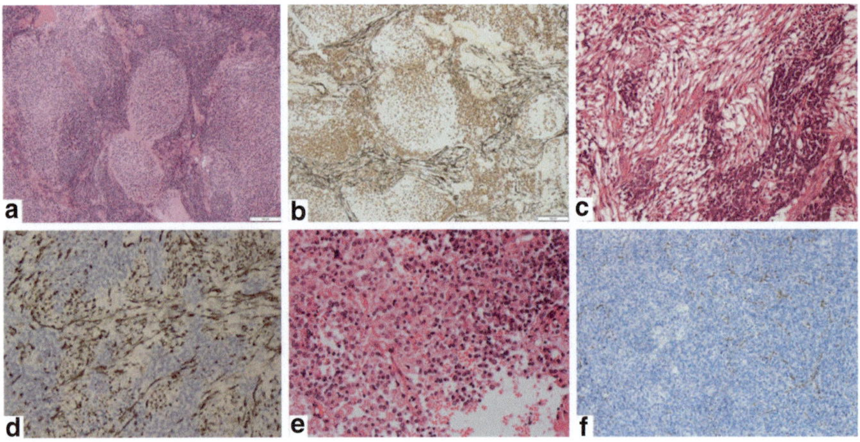


**Fig. 13.1** (**a**) Medulloblastoma, desmoplastic/nodular type, showing large pale nodules with neurocytic differentiation (Hematoxylin and Eosin, x100), (**b**) Same case showing reticulin-rich internodular areas (Reticulin stain, x100). (**c**) A case of medulloblastoma showing myogenic differentiation with presence of elongated strap cells indicating skeletal muscle differentiation (Hematoxylin and eosin, x200). (**d**) The rhabdoid cells are positive for desmin (Immunohistochemistry, x200). (**e**) A case of atypical teratoid/rhabdoid tumor showing rhabdoid cells with abundant eosinophilic cytoplasm (Hematoxylin and Eosin, x200). (**f**) The tumor shows loss of INI1 expression, while endothelial cells are positive (Immunohistochemistry, x100)

ules are pale and show extensive neurocytic differentiation, and the stroma is neuropil rich.

(d) **Large cell/anaplastic (LC/A) medulloblastoma:** It accounts for nearly 10% of all MBs. This variant is seen across all ages [4, 6]. This is a highly cellular tumor composed of undifferentiated cells. The cells show significant nuclear pleomorphism. They show features of anaplasia, such as nuclear molding, cytoplasmic inclusions, and cell wrapping. Tumors with large cell morphology are composed of more uniform large cells. Both types show very high mitotic and apoptotic activity. In addition, medulloblastoma can show myogenic or melanocytic differentiation (Fig. 13.1c and d).

**Medulloblastoma, molecularly defined** Medulloblastoma shows wide molecular alterations. The different molecular subtype of MB shows different clinical behavior and correlates with histological subtypes. DNA methylation profiling is required for the accurate molecular classification of MBs. The following molecular subtypes of MBs have been described:

(a) **Medulloblastoma, WNT-activated:** It comprises of nearly 10% of all MBs. It is seen in children aged between 7 and 14 years [7]. Most of the cases show classic morphology and harbor somatic mutations in exon 3 of the *CTNNB1* gene [8]. The tumor cells show patchy or diffused nuclear expression for beta-catenin [9]. Children with WNT-activated medulloblastoma show excellent outcome with nearly 100% overall survival with surgery and adjuvant therapy [7].

(b) **Medulloblastoma, SHH-activated:** SHH-activated MBs are further classified based on the presence of TP53 mutation.

**b.1. Medulloblastoma, SHH-activated, and TP53-wildtype:** MBs in this group show sonic hedgehog pathway (SHH) signaling activation with wildtype TP53 gene. It is usually seen in infants and adults [10]. Most of the cases show desmoplastic/nodular or MBEN morphology. The tumor cells show positivity for YAP1 and GAB1. They show cytoplasmic (not nuclear) positivity for beta-catenin. TP53 expression is focal (wildtype) [9, 11].

These tumors show germline mutations in the genes involved in the SHH signaling pathway, which leads to SHH pathway activation. The commonly involved genes include *PTCH1* (40%) and *SMO* (10%) [1]. Four provisional subgroups of SHH-activated MBs have been described based on DNA methylation or transcriptome profiling [12]. The prognosis in this group is intermediate between WNT-activated and group 3 medulloblastoma [9].

**b.2. Medulloblastoma, SHH-activated, and TP53-mutant:** This group of MB shows concurrent activation of the SHH pathway and a mutant TP53 gene. It comprises 10–15% of SHH-activated MBs [13, 14].

These cases show large cell/anaplastic morphology. Most of the cases are associated with *MYCN* amplification and associated with a poor outcome [9].

(c) **Medulloblastoma, non-WNT/ non-SHH:** This largest subgroup of MB (also known as group 3 or 4) carries poor prognosis [4, 9].

Most of these cases demonstrate classic or large cell/anaplastic morphology [9]. The commonest molecular alteration in group 3 MB is *MYC* amplification [15]. Group 4 MB shows a wide spectrum of molecular alterations. Based on the methylation profile, this group of MB is further divided into eight molecular subgroups (group 3/4 subgroups 1–8) [16].

### 13.1.2 Atypical Teratoid and Rhabdoid Tumor (AT/RT)

It is a high-grade (grade 4) CNS tumor in children, characterized by the presence of variable rhabdoid cells. It is mostly seen under 2 years of age [1, 17].

Histology: AT/RT shows large morphological heterogeneity. Most cases show undifferentiated embryonal components, admixed with rhabdoid cells, mesenchymal and epithelial elements, in varying proportions. Rhabdoid cells are large and round to polygonal and contain eccentrically placed nuclei and abundant eosinophilic cytoplasm and intracytoplasmic globular eosinophilic inclusions (Fig. 13.1e and f). The mesenchymal elements are composed of spindle cells, arranged in fascicles. Sometimes, glial differentiation is also evident. The undifferentiated and the rhabdoid components show high proliferative activity [18, 19].

Immunophenotype: AT/RT shows polyphenotypic differentiation. The tumor cells show nuclear loss of SMARCB1 (INI1), which is a very specific marker of AT/RT. [20, 21] The rhabdoid cells show variable positivity for vimentin, GFAP, cytokeratin, synaptophysin, EMA, and smooth muscle actin.

Genetics: AT/RT is characterized by mutation or loss of the SMARCB1 gene (>95% cases), located at chromosome 22q11.2 [22, 23]. Around 5% of cases show the inactivation of SMARCA4 protein. Based on methylation profiling, AT/RTs are classified into three molecular subgroups- AT/RT-TYR, AT/RT-SHH, and AT/RT-MYC [24].

### 13.1.3 Cribriform Neuroepithelial Tumor (CRINET)

CRINET is an uncommon tumor, seen in young children (median age of 20 months). It is located predominantly in the periventricular region [25].

Histopathology: It is a cellular tumor, composed of cribriform patterns, ribbons, and nests of tumor cells. The tumor cells are oval to elongated with hyperchromatic nuclei. Rosettes may be seen [26].

The tumor cells express epithelial membrane antigen (EMA), with variable expression for synaptophysin, vimentin, and GFAP. They show characteristic loss of INI1 expression. Ki-67 proliferation index is variable (5–30%) [26, 27]. It behaves better than AT/RT. [26]

### 13.1.4 Embryonal Tumor with Multi-Layered Rosettes (ETMR)

It is an embryonal tumor (grade 4) showing a wide spectrum of morphology. These tumors show multi-layered rosettes and the presence of C19MC amplification. Most cases are reported under four years of age [28].

Histology: ETMR shows a wide morphological spectrum; however, they are unified by the presence of multi-layered rosettes. These rosettes are composed of round to oval embryonal cells (neuroepithelium), arranged in multiple layers around a central lumen. These rosettes have a well-defined internal limiting membrane. The neuroepithelial component shows a high mitotic and apoptotic activity [29, 30]. Depending on the nature of the rosettes and the associated stroma, three morphological subtypes of ETMR are recognized: embryonal tumors with abundant neuropil and true rosettes [31], ependymoblastoma, and medulloepithelioma.

The embryonal cells show expression for vimentin and nestin, with variable expression for synaptophysin, EMA, and CD99. The embryonal cells show diffuse cytoplasmic positivity for LIN28A, which is a surrogate marker for C19MC alteration [29, 32].

Molecular pathology: The majority of cases harbor alteration involving a microRNA cluster on chromosome 19q13.42 (C19MC), including proliferation and fusion [33, 34]. Rare tumors (around 5%) show *DICER1* mutation, as a part of *DICER1* genetic tumor syndrome [35].

### 13.1.5 CNS Neuroblastoma, FOXR2 Activated

It is a grade 4 embryonal tumor showing the presence of variable neuroblastic and neuronal differentiation and structural rearrangement of transcription factor FOXR2 [1].

It is a rare tumor, usually seen in children [36].

Histology: It shows sheets of undifferentiated embryonal cells. These cells have a high N:C ratio, hyperchromatic nuclei and show frequent mitosis. Rare cases show the presence of ganglionic cells in clusters (ganglioneuroblastoma) [37].

The tumor cells show positivity for synaptophysin (usually patchy) and OLIG2. They are negative for GFAP. KI-67 index is high.

Genetics: Most cases show complex rearrangement of the FOXR2 gene [36, 38].

### 13.1.6 CNS Tumors with BCOR Internal Tandem Duplication

This is a rare, high-grade CNS tumor, usually seen in children. It is a molecularly defined tumor, characterized by internal tandem duplication in exon 15 of the *BCOR* gene [36].

Histology: This is a cellular tumor. The tumor cells are round to elongated and have coarse chromatin and moderate eosinophilic cytoplasm. The cells are arranged in a fibrillary background. Many capillary channels are distributed throughout the tumor. The cells show a perivascular (ependymoma-like) arrangement. Mitotic activity is brisk [39–41].

The tumor cells show diffuse positivity for vimentin and CD56 and patchy expression for GFAP, OLIG2, and S100. BCOR shows diffuse and strong nuclear expression [39].

## 13.2 Pediatric-Type Diffuse High-Grade Gliomas

A wide spectrum of glial tumors occurs in the pediatric age group. It can be high-grade as well as low-grade type. In this chapter, we are briefly discussing the pediatric-type diffuse high-grade glioma.

This group comprises the following entities, which have characteristic clinical, histological, and molecular features.

### 13.2.1 Diffuse Midline Glioma, H3K27-Altered

It is a grade 4, infiltrative glioma, located in the midline, and shows loss of H3p.K28me3 (K27me3).

Diffuse midline glioma (DMG) mostly occurs in children. It represents 10–20% of childhood brain tumors. In children, DMG mostly occurs in the pons (also known as diffuse intrinsic pontile glioma), brainstem, or thalamus (often bilateral), whereas in adolescents and adults, they mostly arise from the thalamus (unilaterally) or spinal cord [42, 43].

Histology: DMG shows an infiltrative growth pattern. It is composed of small uniform cells, although atypia may be seen in some cases (Fig. 13.2a). Mitosis is brisk. Necrosis and microvascular proliferation are commonly observed but may be absent in some cases [44–46].

DMGs express S100, OLIG2, and MAP 2, while GFAP expression is variable. They show loss of H3K27me3 protein and express H3K27M mutant protein (Fig. 13.2b and c). This combination of H3K27me3 and H3K27M is highly diagnostic of DMG [46, 47].

Genetics: DMG is characterized by heterozygous mutations in the Histone (H3.1, H3.2, or H3.3) genes, causing loss of H3p.K28me3 (K27me3) on wildtype histone 3. Based on the molecular profiles, DMGs are further classified into four molecular subgroups [48, 49].

### 13.2.2 Diffuse Hemispheric Glioma, H3G34-Mutant

It is an infiltrative high-grade (grade 4) glioma in the younger age group that affects the cerebral hemispheres and is characterized by a missense mutation in the 34th codon of the H3F3A gene. It affects mainly adolescents and young adults (median age of 19 years) [50–52].

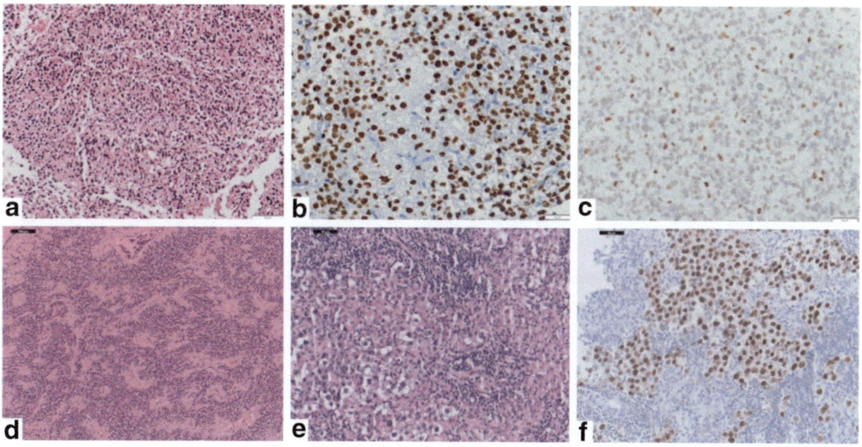

**Fig. 13.2** (**a**) Diffuse midline glioma showing a cellular tumor with frequent mitosis (Hematoxylin and eosin, x100). It shows a diffuse nuclear expression of H3K27m (**b**, Immunohistochemistry, x200) and loss of H3K27me3 (**c**, Immunohistochemistry, x200). (**d**) A case of ependymoma showing perivascular pseudorosettes (Hematoxylin and eosin, x100). (**e**) A case of germinoma showing many large atypical cells with the presence of lymphoid cells in the background (Hematoxylin and eosin, x200). (**f**) The tumor cells show nuclear expression for SALL4 (Immunohistochemistry, x200)

Histology: It shows a cellular astrocytic tumor with a diffusely infiltrating pattern. Frequent mitosis, necrosis, and microvascular proliferation are common. It can show areas resembling oligodendroglioma and undifferentiated small round cell morphology [53, 54].

The tumor cells show variable GFAP expression and lack OLIG2 expression. They show loss of ATRX and diffuse TP53 positivity. IHC for H3G34 mutant proteins can be useful to identify the mutant variants [53, 54].

Genetics: Heterozygous mutation at codon 35 (34) of the H3F3A gene is characteristic of this entity [51, 54].

### 13.2.3 Diffuse Pediatric Type High-Grade Glioma, H3-Wildtype and IDH-Wildtype

This is a heterogeneous group of pediatric HGG. It lacks both IDH and H3 mutations [1]. The median age of presentation is around 10 years. They resemble glioblastoma or an undifferentiated tumor in morphology.

## 13.3 Ependymoma

Ependymoma is a neuroepithelial tumor that is seen mostly in the intra- or periventricular regions. It is seen in children and adults, both in the supra and infratentorial locations.

Microscopically, ependymomas are relatively circumscribed tumors, composed of oval to elongated glial cells arranged predominantly around the blood vessels. The cell process radiates from the basement membrane of the vessels, producing the appearance of perivascular pseudorosette (Fig. 13.2d). The intervening area shows variable cellularity. True ependymal rosettes or canals may be seen. The tumor cells express GFAP and perinuclear dot-like positivity for EMA. L1CAM can act as a surrogate IHC marker for supratentorial ependymomas with *C11orf95* rearrangement [1, 55].

Ependymomas were traditionally classified as WHO grades 1, 2, and 3, depending on the histological criteria, such as mitosis and necrosis. However, as per the current WHO classification [1], ependymomas are now classified according to their location and molecular alteration, as follows:

1. Supratentorial ependymoma (ST-EP)
   (a) ST-EP, *ZFTA* fusion-positive
   (b) ST-EP, *YAP1* fusion-positive
   (c) ST-EP, grade 2/3
2. Posterior fossa ependymoma (PF-EP)
   (a) PF-EP, group A
   (b) PF-EP, group B
   (c) PF-EP, grade 2/3
3. Spinal ependymomas
   (a) Spinal ependymoma, *MYCN*-amplified
   (b) Myxopapillary ependymoma, grade 2
   (c) Spinal ependymoma, grade 2/3
4. Subependymoma, grade 1

   The posterior fossa ependymomas (PF-EP groups A and B) show different methylation profiles and group A lacks H3K27me3 expression. *MYCN* amplification in spinal ependymomas are associated with an adverse outcome [56, 57].

## 13.4 Choroid Plexus Tumors

Choroid plexus tumors include choroid plexus papilloma (CPP, grade 1), atypical choroid plexus papilloma (grade 2), and choroid plexus carcinoma (CPC, grade 3). They arise in the ventricles, the most common site being the lateral ventricle. CPP arises in children and adults, while CPC arises mostly in children [58].

Histologically, CPP shows the papillary architecture, which is lined by cuboidal cells with mild nuclear pleomorphism. Mitosis is low (<2/10 HPF). Atypical CPP shows increased mitosis (≥2/10 HPF). CPC shows fusion of the papillae, increased cellularity, high mitosis (>5/10 HPF), necrosis, and brain invasion. On immunohistochemistry, choroid plexus tumors are positive for CK7, EMA, Kir7.1, and focally for GFAP [59, 60].

## 13.5 Germ Cell Tumors

A wide spectrum of germ cell tumors (GCTs) arises in the brain. They mostly affect children and young adults and commonly involve the midline structures (pineal gland, sellar, and suprasellar region are the most common sites) [61, 62].

Histologically, GCTs show similar morphology to their gonadal counterpart (Fig. 13.2e and f).

## 13.6 Pineal Tumors

Pineal region tumors in children include pineal parenchymal tumors, ependymomas, germ cell tumors, etc. Among the pineal parenchymal tumors include pineocytoma, pineal parenchymal tumor in intermediate differentiation (PPTID), pineoblastoma, and the papillary tumor of the pineal region (PTPR) [1]. Pineoblastoma occurs mostly in children [63]. It is a grade 4 undifferentiated tumor. It is composed of sheets of embryonal cells with a high N:C ratio, showing high mitotic activity. Necrosis is commonly encountered. Homer Wright and Flexner-Wintersteiner rosettes are observed. A rare variant of pineoblastoma shows neuroectodermal (melanocytic) and heterologous ectomesenchymal components, known as pineal anlage tumor [64, 65]. Pineocytoma is a low-grade (grade 1) tumor with low cellularity, infrequent mitosis, and the presence of pineocytomatous rosettes. PPTID (grades 2 and 3) shows feature intermediate between pineocytoma and pineoblastoma [66, 67]. The pineal parenchymal tumors express synaptophysin. Neurofilament protein expression is variable. They usually do not express GFAP and NeuN. Pineoblastoma commonly shows mutation and copy number variation involving *DICER1* gene [68].

## References


1. WHO Classification of Tumours Editorial Board. Central nervous system tumours, WHO classification of tumours series, vol. 6. 5th ed. Lyon: International Agency for Research on Cancer; 2021. https://publications.iarc.fr/601
2. Eberhart CG, Kepner JL, Goldthwaite PT, Kun LE, Duffner PK, Friedman HS, Strother DR, Burger PC. Histopathologic grading of medulloblastomas: a Pediatric Oncology Group study. Cancer. 2002;94(2):552–60.
3. Ellison DW. Childhood medulloblastoma: novel approaches to the classification of a heterogeneous disease. Acta Neuropathol. 2010 Sep;120(3):305–16.
4. Kool M, Korshunov A, Remke M, Jones DT, Schlanstein M, Northcott PA, et al. Molecular subgroups of medulloblastoma: an international meta-analysis of transcriptome, genetic aberrations, and clinical data of WNT, SHH, group 3, and group 4 medulloblastomas. Acta Neuropathol. 2012 Apr;123(4):473–84.
5. Korshunov A, Sahm F, Okonechnikov K, Ryzhova M, Stichel D, Schrimpf D, Casalini B, Sievers P, Meyer J, Zheludkova O, Golanov A, Lichter P, Jones DTW, Pfister SM, Kool M, von Deimling A. Desmoplastic/nodular medulloblastomas (DNMB) and medulloblastomas with extensive nodularity (MBEN) disclose similar epigenetic signatures but different transcriptional profiles. Acta Neuropathol. 2019 Jun;137(6):1003–15.

6. Taylor MD, Northcott PA, Korshunov A, Remke M, Cho YJ, Clifford SC, Eberhart CG, Parsons DW, Rutkowski S, Gajjar A, Ellison DW, Lichter P, Gilbertson RJ, Pomeroy SL, Kool M, Pfister SM. Molecular subgroups of medulloblastoma: the current consensus. Acta Neuropathol. 2012 Apr;123(4):465–72.
7. Ellison DW, Onilude OE, Lindsey JC, Lusher ME, Weston CL, Taylor RE, Pearson AD, Clifford SC. United Kingdom children's Cancer Study Group Brain Tumour Committee. Beta-catenin status predicts a favorable outcome in childhood medulloblastoma: the United Kingdom children's Cancer Study Group Brain Tumour Committee. J Clin Oncol. 2005;23(31):7951–7.
8. Clifford SC, Lusher ME, Lindsey JC, Langdon JA, Gilbertson RJ, Straughton D, Ellison DW. Wnt/wingless pathway activation and chromosome 6 loss characterize a distinct molecular sub-group of medulloblastomas associated with a favorable prognosis. Cell Cycle. 2006 Nov;5(22):2666–70.
9. Ellison DW, Dalton J, Kocak M, Nicholson SL, Fraga C, Neale G, Kenney AM, Brat DJ, Perry A, Yong WH, Taylor RE, Bailey S, Clifford SC, Gilbertson RJ. Medulloblastoma: clinicopathological correlates of SHH, WNT, and non-SHH/WNT molecular subgroups. Acta Neuropathol. 2011 Mar;121(3):381–96.
10. Northcott PA, Jones DT, Kool M, Robinson GW, Gilbertson RJ, Cho YJ, Pomeroy SL, Korshunov A, Lichter P, Taylor MD, Pfister SM. Medulloblastomics: the end of the beginning. Nat Rev Cancer. 2012;12(12):818–34.
11. Kaur K, Kakkar A, Kumar A, Mallick S, Julka PK, Gupta D, Suri A, Suri V, Sharma MC, Sarkar C. Integrating molecular subclassification of medulloblastomas into routine clinical practice: a simplified approach. Brain Pathol. 2016 May;26(3):334–43.
12. Cavalli FMG, Remke M, Rampasek L, Peacock J, Shih DJH, Luu B, et al. Intertumoral heterogeneity within medulloblastoma subgroups. Cancer Cell. 2017;31(6):737–754.e6.
13. Kool M, Jones DT, Jäger N, Northcott PA, Pugh TJ, Hovestadt V, et al. Genome sequencing of SHH medulloblastoma predicts genotype-related response to smoothened inhibition. Cancer Cell. 2014;25(3):393–405.
14. Zhukova N, Ramaswamy V, Remke M, Pfaff E, Shih DJ, Martin DC, et al. Subgroup-specific prognostic implications of TP53 mutation in medulloblastoma. J Clin Oncol. 2013;31(23):2927–35.
15. Northcott PA, Shih DJ, Peacock J, Garzia L, Morrissy AS, Zichner T, et al. Subgroup-specific structural variation across 1,000 medulloblastoma genomes. Nature. 2012;488(7409):49–56.
16. Sharma T, Schwalbe EC, Williamson D, Sill M, Hovestadt V, Mynarek M, et al. Second-generation molecular subgrouping of medulloblastoma: an international meta-analysis of group 3 and group 4 subtypes. Acta Neuropathol. 2019 Aug;138(2):309–26.
17. Ostrom QT, Chen YM, de Blank P, Ondracek A, Farah P, Gittleman H, et al. The descriptive epidemiology of atypical teratoid/rhabdoid tumors in the United States, 2001-2010. Neuro-Oncology. 2014;16(10):1392–9.
18. Burger PC, Yu IT, Tihan T, Friedman HS, Strother DR, Kepner JL, Duffner PK, Kun LE, Perlman EJ. Atypical teratoid/rhabdoid tumor of the central nervous system: a highly malignant tumor of infancy and childhood frequently mistaken for medulloblastoma: a Pediatric Oncology Group study. Am J Surg Pathol. 1998 Sep;22(9):1083–92.
19. Rorke LB, Packer RJ, Biegel JA. Central nervous system atypical teratoid/rhabdoid tumors of infancy and childhood: definition of an entity. J Neurosurg. 1996 Jul;85(1):56–65.
20. Haberler C, Laggner U, Slavc I, Czech T, Ambros IM, Ambros PF, Budka H, Hainfellner JA. Immunohistochemical analysis of INI1 protein in malignant pediatric CNS tumors: lack of INI1 in atypical teratoid/rhabdoid tumors and in a fraction of primitive neuroectodermal tumors without rhabdoid phenotype. Am J Surg Pathol. 2006;30(11):1462–8.
21. Judkins AR, Mauger J, Ht A, Rorke LB, Biegel JA. Immunohistochemical analysis of hSNF5/INI1 in pediatric CNS neoplasms. Am J Surg Pathol. 2004 May;28(5):644–50.
22. Biegel JA, Zhou JY, Rorke LB, Stenstrom C, Wainwright LM, Fogelgren B. Germ-line and acquired mutations of INI1 in atypical teratoid and rhabdoid tumors. Cancer Res. 1999;59(1):74–9.

23. Versteege I, Sévenet N, Lange J, Rousseau-Merck MF, Ambros P, Handgretinger R, Aurias A, Delattre O. Truncating mutations of hSNF5/INI1 in aggressive paediatric cancer. Nature. 1998;394(6689):203–6.
24. Johann PD, Erkek S, Zapatka M, Kerl K, Buchhalter I, Hovestadt V, et al. Atypical Teratoid/Rhabdoid tumors are comprised of three epigenetic subgroups with distinct enhancer landscapes. Cancer Cell. 2016;29(3):379–93.
25. Hasselblatt M, Oyen F, Gesk S, Kordes U, Wrede B, Bergmann M, et al. Cribriform neuroepithelial tumor (CRINET): a nonrhabdoid ventricular tumor with INI1 loss and relatively favorable prognosis. J Neuropathol Exp Neurol. 2009;68(12):1249–55.
26. Johann PD, Hovestadt V, Thomas C, Jeibmann A, Heß K, Bens S, et al. Cribriform neuroepithelial tumor: molecular characterization of a SMARCB1-deficient non-rhabdoid tumor with favorable long-term outcome. Brain Pathol. 2017 Jul;27(4):411–8.
27. Gessi M, Japp AS, Dreschmann V, Zur Mühlen A, Goschzik T, Dörner E, et al. High-resolution genomic analysis of cribriform Neuroepithelial tumors of the central nervous system. J Neuropathol Exp Neurol. 2015;74(10):970–4.
28. Lambo S, von Hoff K, Korshunov A, Pfister SM, Kool M. ETMR: a tumor entity in its infancy. Acta Neuropathol. 2020 Sep;140(3):249–66.
29. Korshunov A, Sturm D, Ryzhova M, Hovestadt V, Gessi M, Jones DT, et al. Embryonal tumor with abundant neuropil and true rosettes (ETANTR), ependymoblastoma, and medulloepithelioma share molecular similarity and comprise a single clinicopathological entity. Acta Neuropathol. 2014 Aug;128(2):279–89.
30. Judkins AR, Ellison DW. Ependymoblastoma: dear, damned, distracting diagnosis, farewell!*. Brain Pathol. 2010 Jan;20(1):133–9.
31. Gessi M, Giangaspero F, Lauriola L, Gardiman M, Scheithauer BW, Halliday W, et al. Embryonal tumors with abundant neuropil and true rosettes: a distinctive CNS primitive neuroectodermal tumor. Am J Surg Pathol. 2009 Feb;33(2):211–7.
32. Spence T, Sin-Chan P, Picard D, Barszczyk M, Hoss K, Lu M, et al. CNS-PNETs with C19MC amplification and/or LIN28 expression comprise a distinct histogenetic diagnostic and therapeutic entity. Acta Neuropathol. 2014 Aug;128(2):291–303.
33. Lambo S, Gröbner SN, Rausch T, Waszak SM, Schmidt C, Gorthi A, et al. The molecular landscape of ETMR at diagnosis and relapse. Nature. 2019;576(7786):274–80.
34. Kleinman CL, Gerges N, Papillon-Cavanagh S, Sin-Chan P, Pramatarova A, Quang DA, et al. Fusion of TTYH1 with the C19MC microRNA cluster drives expression of a brain-specific DNMT3B isoform in the embryonal brain tumor ETMR. Nat Genet. 2014;46(1):39–44.
35. de Kock L, Priest JR, Foulkes WD, Alexandrescu S. An update on the central nervous system manifestations of DICER1 syndrome. Acta Neuropathol. 2020;139(4):689–701.
36. Sturm D, Orr BA, Toprak UH, Hovestadt V, Jones DTW, Capper D, et al. New brain tumor entities emerge from molecular classification of CNS-PNETs. Cell. 2016;164(5):1060–72.
37. Holsten T, Lubieniecki F, Spohn M, Mynarek M, Bison B, Löbel U, et al. Detailed clinical and histopathological description of 8 cases of molecularly defined CNS neuroblastomas. J Neuropathol Exp Neurol. 2021;80(1):52–9.
38. Poh B, Koso H, Momota H, Komori T, Suzuki Y, Yoshida N, et al. Foxr2 promotes formation of CNS-embryonal tumors in a Trp53-deficient background. Neuro-Oncology. 2019;21(8):993–1004.
39. Yoshida Y, Nobusawa S, Nakata S, Nakada M, Arakawa Y, Mineharu Y, et al. CNS high-grade neuroepithelial tumor with BCOR internal tandem duplication: a comparison with its counterparts in the kidney and soft tissue. Brain Pathol. 2018 Sep;28(5):710–20.
40. Appay R, Macagno N, Padovani L, Korshunov A, Kool M, André N, et al. HGNET-BCOR tumors of the cerebellum: clinicopathologic and molecular characterization of 3 cases. Am J Surg Pathol. 2017;41(9):1254–60.
41. Ferris SP, Velazquez Vega J, Aboian M, Lee JC, Van Ziffle J, Onodera C, e al. High-grade neuroepithelial tumor with BCOR exon 15 internal tandem duplication-a comprehensive clinical, radiographic, pathologic, and genomic analysis. Brain Pathol. 2020;30(1):46–62.

42. Roux A, Pallud J, Saffroy R, Edjlali-Goujon M, Debily MA, Boddaert N, et al. High-grade gliomas in adolescents and young adults highlight histomolecular differences from their adult and pediatric counterparts. Neuro-Oncology. 2020;22(8):1190–202.
43. Meyronet D, Esteban-Mader M, Bonnet C, Joly MO, Uro-Coste E, Amiel-Benouaich A, et al. Characteristics of H3 K27M-mutant gliomas in adults. Neuro-Oncology. 2017;19(8):1127–34.
44. Castel D, Philippe C, Calmon R, Le Dret L, Truffaux N, Boddaert N, et al. Histone H3F3A and HIST1H3B K27M mutations define two subgroups of diffuse intrinsic pontine gliomas with different prognosis and phenotypes. Acta Neuropathol. 2015;130(6):815–27.
45. Buczkowicz P, Hoeman C, Rakopoulos P, Pajovic S, Letourneau L, Dzamba M, et al. Genomic analysis of diffuse intrinsic pontine gliomas identifies three molecular subgroups and recurrent activating ACVR1 mutations. Nat Genet. 2014;46(5):451–6.
46. Solomon DA, Wood MD, Tihan T, Bollen AW, Gupta N, Phillips JJ, et al. Diffuse midline gliomas with histone H3-K27M mutation: a series of 47 cases assessing the spectrum of morphologic variation and associated genetic alterations. Brain Pathol. 2016;26(5):569–80.
47. Huang T, Garcia R, Qi J, Lulla R, Horbinski C, Behdad A, et al. Detection of histone H3 K27M mutation and post-translational modifications in pediatric diffuse midline glioma via tissue immunohistochemistry informs diagnosis and clinical outcomes. Oncotarget. 2018;9(98):37112–24.
48. Lewis PW, Müller MM, Koletsky MS, Cordero F, Lin S, Banaszynski LA, et al. Inhibition of PRC2 activity by a gain-of-function H3 mutation found in pediatric glioblastoma. Science. 2013;340(6134):857–61.
49. Bender S, Tang Y, Lindroth AM, Hovestadt V, Jones DT, Kool M, et al. Reduced H3K27me3 and DNA hypomethylation are major drivers of gene expression in K27M mutant pediatric high-grade gliomas. Cancer Cell. 2013;24(5):660–72.
50. Schwartzentruber J, Korshunov A, Liu XY, Jones DT, Pfaff E, Jacob K, et al. Driver mutations in histone H3.3 and chromatin remodelling genes in paediatric glioblastoma. Nature. 2012;482(7384):226–31.
51. Mackay A, Burford A, Carvalho D, Izquierdo E, Fazal-Salom J, Taylor KR, et al. Integrated molecular meta-analysis of 1,000 pediatric high-grade and diffuse intrinsic pontine glioma. Cancer Cell. 2017;32(4):520–537.e5.
52. Kasper LH, Baker SJ. Invited review: emerging functions of histone H3 mutations in paediatric diffuse high-grade gliomas. Neuropathol Appl Neurobiol. 2020;46(1):73–85.
53. Leske H, Dalgleish R, Lazar AJ, Reifenberger G, Cree IA. A common classification framework for histone sequence alterations in tumours: an expert consensus proposal. J Pathol. 2021;254(2):109–20.
54. Korshunov A, Capper D, Reuss D, Schrimpf D, Ryzhova M, Hovestadt V, et al. Histologically distinct neuroepithelial tumors with histone 3 G34 mutation are molecularly similar and comprise a single nosologic entity. Acta Neuropathol. 2016;131(1):137–46.
55. Andreiuolo F, Varlet P, Tauziède-Espariat A, Jünger ST, Dörner E, Dreschmann V, et al. Childhood supratentorial ependymomas with YAP1-MAMLD1 fusion: an entity with characteristic clinical, radiological, cytogenetic and histopathological features. Brain Pathol. 2019;29(2):205–16.
56. Pajtler KW, Witt H, Sill M, Jones DT, Hovestadt V, Kratochwil F, et al. Molecular classification of ependymal tumors across all CNS compartments, histopathological grades, and age groups. Cancer Cell. 2015;27(5):728–43.
57. Ghasemi DR, Sill M, Okonechnikov K, Korshunov A, Yip S, Schutz PW, et al. MYCN amplification drives an aggressive form of spinal ependymoma. Acta Neuropathol. 2019;138(6):1075–89.
58. Cannon DM, Mohindra P, Gondi V, Kruser TJ, Kozak KR. Choroid plexus tumor epidemiology and outcomes: implications for surgical and radiotherapeutic management. J Neuro-Oncol. 2015;121(1):151–7.
59. Jeibmann A, Hasselblatt M, Gerss J, Wrede B, Egensperger R, Beschorner R, et al. Prognostic implications of atypical histologic features in choroid plexus papilloma. J Neuropathol Exp Neurol. 2006;65(11):1069–73.

60. Siegfried A, Morin S, Munzer C, Delisle MB, Gambart M, Puget S, et al. A French retrospective study on clinical outcome in 102 choroid plexus tumors in children. J Neuro-Oncol. 2017;135(1):151–60.
61. Takami H, Fukuoka K, Fukushima S, Nakamura T, Mukasa A, Saito N, et al. Integrated clinical, histopathological, and molecular data analysis of 190 central nervous system germ cell tumors from the iGCT consortium. Neuro-Oncology. 2019;21(12):1565–77.
62. Takami H, Perry A, Graffeo CS, Giannini C, Narita Y, Nakazato Y, et al. Comparison on epidemiology, tumor location, histology, and prognosis of intracranial germ cell tumors between Mayo Clinic and Japanese consortium cohorts. J Neurosurg. 2020;31:1–11.
63. Liu APY, Li BK, Pfaff E, Gudenas B, Vasiljevic A, Orr BA, et al. Clinical and molecular heterogeneity of pineal parenchymal tumors: a consensus study. Acta Neuropathol. 2021;141(5):771–85.
64. Ahuja A, Sharma MC, Suri V, Sarkar C, Sharma BS, Garg A. Pineal anlage tumour—a rare entity with divergent histology. J Clin Neurosci. 2011;18(6):811–3.
65. Uppal DK, Madan R, Chatterjee D, Mohindra S, Bhatia V, Goyal S. Pineal anlage tumor: a case report and clinico-pathological review. Clin Neurol Neurosurg. 2021;206:106629. https://doi.org/10.1016/j.clineuro.2021.106629. Epub 2021 May 5
66. Chatterjee D, Lath K, Singla N, Kumar N, Radotra BD. Pathologic prognostic factors of pineal parenchymal tumor of intermediate differentiation. Appl Immunohistochem Mol Morphol. 2019;27(3):210–5.
67. Lu VM, Luther EM, Eichberg DG, Morell AA, Shah AH, Komotar RJ, et al. Prognosticating survival of pineal parenchymal tumors of intermediate differentiation (PPTID) by grade. J Neuro-Oncol. 2021;155(2):165–72.
68. de Kock L, Sabbaghian N, Druker H, Weber E, Hamel N, Miller S, et al. Germ-line and somatic DICER1 mutations in pineoblastoma. Acta Neuropathol. 2014;128(4):583–95.

# Pathological Aspects and Recent Advances in Pathology (Hematopathology)

14

Harpreet Virk and Pulkit Rastogi

## 14.1 Introduction

In the current era, the hemato-pathology laboratory deals with the various aspects of diagnostic and prognostic tests for benign and malignant blood disorders. With the advancement in the understanding of disease biology of hematological disorders, there have been refinements in the diagnostic criteria for known entities, the inclusion of newer entities, and the identification of disease biomarkers of diagnostic and prognostic relevance. The chapter details the pathological aspects of hematological neoplasms commonly encountered in pediatric radiation oncology practice, emphasizing the recent updates.

## 14.2 Classification of Hematological Neoplasms

The hematological neoplasms are broadly classified as per the World Health Organization (WHO) 2017 update according to the lineage: myeloid, lymphoid, or histiocytic/dendritic cells and further as per the cell of origin: precursor (leukemia) or mature neoplasms (lymphoma) [1]. Since there are more than a hundred entities spanning all the above categories, only the ones that are relevant to the pediatric radiation oncology practice have been discussed further (table 14.1).

H. Virk · P. Rastogi (✉)
Department of Hematology, Post Graduate Institute of Medical Education and Research, Chandigarh, India





R. Madan et al. (eds.), *Evidence Based Practice in Pediatric Radiation Oncology*, https://doi.org/10.1007/978-981-96-4872-6_14

**Table 14.1** The common hematological malignancies in the pediatric population

| | |
|---|---|
| Myeloproliferative neoplasms | (a) Chronic myeloid leukemia |
| Precursor neoplasm | (a) B-lymphoblastic leukemia/lymphoma<br>(b) T-lymphoblastic leukemia/lymphoma<br>(c) Acute myeloid leukemia |
| Mature B cell lymphoma | (a) Burkitt lymphoma<br>(b) Diffuse large B cell lymphoma<br>(c) Primary mediastinal (thymic) large B-cell lymphoma |
| Mature T- and NK-cell lymphoma | (a) Anaplastic large-cell lymphoma, ALK type<br>(b) Peripheral T-cell lymphoma, NOS<br>(c) Aggressive NK-cell leukemia<br>(d) Hepatosplenic T-cell lymphoma |
| Hodgkin lymphoma | (a) Classic Hodgkin lymphoma<br>(b) Nodular lymphocyte-predominant Hodgkin lymphoma |
| Histiocytic disorders | (a) Langerhans cell histiocytosis<br>(b) Primary hemophagocytic lymphohistiocytosis<br>(c) Rosai-Dorfman disease<br>(d) Juvenile xanthogranuloma |
| Others | (a) Systemic mastocytosis<br>(b) Myeloid proliferations associated with down syndrome<br>(c) Immunodeficiency-associated lymphoproliferative disorder |

## 14.3 Acute Lymphoblastic Leukemia

A better understanding of genetic and biological basis has revolutionized the molecular taxonomy of acute lymphoblastic leukemia (ALL). Historically ALL is divided into B-lineage and T-lineage, rarely NK-lymphoblastic leukemia.

### 14.3.1 B-Lineage Acute Lymphoblastic Leukemia

B-ALL is a malignancy of precursor lymphoid cells committed to the B-lineage. Morphologically, the blasts of B-ALL are small to medium in size, with a high N:C ratio, moderately clumped chromatin, inconspicuous nucleoli, and scanty agranular cytoplasm. The blasts are usually confined to bone marrow (BM) or peripheral blood (PB); however, if it involves only the nodal or extra-nodal sites (spleen, liver, testis, and central nervous system), the term B-Lymphoblastic lymphoma (B-LBL) is more appropriate. B-ALL is primarily a childhood disease, with more than 75% of cases occurring in children under 6 years of age. The estimated annual incidence worldwide is 1–4.75 cases per 100,000 population [2].

The risk factors implicated for B-ALL/LBL are Down syndrome and other constitutional genetic disorders, single nucleotide polymorphisms (SNP) in genes like *GATA3*, *IKZF1*, *CDKN2A/2B,* and *ARID5B*. In the work-up, the basic cytochemistry is important with myeloperoxidase (MPO) stain, which is usually negative. The blasts can show dot and block positivity with periodic acid Schiff stain (PAS) [3]. On multiparameter flow cytometry, the blasts show strong positivity with B-cell markers (CD19, cCD79a, and cCD22). They are also positive for CD10, surface CD22, CD24, PAX5, and TdT in most cases.

Cytogenetic abnormalities can be identified in most cases of B-ALL, and some of these represent specific entities (B-ALL with recurrent genetic abnormalities) having unique phenotypic and prognostic features. The recurrent genetic abnormalities include iAMP21, *BCR::ABL1* fusion, *KMT2A* rearrangements, *ETV6::RUNX1* fusion, *TCF3::PBX1* fusion or *IGH::IL3* fusion. More recently, Ph-like ALL, *DUX4*, *ZNF384*, *MEF2D*, and *NUTM1* rearrangements have been defined with relevant prognostic significance. Overall, B-ALL is considered a good prognosis in children compared to adults. The specific genetic abnormalities mentioned above have specific prognostic implications [4].

### 14.3.2 T-Lineage Acute Lymphoblastic Leukemia

T-lymphoblastic leukemia/lymphoma is a neoplasm of lymphoblasts committed to the T-cell lineage involving bone marrow and blood (T-acute lymphoblastic leukemia, T-ALL) or presenting with primary involvement of thymus, nodal or extranodal sites (T-lymphoblastic lymphoma, T-LBL) and accounts for about 15% of childhood ALL cases. It is more common in adolescents than in younger children and is more common in males than in females. Mediastinal (thymic) involvement is frequently seen in the form of a mediastinal mass, rest of the symptoms and signs overall with B-ALL. T-ALL usually present with high leukocyte counts, although morphologically, the blasts are indistinguishable from B-ALL lymphoblasts. The lymphoblasts in T-ALL are usually TdT-positive and variably express CD1a, CD2, CD3, CD4, CD5, CD7, and CD8. Early T-cell Precursor (ETP) leukemias have been recently recognized as a form of T-ALL with a poor prognosis. By definition, blasts in ETP ALL express CD7 but lack CD1a and CD8 and are positive for one or more of the myeloid/stem cell markers CD34, CD117, HLA-DR, CD13, CD33, CD11b, or CD65 [5].

## 14.4 Hodgkin Lymphoma

It is the clonal, malignant lymphoproliferation originating from germinal-center B-cells. The malignant cells usually represent only a small minority (0.1–2%) of the total cellular population of involved tissues, which predominantly includes the reactive background. WHO 2017 classifies Hodgkin lymphoma (HL) into two major sub-categories, the classic HL (CHL) which is the commoner and the nodular lymphocyte-predominant Hodgkin lymphoma (NLPHL) which is rarely encountered in children.

CHL constitutes 90% of all HLs. It is sub-classified as nodular-sclerosis CHL (NSCHL), mixed-cellularity CHL (MCCHL), lymphocyte-depleted HL, and lymphocyte-rich HL. Infiltration of the bone marrow at diagnosis is uncommon (3% NSHL, 10% MCCHL, LDHL 50–75%), usually focal, and almost always

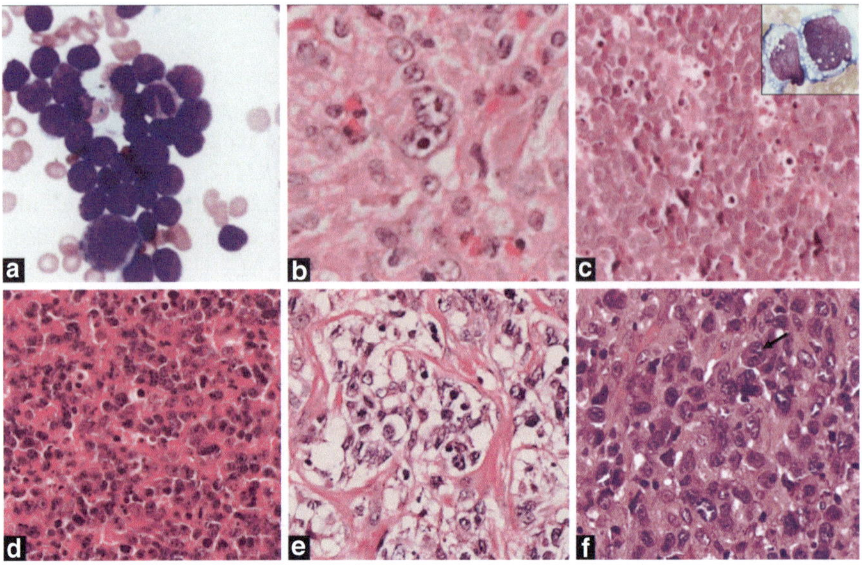


**Fig. 14.1** (**a**) The morphology of myeloblasts (black arrow showing myeloblast with fine granules and an Auer rod; May-Grünwald-Giemsa stain, 1000x). (**b**) Case of Hodgkin lymphoma showing Reed-Sternberg (RS) cell surrounded by eosinophils and histiocytes (hematoxylin and eosin stain, 1000x). (**c**) Case of Burkitt lymphoma showing intermediate-sized lymphoid cells with apoptotic debris around them (hematoxylin and eosin stain, 400x; inset shows bone marrow infiltrate of Burkitt lymphoma cells). (**d**) Histopathology of diffuse large B-cell lymphoma showing large-sized lymphoid cells, the centroblasts with 2–3 membrane bound nucleoli, and moderate cytoplasm (hematoxylin and eosin stain, 600x). (**e**) Case of primary mediastinal (thymic) large B-cell lymphoma showing large-sized lymphoid cells surrounded by fine fibrotic septe (hematoxylin and eosin stain, 600x). (**f**) Case of anaplastic large-cell lymphoma showing large pleomorphic cells (black arrow pointing to embryo shaped nucleus; hematoxylin and eosin stain, 600x)

associated with extensive disease, systemic symptoms, and unfavorable histology. Classical histopathology shows scattered Reed-Sternberg cells (RS cells) in a polymorphous reactive background composed of eosinophils, lymphocytes, macrophages, neutrophils, and fibroblasts (Fig. 14.1). These RS cells show positivity with CD30 and CD15 and weaker expression of B cell-associated antigens like PAX-5 on immunohistochemistry [6–7].

## 14.5 Burkitt Lymphoma

It is an aggressive B-cell lymphoma with a mature B-cell phenotype. Histologically, it is composed of monomorphic medium-sized transformed cells with a high degree of proliferation (Ki-67 index approaching 100%). These cells have round nuclei with finely clumped chromatin, multiple basophilic medium-sized centrally located nucleoli with deeply basophilic cytoplasm showing coarse vacuoles which stain with Oil red O stain (Fig. 14.1). Deregulation of the *c-MYC* gene is most often seen owing to t(8;14)(q24.1;q32). Three clinical variants have been described: endemic, sporadic, and immunodeficiency-associated, with variable associations with EBV infection. The abnormal cells show immunophenotype of germinal center B cells with CD10, CD19, CD20, CD22, CD79a, BCL-6, and PAX5 positivity but negativity for BCL-2. Monotypic bright surface IgM with light chain restriction is seen. Fluorescent in situ hybridization (FISH) analysis, using probes help to identify fusion of *IGH* with *MYC* due to a t(8, 14)(q24;q32) translocation.

## 14.6 Diffuse Large B-Cell Lymphoma

The DLBCL is a heterogeneous group of aggressive lymphomas of large, transformed B-cells. It is one of the most common B-cell lymphoid neoplasm in adults, although it can be frequently seen in the pediatric population with a male predominance. It can arise as a de novo malignancy or may transform from a low-grade lymphoma, such as small lymphocytic lymphoma or follicular lymphoma. The typical presentation is rapidly enlarging, symptomatic lymphoid masses with B symptoms. Both nodal and extra-nodal involvement (GIT, testis, bone, thyroid, salivary glands, skin, liver, breast, nasal cavity, paranasal sinuses, and CNS) are observed. Histologically, there is diffuse effacement of the nodal architecture by large-sized lymphoid cells (Fig. 14.1). Bone marrow involvement is seen in 11–27% of cases. The molecular subtypes include the Germinal center B-cells (GCB) and activated B-cells (ABC) subtypes with prognostic relevance. GCB subtype DLBCL harbors a gene expression profile similar to germinal center B-cells, while the ABC-DLBCLs are derived from B-cells that have traversed through the germinal center and are committed to plasmablastic differentiation. Patients with ABC-DLBCLs have reported less favorable responses to standard therapy than those with the GCB-DLBCL subtype [8–9].

## 14.7 Primary Mediastinal (Thymic) Large-Cell Lymphoma

Primary mediastinal (thymic) large B-cell lymphoma (PMBL) is a mature aggressive large B-cell lymphoma of putative thymic B-cell origin arising in the mediastinum, with distinctive clinical, immunophenotypic, genotypic, and molecular features. Usually seen in young children and adults, the majority of these patients present with a localized mediastinal mass in the thymic area. Histopathologically, the lesion shows a diffuse growth pattern, commonly associated with compartmentalizing alveolar fibrosis (Fig. 14.1) [10]. The neoplastic cells are usually medium-sized with a round to oval nuclei and express B-cell-lineage antigens such as CD19, CD20, CD22, and CD79 and may express CD30. Unlike most cases of DLBCL, approximately 70% of PMBL express CD23, MAL antigen, and programmed cell death ligands PDL1 and PDL2. The prognosis of this entity is relatively better than the DLBCL.

## 14.8 Anaplastic Large-Cell Lymphoma

Anaplastic large-cell lymphoma (ALCL) is considered an aggressive T-cell lymphoma. Two subtypes have been recognized for ALCL based on ALK positivity, of which ALK-positive ALCL are common in children with male predominance. Extra-nodal involvement is common in skin, soft tissue, bone, and lungs and has an overall favorable prognosis. Histologically, the tumor tends to grow cohesively with a propensity for invading lymph node sinuses. ALCL is characterized by the presence of large, atypical "hallmark cells" which have a pleomorphic, horseshoe, or wreath-shaped nucleus and abundant cytoplasm (Fig. 14.1). Multi-lobated nuclei may be present, and hallmark cells may resemble the RS-cells of classic Hodgkin lymphoma [11]. Immunophenotypic features include positivity for CD45, CD30 (membranous and paranuclear pattern), and T-cell markers (CD2, CD4) and negativity for B-cell markers. In addition, tumor cells show positivity for EMA. ALK immunohistochemistry is positive in 50–60% of ALCLs. ALK positivity can be combined nuclear and cytoplasmic, only cytoplasmic or membranous depending on the fusion partner with *the ALK* gene [12].

## 14.9 Role of Flow Cytometry in Hematological Malignancies

Multiparametric flow cytometry (FCM) is a state-of-the-art technology that assesses cells' antigenic profile of leukemia/lymphoma cells using fluorochrome labelled antibodies. Flow cytometry can be performed on peripheral blood and bone marrow as well as effusion fluids (pleural, pericardial, ascetic, etc.). The detailed antibody panels are used to determine the presence of B-cell, T-cell, or myeloid markers and to further delineate the stage of leukemia/lymphoma cell differentiation. This is important for diagnosis and allows diagnostic molecular and/or FISH algorithms to be rationally carried out to fulfil clinical needs according to modern standards [13]. In addition, flow cytometry can be used to identify the expression of targets for potential antibody-directed therapy and provide some additional prognostic information as indicated by the expression of certain markers [14]. Besides, the FCM has now become the preferred technique to assess response to therapy at different time points of the treatment phase. The measurable residual disease (MRD) analysis, which is particularly useful in acute leukemia, is usually done post-induction, post-consolidation, during maintenance, and after the end of therapy. Monitoring treatment response by MRD allows stratification of patients into various risk groups and thus a lower risk of treatment-related morbidity and mortality. MRD detection is also used for monitoring disease burden in the setting of stem cell transplantation and for early recognition of impending relapse [15].

## 14.10 Role of Molecular Techniques in Hematological Malignancies

Many molecular techniques are available that help in the analysis of complex genomic profiles of hematological malignancies, including mutations, translocations, karyotypic rearrangements, and post-translational modifications. Using polymerase chain reaction (PCR), karyotype analysis, fluorescence in situ hybridization (FISH), multiplex ligation probe amplification (MLPA), droplet-digital PCR (ddPCR), and next-generation sequencing (NGS), it is possible to design better risk stratification categories and determination of molecular MRD. These methods generally include extraction and isolation of nucleic acids and further separation into DNA, RNA, and proteins [16].

## 14.11 Challenges in Diagnosis of Hematological Malignancies in Resource-Constrained Settings

With the advances in disease understanding, the modalities of diagnostic tests and their further applications at various time points of disease management are increasing day by day. To meet this rising demand, pathology laboratories in the developing world face challenges in incorporating these advanced techniques into routine reporting practice. The limitations are inadequate finances, lack of trained personnel, and quality control issues for these tests. However, WHO has recently come up with the newer classification of hematopoietic neoplasms, where these limitations have been addressed [17]. A hierarchical approach has been adopted to classify a tumor with a certain set of criteria which are "essential" and some others being "desirable," usually requiring advanced techniques. This will help laboratories to give a diagnosis label to the entities as per their available expertise and will also urge them to incorporate newer techniques in their laboratories.

**Conflict(s) of Interests** All authors declare that they do not have any conflict(s) of interest(s) to declare.

## References

1. Arber DA, Orazi A, Hasserjian RP, et al. Introduction and overview of classification of myeloid neoplasm. Revised 4th ed, Lyon, International Agency for Research on Cancer. 2017; pp. 16–27.
2. Borowitz MJ, Chan JKC, Downing JR, et al. B-lymphoblastic leukaemia/lymphoma, not otherwise specified (NOS). Revised 4th ed, Lyon, International Agency for Research on Cancer. 2017; pp. 200–202.
3. Brown P, Inaba H, Annesley C, et al. Pediatric acute lymphoblastic leukemia, version 2.2020, NCCN Clinical Practice Guidelines in Oncology. J Natl Compr Cancer Netw. 2020;18(1):81–112.
4. Luca DC. Update on lymphoblastic leukemia/lymphoma. Clin Lab Med. 2021;41(3):405–16.

5. Chandra D, Singh MK, Gupta R, et al. Clinicopathological and immunophenotypic features of early T cell precursor acute lymphoblastic leukaemia: a flow cytometry score for the initial diagnosis. Int J Lab Hematol. 2021;43(6):1417–23.
6. Connors JM, Cozen W, Steidl C, et al. Hodgkin lymphoma. Nat Rev Dis Primers. 2020;6(1):61.
7. Brice P, de Kerviler E, Friedberg JW. Classical Hodgkin lymphoma. Lancet. 2021;398(10310):1518–27.
8. Li S, Young KH, Medeiros LJ. Diffuse large B-cell lymphoma. Pathology. 2018;50(1):74–87.
9. Chapuy B, Stewart C, Dunford AJ, et al. Molecular subtypes of diffuse large B cell lymphoma are associated with distinct pathogenic mechanisms and outcomes. Nat Med. 2018;24:679–90.
10. Ahmed Z, Afridi SS, Shahid Z, et al. Primary mediastinal B-cell lymphoma: a 2021 update on genetics, diagnosis, and novel therapeutics. Clin Lymphoma Myeloma Leuk. 2021;21(11):e865–75.
11. Leventaki V, Bhattacharyya S, Lim MS. Pathology and genetics of anaplastic large cell lymphoma. Semin Diagn Pathol. 2020;37(1):57–71.
12. Tsuyama N, Sakamoto K, Sakata S, et al. Anaplastic large cell lymphoma: pathology, genetics, and clinical aspects. J Clin Exp Hematop. 2017;57(3):120–42.
13. Cools J, Vandenberghe P. New flow cytometry in hematologic malignancies. Haematologica. 2009;94(12):1639–41.
14. DiGiuseppe JA, Wood BL. Applications of flow cytometric immunophenotyping in the diagnosis and posttreatment monitoring of B and T lymphoblastic leukemia/lymphoma. Cytometry B Clin Cytom. 2019;96(4):256–65.
15. Theunissen P, Mejstrikova E, Sedek L, van der Sluijs-Gelling AJ, et al. EuroFlow consortium. Standardized flow cytometry for highly sensitive MRD measurements in B-cell acute lymphoblastic leukemia. Blood. 2017;129(3):347–57.
16. Koutsi A, Vervesou EC. Diagnostic molecular techniques in haematology: recent advances. Ann Transl Med. 2018;6(12):242.
17. Alaggio R, Amador C, Anagnostopoulos I, et al. The 5th edition of the World Health Organization classification of haematolymphoid tumours: lymphoid neoplasms. Leukemia. 2022;36(7):1720–48.

# 15 Pathological Aspects and Recent Advances in Pathology-Renal and Suprarenal Tumors

Lavleen Singh

## 15.1 Renal Tumors in Children

Renal tumors form 7% of all pediatric tumors. These are the commonest abdominal tumors in pediatric age group. The most common being the Wilms tumor(WT), followed by congenital mesoblastic nephroma (CMN), clear cell sarcoma of the kidney (CCSK), malignant rhabdoid tumor (MRT), and variants of renal cell carcinoma (RCC) [1, 2].

## 15.2 Wilms Tumor

### 15.2.1 Epidemiology

The incidence is around 1 in 8000 children. The mean age at diagnosis is around 3 years. Its occurrence is rare in children younger than 3 months and older than 6 years [3].

### 15.2.2 Clinical Features

Most commonly presents as an abdominal mass, followed by hematuria, pain, hypertension, and traumatic rupture in some rare cases [4].

It can have both sporadic presentations and syndromic associations. The most commonly associated syndromes are WAGR (Wilms tumor, aniridia, genitourinary anomalies, and mental retardation) syndrome, which is associated with deletion of 11p13. Denys Drash syndrome (gonadal dysgenesis, nephropathy, and Wilms

L. Singh (✉)
Department of Pathology, AIIMS, New Delhi, India



R. Madan et al. (eds.), *Evidence Based Practice in Pediatric Radiation Oncology*,
https://doi.org/10.1007/978-981-96-4872-6_15

tumor) is associated with a point mutation in the WT1 gene. Beckwith Weidman syndrome (overgrowth syndrome) is also seen associated with 11p15.5 locus on the WT 2 gene, which contains gene for insulin growth factor II.

### 15.2.3 Morphology

#### 15.2.3.1 Gross

It classically presents as a unicentric circumscribed lobulated mass, distinctly demarcated from the rest of the renal parenchyma. On the cut section, it has a pale grey appearance with cystic change along with areas of hemorrhage and necrosis seen in some cases. Multicentricity is noted in around 7% of cases and warrants a thorough assessment and nephrectomy sample. Pathologists should always be on the lookout for any distinct-looking pale areas; these should be sampled to rule out foci of nephrogenic rests (NR) [5]. The NR are associated with an increased risk of recurrence in cases of partial nephrectomy and also the presence of contralateral tumors.

It is of utmost importance for the tumor not to be bivalved by the surgeon as it alters the tumor relation to the capsule due to its retraction and thus may alter the staging. It is also advised to take precautions to not strip the renal capsule or Gerota's fascia during surgical resection for the same reason. One section per centimeter of tumor is processed for adequate assessment of the heterologous tumor morphology. In cases of multicentric nodule, each nodule is processed extensively. Other important sections include a section from the periphery for capsular involvement, a section from Gerota's fascia, a section from renal sinus and any palpable sinus node, normal kidney, and renal vein for possible vascular involvement [6].

### 15.2.4 Microscopy

Wilms tumor has a triphasic appearance comprising blastemal, stromal, and epithelial components that can be seen up to variable degrees. Monophasic and biphasic lesions are also seen [7].

Anaplasia in Wilms tumor is the most important prognostic factor. It is defined by three criteria: (i) the presence of enlarged nuclei that is up to three times the size of adjacent normal nuclei, (ii) multipolar mitotic figures, and (iii) obvious hyperchromasia. Anaplasia shows a strong association with TP53 mutation and is therefore associated with an unfavorable prognosis [6].

Children Oncology Group (COG) classifies Wilms tumor as those with (i) focal anaplasia and (ii) diffuse anaplasia.

### 15.2.5 Immunohistochemistry

The immunohistochemistry (IHC) profile is dependent on the various components present. Nuclear WT1 expression is seen on 80% of epithelial and blastemal components. The epithelial component shows keratin and epithelial membrane antigen expression. Mesenchymal expression is dependent on the type of differentiation. Other IHC markers include PAX8 and CD56 [8].

### 15.2.6 Genetic Profile

The frequent genetic loci predisposing for Wilms tumor are WTI and WT2 located at 11p.13 and 11p.15, respectively. WT1 gene encodes for a zinc finger transcription factor involved in the early development of the urogenital system. Point mutation and deletion at these loci are seen in Denys Drash syndrome and WAGR syndrome, respectively. WTX inactivation is also seen in 6–30% of Wilms tumors. *TP53* mutation is a well-established poor prognostic marker due to its strong association with anaplasia [9].

### 15.2.7 Prognosis

The majority of Wilms tumor cases are managed according to established protocols, primarily those developed by the international society of Pediatric oncology(SIOP) and Childrens oncology group(COG). The COG guidelines advocate primary resection of tumors followed by therapy [10]. It is important to recognize a prognostic factor that is predictive of outcome with one treatment approach that may not necessarily have the same prognostic value with another treatment approach.

The COG studies determine prognosis based on stage, histology (anaplasia vs favorable histology), patient age, tumor weight, lung nodule response, and loss of heterozygosity (LOH) at chromosomes 1p and 16q to assign treatment groups [10]. Studies are underway to assess role of 11p15 methylation status to select patients' eligible for treatment without adjuvant chemotherapy in COG protocol.

In the SIOP system, tumor stage, histology, response to preoperative chemotherapy, and tumor volume are used for risk stratification. Molecular markers have not been used for treatment stratification to date in SIOP protocol [10].

## 15.3 Nephrogenic Rest (NR) and Nephroblastomatosis

Nephrogenic rests are persistent embryonal tissue that represents the precursor lesion of the Wilms tumor.

### 15.3.1 Morphology

Based on the topographic location of these, NR are divided into intralobar and perilobar categories. The perilobar NR are usually present at the periphery and show clear demarcation between the tumor and the normal renal parenchyma. The intralobar NR presents as a single or sparse epithelial element interspersed within the lobe. These nephrogenic rests can progress in three ways: (i) dormant NR (remains unchanged as a microscopic focus), (ii) sclerosing or obsolescent NR (undergo maturation, sclerosis, and eventual disappearance), and (iii) hyperplastic NR (non-clonal proliferation of cells that can either progress to form Wilms tumor or may undergo arrest and regression) [11].

### 15.3.2 Prognosis

The presence of these NRs indicate an increased risk for recurrence of Wilms tumor in the remanent renal parenchyma and tumor in contralateral kidney [12].

## 15.4 Cystic Partially Differentiated Nephroblastoma

Cystic partially differentiated nephroblastoma (CPDN) is a multilocular cystic neoplasm with thin non-expansile septae containing nephroblastomatous elements.

### 15.4.1 Epidemiology

The majority of the patients are less than 2 years of age with incidence higher in males than in females.

### 15.4.2 Clinical Features

It presents as an abdominal mass. On imaging, it presents as a large cystic mass (mean diameter of 10 cm) with thin septation and no solid areas.

### 15.4.3 Morphology

It is a well-circumscribed multi-locular cystic mass with thin non-expansile septae. At no occasion, solid expansile area must be seen as its presence indicates towards diagnosis of a cystic Wilms tumor.

On microscopy, the cysts are lined by flattened, cuboidal, and/or hobnail epithelium. The septa show admixture of different tissue like fibrous, muscular, cartilaginous, fatty, blastemal and epithelial component. In some cases, papillary infoldings may also be seen [13].

### 15.4.4 Prognosis

Surgical resection is always curative.

## 15.5 Pediatric Cystic Nephroma

Pediatric cystic nephroma is a multilocular cystic neoplasm with thin non-expansile septae containing fibrous tissue and differentiated tubules.

### 15.5.1 Epidemiology

The majority of the patients are less than 2 years of age with incidence higher in males than in females.

### 15.5.2 Clinical Features

They commonly present as an abdominal mass and uncommonly as ureteral obstruction caused by the mass.

### 15.5.3 Morphology

It is a well-circumscribed large cystic mass of variable size. The septa are thin with no solid areas seen.

Microscopy shows cysts lined by flattened, cuboidal, and hobnail epithelium. The septa are made of fibrous tissue with well-differentiated tubules and focal cellular condensations. No immature nephroblastic elements should be seen to make the diagnosis of cystic nephroma.

### 15.5.4 Molecular

They harbor DICER1 mutation and are a distinct category from adult cystic nephroma. Familial cystic nephroma is frequently bilateral and associated with pleuropulmonary blastoma. Cystic nephroma and pleuropulmonary blastoma have similar DICER1 loss of function and "hotspot" missense mutation rates, which involve specific amino acids in the RNase IIIb domain [14]. Cystic nephroma to

DICER1-anaplastic sarcoma of kidney progression is considered to be akin to type I to type II/III malignant progression of pleuropulmonary blastoma.

### 15.5.5 Prognosis

Surgical resection is curative.

## 15.6 Congenital Mesoblastic Nephroma (CMN)

Congenital mesoblastic nephroma (CMN) is an infantile monomorphic spindle cell tumor, associated with a good prognosis. It has two subtypes classical and cellular. The latter subtype is associated with a specific chromosomal translocation, t(12;15)(p13;q25), which results in a fusion of the ETV6 and NTRK3 [14].

### 15.6.1 Epidemiology

It constitutes 2–4% of all childhood renal tumors, with 90% of cases presenting in the 1st year of life [15].

### 15.6.2 Clinical Features

It presents as an abdominal mass.

### 15.6.3 Morphology

It is a unicentric tumor usually arising near the renal sinus. Depending on the tumor cellularity, it can have a whorled leiomyoma-like gross appearance to a more friable and variegated appearance in cellular lesions.

The histomorphology is divided into the classic type and cellular type. The classic CMN (24%) shows fibromatosis-like morphology with low cellular density and low to moderate mitosis. The cellular CMN (66%) shows densely packed spindle cells with high mitotic activity and pushing type borders along with areas of necrosis.

### 15.6.4 Genetic Profile

Cellular CMN has a recurrent chromosomal translocation, t(12;15)(p13;q25), which results in a fusion of the ETV6 and NTRK3 genes.

### 15.6.5 Prognosis

When completely excised, it shows an excellent prognosis. In rare cases, metastasis to the lung and brain may be seen [7].

## 15.7 Clear Cell Sarcoma of the Kidney

Clear cell sarcoma characteristically shows uniform round cells with clear cytoplasm and finely distributed chromatin separated by fine vascular septae. It is characterized molecularly by *BCOR* genetic alterations or *YWHAE::NUTM2 gene fusion.*

### 15.7.1 Epidemiology

It accounts for approximately 3% of pediatric malignant renal tumors. It is most commonly diagnosed by the 2nd or 3rd year of life and is a relatively slow-growing tumor. There is a clear male preponderance [16].

### 15.7.2 Morphology

It presents as a unicentric, unencapsulated, circumscribed tumor centered in the medulla. The cut surface appears variegated with a solid, glistening gelatinous appearance.

The classic microscopic pattern shows cells in cords and nests separated by thin-walled vascular septa. Tumor cells have clear cytoplasm with indistinct cell margins, round nucleus, granular chromatin, and inconspicuous nucleoli. Mitosis is usually low to moderate.

The immunoreactivity for cyclin D1 and BCOR aids in diagnosing CCSK. Additional positive markers include vimentin, SATB2, BCL2 and TLE1. CCSK with BCOR::CCNB3 fusion exhibits Cyclin B3 immunoepression.

### 15.7.3 Prognosis

Perirenal lymph node metastasis is seen in up to 30% cases at the time of diagnosis. However, survival outcome has improved to up to 70% due to newer chemotherapeutic protocols.

## 15.8 Rhabdoid Tumor of the Kidney (RTK)

Rhabdoid tumor of kidney is an aggressive pediatric renal tumor composed of cells with vesicular chromatin, prominent nucleoli, and hyaline intracytoplasmic inclusion.

### 15.8.1 Epidemiology

RTK accounts for approximately 2% of all the renal tumors. It is rarely seen in children more than 3 years age. Infants are commonly affected with a median age at diagnosis being 13 months [7].

### 15.8.2 Clinical Features

Patients usually present at advanced stage (stage III or IV) of disease. Approximately 15% children develop central nervous system counterpart of rhabdoid tumor, that is, AT/RT.

### 15.8.3 Morphology

Grossly they are solid tumors with indistinct tumor margin and are almost always seen associated with hemorrhage and necrosis. Tumor cells are large, round to polygonal with abundant eosinophilic to amphophilic cytoplasm and cytoplasmic inclusions. They have large vesicular nuclei with prominent nucleoli. Loss of INI1 protein on IHC is a sensitive and fairly specific marker of RTK.

### 15.8.4 Genetic Profile

These tumors show a strong association with the inactivation of the Hsnf1/INI1 gene on chromosome 22. RTK is known to be associated with AT/RT showing germline mutation in the SMARCB1 gene. This group of diseases is also termed "rhabdoid tumor predisposition syndrome type 1." When associated with SMARCA4/BRG1 gene, it is termed "rhabdoid tumor predisposition syndrome type 2." [17].

### 15.8.5 Prognosis

RTK has high morbidity due to its aggressive nature and early lymphovascular spread with >80% dying within 2 years of diagnosis.

## 15.9 Suprarenal Tumors in Children

The most common childhood adrenal tumor is neuroblastoma accounting to 8–10% of childhood cancers. Other rarer suprarenal tumors may include pheochromocytoma, adrenocortical carcinoma and extra lobar pulmonary sequestration in infants.

## 15.10 Neuroblastoma

It belongs to the group of tumors of ganglion cell origin arising from primordial neural crest cells. This group comprises of neuroblastoma, ganglioneuroblastoma, and ganglioneuroma. It is the third most common childhood neoplasm following leukemia and CNS tumors. It is the most common extracranial solid tumor during the first 2 years of life.

### 15.10.1 Epidemiology

Around 90% of cases are diagnosed before 5 years of age with male to female ratio of 1.2:1.

About 40% of peripheral neuroblastoma is seen located in adrenal glands [7].

### 15.10.2 Clinical Features

Patients most commonly present as abdominal mass leading to abdominal distention and respiratory distress in some cases due to its large size. Other presentations may be secondary to metastasis to distant organs. Some cases are also known to be associated with paraneoplastic syndromes like Horner's syndrome, WDHA syndrome, etc.

### 15.10.3 Morphology

They present as a solid, soft greyish tan mass, with or without necrosis and calcification. It can present as an encapsulated or invasive mass. The diagnosis of neuroblastoma should be made on incisional or core needle biopsy with proper risk stratification. The tumor is made of neuroblastic cells arranged in groups or nests separated by thin fibrovascular stromal septa. Three subtypes are recognized: (i) undifferentiated, (ii) poorly differentiated, and (iii) differentiated based on the relative percentage of neuroblasts, neuropil, Schwannian stroma, and ganglion cells.

Neuroblastoma shows positivity for neuronal markers, namely, synaptophysin, chromogranin, CD 56, NFP, and neuroblastoma marker NB-84. Neural crest markers tyrosine hydroxylase and PHOXB2 positivity is also seen along with MYCN protein expression.

### 15.10.4 Genetic Profile

#### 15.10.4.1 MYCN Amplification

MYCN is the most prognostically relevant genetic alteration in neuroblastoma. *MYCN* amplification is associated with poor patient prognosis and an important ancillary test for risk stratification [18].

#### 15.10.4.2 DNA Index

Hyperdiploid (near triploid) tumors have a better prognosis. The tumors in the near diploid/tetraploid range have poorer outcomes. Thus, DNA index determination by flowcytometry is an important investigation for risk stratification. [19].

#### 15.10.4.3 ALK Mutation and Amplification

ALK mutation and amplification are all associated with higher risk and worse prognosis. ALK immunohistochemistry does not always correlate with expression status. In treatment refractory cases, ALK gene sequencing may be performed to identify candidates who can benefit from tyrosine kinase inhibitor therapy. [20].

#### 15.10.4.4 ATRX

The ATRX gene mutation is found in 2–3% of all neuroblastic tumors, majority of which are high-stage tumors in older children and adolescents [21].

#### 15.10.4.5 Structural Chromosomal Alterations

Segmental chromosomal aberrations (especially 1p deletion, 11q deletion, and/or 17q gain) are associated with high-risk tumors, whereas alterations in the number of whole chromosomes are associated with lower-risk tumors [22].

#### 15.10.4.6 Prognosis

The COG gives guidelines for risk stratification in these tumors based on age, MYCN status, DNA ploidy, and histologic group into low, intermediate, and high-risk groups [23].

## References


1. Hewitt M, Weiner SL, Simone JV. Institute of Medicine (US) and National Research CouInstitute of Medicine (US) and National Research Council (US) National Cancer Policy Board. The Trajectory of Childhood Cancer Care
2. Nakata K, Colombet M, Stiller CA, Pritchard-Jones K, Steliarova-Foucher E. IICC-3 Contributors. Incidence of childhood renal tumours: an international population-based study. Int J Cancer. 2020;147(12):3313–27.
3. Breslow N, Olshan A, Beckwith JB, Green DM. Epidemiology of Wilms tumor. Med Pediatr Oncol. 1993;21(3):172–81.
4. Birch JM, Breslow N. Epidemiologic features of Wilms tumor. Hematol Oncol Clin North Am. 1995;9(6):1157–78.
5. Hoda RS, Hoda SA. Grossing, staging, and reporting—an integrated manual of modern surgical pathology. Adv Anatom Pathol. 2021;28(6):446.
6. College of American Pathologists. Protocol for the examination of specimens from patients with wilms and other pediatric renal tumors. Version: WilmsTumor 3.2.0.1CAP; 2016.
7. Urinary and male genital tumors. (2022). Lyon: International Agency for Research on Cancer.
8. Vasei M, Moch H, Mousavi A, Kajbafzadeh AM, Sauter G. Immunohistochemical profiling of Wilms tumor: a tissue microarray study. Appl Immunohistochem Mol Morphol. 2008;16(2):128–34.
9. Lahoti C, Thorner P, Malkin D, Yeger H. Immunohistochemical detection of p53 in Wilms tumors correlates with unfavorable outcome. Am J Pathol. 1996;148(5):1577–89.

10. Aldrink JH, Heaton TE, Dasgupta R, Lautz TB, Malek MM, Abdessalam SF, Weil BR, Rhee DS, Baertschiger R, Ehrlich PF. American Pediatric Surgical Association Cancer Committee. Update on Wilms tumor. J Pediatr Surg. 2019;54(3):390–7.
11. Beckwith JB. Children at increased risk for Wilms tumor: monitoring issues. J Pediatr. 1998;132(3):377–9.
12. Beckwith JB, Kiviat NB, Bonadio JF. Nephrogenic rests, nephroblastomatosis, and the pathogenesis of Wilms' tumor. Pediatr Pathol. 1990;10(1–2):1–36.
13. Doros LA, Rossi CT, Yang J, Field A, Williams GM, Messinger Y, Cajaiba MM, Perlman EJ, Schultz A, K, Cathro HP, Legallo RD. DICER1 mutations in childhood cystic nephroma and its relationship to DICER1-renal sarcoma. Mod Pathol. 2014;27(9):1267–80.
14. Vokuhl C, Nourkami-Tutdibi N, Furtwängler R, Gessler M, Graf N, Leuschner I. ETV6–NTRK3 in congenital mesoblastic nephroma: a report of the SIOP/GPOH nephroblastoma study. Pediatr Blood Cancer. 2018;65(4):e26925.
15. England RJ, Haider N, Vujanic GM, Kelsey A, Stiller CA, Pritchard-Jones K, Powis M. Mesoblastic nephroma: a report of the United Kingdom Children's Cancer and Leukaemia Group (CCLG). Pediatr Blood Cancer. 2011;56(5):744–8.
16. Argani P, Perlman EJ, Breslow NE, Browning NG, Green DM, D'Angio GJ, Beckwith JB. Clear cell sarcoma of the kidney: a review of 351 cases from the National Wilms Tumor Study Group Pathology Center. Am J Surg Pathol. 2000;24(1):4.
17. Sigauke E, Rakheja D, Maddox DL, Hladik CL, White CL, Timmons CF, Raisanen J. Absence of expression of SMARCB1/INI1 in malignant rhabdoid tumors of the central nervous system, kidneys and soft tissue: an immunohistochemical study with implications for diagnosis. Mod Pathol. 2006;19(5):717–25.
18. College of American Pathologists. Protocol for the Examination of resection specimens from patients with neuroblastoma. Version: Neuroblastoma Resection 4.0.0.00. CAP; 2019.
19. Look AT, Hayes FA, Shuster JJ, et al. Clinical relevance of tumor cell ploidy and N-myc gene amplification in childhood neuroblastoma: a Pediatric Oncology Group study. J Clin Oncol. 1991;9(4):581–91.
20. Pugh TJ, Morozova O, Attiyeh EF, et al. The genetic landscape of high-risk neuroblastoma. Nat Genet. 2013;45(3):279–84.
21. Cheung NK, Zhang J, Lu C, et al. Association of age at diagnosis and genetic mutations in patients with neuroblastoma. JAMA. 2012;307(10):1062–71.
22. Schleiermacher G, Mosseri V, London WB, et al. Segmental chromosomal alterations have prognostic impact in neuroblastoma: a report from the INRG project. Br J Cancer. 2012;107(8):1418–22.
23. Peuchmaur M, d'Amore ES, Joshi VV, et al. Revision of the International Neuroblastoma Pathology Classification: confirmation of favorable and unfavorable prognostic subsets in ganglioneuroblastoma, nodular. Cancer. 2003;98(10):2274–81.

# Cancer Genetics

# 16

Abhilash Dagar, Rampukar Bharat, and Supriya Mallick

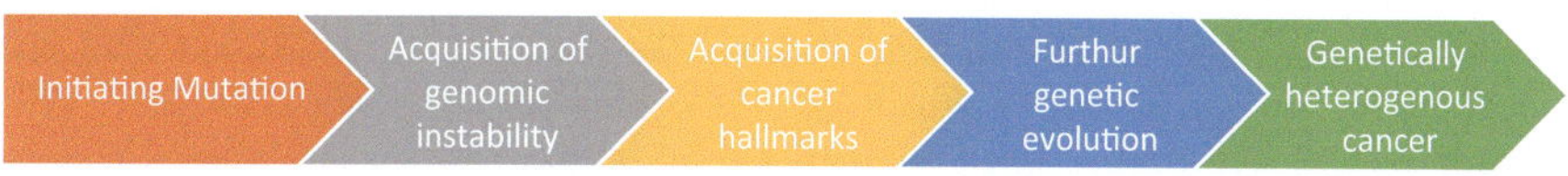
Initiating Mutation
Acquisition of genomic instability
Acquisition of cancer hallmarks
Furthur genetic evolution
Genetically heterogenous cancer

Stepwise acquisition of complementary mutations.

At the heart of carcinogenesis lies the non-lethal damage than normal cells acquire using environmental exposure, germline inheritance, or sporadic means.

A tumor is formed by the clonal expansion of a single precursor cell that has incurred genetic damage. Mutations are heritable and passed onto the next generation resulting in the growth of a colony of cells that have the same mutation.

There are four classes of normal regulatory genes that prevent such kind of transformation

1. Growth-promoting proto-oncogenes.
2. Growth inhibiting tumor-suppressing genes.
3. genes regulating programmed cell death (apoptosis),
4. Genes involved in DNA repair.

Carcinogenesis can be initiated by mutations in any four of these regulatory genes.

Carcinogenesis results from the accumulation of complementary mutations in a stepwise fashion. There are driver mutations that initiate carcinogenesis and passenger mutations that carry forward the tumor.

A. Dagar · R. Bharat
National Cancer Institute, AIIMS, New Delhi, India

S. Mallick (✉)
Department of Radiation Oncology, National Cancer Institute, Jhajjar, Haryana, India

2nd Campus AIIMS, New Delhi, Delhi, India



R. Madan et al. (eds.), *Evidence Based Practice in Pediatric Radiation Oncology*,
https://doi.org/10.1007/978-981-96-4872-6_16

Once the cells acquire these mutations tumors evolve genetically during their growth under the pressure of Darwinian selection (selection of fittest). Initially, the tumor cells are a clonal population, but by the time they become clinically relevant, they become extremely heterogeneous under the pressure of limited resources available for growth. So a single tumor population can harbor multiple subclones. Selection of fittest can also explain the changes in tumor behavior following therapy.

## 16.1 Genetic Syndromes in Brain Tumors

Nervous system tumors represent unique neoplasms that arise within the central and peripheral nervous system. While the vast majority of nervous system neoplasms occur sporadically, most have a hereditary equivalent. There has been a tremendous increase in knowledge of the primary genetic basis of many of the familial cancer syndromes that involve the nervous system, syndromes that are mostly inherited as autosomal dominant traits. Identifying genes associated with familial cancer syndromes have enabled a clinical assessment and allows cancer surveillance for those at risk.

### 16.1.1 Ataxia Telangiectasia

**Incidence**: 1 in 20,000 to 100,000 individuals [1].

**Inheritance**: Autosomal Dominant.

**Genetic pathways involved**: Mutation in the ataxia telangiectasia mutated (ATM) gene located on chromosome 11q22. Gene product is a protein kinase involved in the repair of double DNA breaks. Mutation results in the defective repair of DNA damage resulting in apoptosis and oxidative stress for the cell resulting in malignant transformation [2, 3].

**Clinical Features**: Progressive cerebellar atrophy (ataxia, dysarthria, dysmetria) immunodeficiency, telangiectasias, radiosensitivity, risk of malignancies [4].

**Associated Brain Tumors**: Meningiomas, glioblastomas, pilocytic astrocytomas, and medulloblastomas [5].

**Other Associated Malignancies**: Leukemia, lymphoma, breast, and gastric carcinoma [5].

### 16.1.2 Cowden Syndrome

**Incidence**: 1 in 2,50,000.

**Inheritance**: Autosomal Dominant.

**Genetic Pathways Involved**: Mutation of the PTEN suppressor oncogene, seen at locus 10q23. The PTEN protein product is a negative regulator in the PI3K-AKT and mTOR signaling pathways involved in cell proliferation, cell cycle progression, and apoptosis. Gene mutations result in oncogenesis and malignancies [6].

**Clinical Features**: mucocutaneous papillomatous lesions, multiple hamartomas, and higher risk for follicular thyroid, breast, and endometrial cancers [7].

**CNS Features**: Macrocephaly, Lhermitte-Duclos disease, gliosarcoma [8].

### 16.1.3 Turcot Syndrome

Turcot syndrome is a historical term used to describe the association of primary CNS tumors and two different forms of colorectal polyps: Familial adenomatosis polyposis (FAP) and hereditary non-polyposis-related colorectal cancer (HNPCC) (or Lynch syndrome). CNS malignancies usually manifest at an earlier age, with medulloblastomas typically diagnosed before 10 years of age in FAP and gliomas before 30 years of age in HNPCC [9].

### 16.1.4 FAP (Turcot Syndrome Type 2)

**Inheritance:** Autosomal Dominant.

**Genetic Pathways Involved:** Germline mutations in the APC gene at locus 5q21 are seen in FAP. APC is a large protein complex in the wingless-type (WNT) signaling pathway controlling cell proliferation and differentiation. A defect in APC can cause intranuclear accumulation of b-catenin and is involved in the pathogenesis of medulloblastoma. CNS tumors seen in patients with FAP, especially WNT-subtype medulloblastoma, have been linked to APC gene segment 2 mutations [10].

**Brain Tumors Associated:** FAP has a high association with medulloblastoma and less commonly with astrocytoma and ependymomas [11].

**Other Tumors:** Multiple adenomatous polyposes.

### 16.1.5 HNPCC (Turcot Syndrome Type 1)

**Inheritance:** Autosomal Dominant.

**Genetic Pathways Involved:** Germline mutations in DNA mismatch repair genes (MLH1, MSH2, MSH6, PMS2) in HNPCC. DNA mismatch repair maintains genomic integrity by correcting mismatches during DNA replication, and defective genes can cause microsatellite instability characteristic of HNPCC-associated tumors [10].

**Brain Tumors Associated:** Individuals with HNPCC have a higher risk of developing gliomas, particularly glioblastoma multiforme (GBM).

**Other Tumors:** Colorectal Carcinoma.

### 16.1.6 Gorlin Syndrome

**Incidence:** 1 in 57,000 to 164,000 [12].

**Inheritance:** Autosomal Dominant [13].

**Genetic Pathways Involved:** Germline mutations in the human homolog PTCH of the Drosophila gene patched, at locus 9q22.3- q31. This gene encodes a transmembrane glycoprotein that is a binding site for sonic hedgehog ligand (SHH) (gene, SHH), forming a complex that inhibits another transmembrane protein, smoothened (gene, SMO), which is involved in a pathway involved in cellular proliferation. Mutations lead to unregulated growth promotion and subsequent neoplasm development. Loss-of-function mutation in the suppressor of fused homolog gene SUFU at locus 10q24 has also been observed in patients with Gorlin Syndrome [14, 15].

**Brain Tumor Associated:** Medulloblastoma, mostly the desmoplastic subtype (SHH subtype) up to 20 times higher risk of getting Medulloblastoma. Other CNS tumors such as meningioma, oligodendroglioma, and craniopharyngioma have been identified less commonly in GS [16].

**Other Features:** Other intracranial findings include dural and/or falcine calcifications, bridging of the sella, eye anomalies, macrocephaly, and congenital facial malformations such as cleft lip/palate, frontal bossing coarse facies, and moderate or severe hypertelorism. The most common non-CNS tumors include multiple basal cell carcinomas, odontogenic keratocyst cardiac fibroma, and ovarian fibroma [17].

### 16.1.7 Li-Fraumeni Syndrome

**Incidence:** 1 in 5000 individuals [18].

**Inheritance:** Autosomal dominant [18].

**Genetic Pathways Involved:** Loss-of-function germline mutation in the p53 gene located at locus 17p13 and encodes the tumor suppressor gene TP53, which can promote cell cycle arrest, DNA damage repair, and apoptosis.

**Brain Tumors Associated:** Gliomas, primitive neuroectodermal tumors, medulloblastomas, and choroid plexus carcinomas are commonly identified in LFS and manifest at an earlier age (average, 25 years) [19].

**Other Features:** Adrenocortical carcinoma, bone and/or soft-tissue sarcomas, and breast cancer are other common extracranial tumor manifestations.

### 16.1.8 Multiple Endocrine Neoplasia Syndrome Type 1(MEN 1)

**Incidence:2 in 1,00,000** [20].

**Inheritance: Autosomal Dominant.**

**Genetic Pathways Involved:** Germline-inactivating mutation in the tumor suppressor MEN1 gene, present on the long arm of chromosome 11 and encoding the protein menin [21].

**Brain Tumors Associated:** The most common type of pituitary adenoma in MEN1 is a prolactin-producing adenoma, and those adenomas in MEN1 patients are more likely to be macroadenomas and be more resistant to treatment than their non-MEN1 counterparts. Approximately 15%–20% of patients with MEN1 have been found to have clinically apparent pituitary adenomas when evaluated at imaging [22].

**Other Associated Tumors**: Tumors of the pancreas, and parathyroid glands, tumors of the duodenum (including carcinoid tumors, gastrinomas, and others), and adrenal gland.

### 16.1.9 Neurofibromatosis Type 1 (NF 1)

**Incidence:** 1 in 2500–3000 people worldwide [23].

**Inheritance: Autosomal Dominant.**

**Genetic Pathways Involved:** Mutation in the NF1 tumor suppressor gene, located at locus 17q11.2 and encoding the cytoplasmic protein neurofibromin type 1. This protein is a negative regulator of the Ras proto-oncogene [23, 24].

**Associated Brain Tumors:** NF1 confers at least a fivefold increased risk for developing gliomas, including glioblastomas. Glioblastomas usually occur in young adults, in whom the overall prognosis is poor. About 15%–20% of individuals with NF1 will develop low-grade (WHO grade I) glial neoplasms, 80% in the optic pathway and about 15% in the brainstem. As with optic nerve gliomas, brainstem gliomas are usually pilocytic astrocytomas but manifest at a later age [23, 25].

**Other Tumors:** Neurofibromas are benign tumors composed of Schwann cells as well as a mix of nonneoplastic fibroblasts, mast cells, macrophages, endothelial cells, pericytes, and perineural cells. There are four subtypes of neurofibroma: cutaneous, subcutaneous, nodular or diffuse plexiform, and spinal [26].

### 16.1.10 Neurofibromatosis Type 2 (NF 2)

**Incidence:** 1 in 25,000 individuals.

**Inheritance:** Autosomal Dominant.

**Genetic Pathways Involved:** Abnormalities on chromosome 22, namely the NF2 gene (locus 22q12), which normally produces merlin, also known as schwannoma, a cell membrane-related protein that acts as a tumor suppressor gene. Abnormalities include inframe deletions or frameshift, nonsense, or missense mutations and are identified in approximately 93% of the families affected with NF2 [27].

**Associated Brain Tumors:** Bilateral vestibular schwannomas occur in approximately 90%–95% of NF2 patients, often occurring by 30 years of age most of which are benign and can cause internal auditory canal widening if large. Approximately 45–77% of NF2 patients develop meningiomas, and multiple meningiomas are often present. Most of them are intracranial but spinal have also been reported and are more likely to be atypical and anaplastic variant. Brainstem and spinal intramedullary ependymomas can also be seen in NF2 patients but the incidence is low around 6% [28].

### 16.1.11 Tuberous Sclerosis (TSC)

**Incidence:** 1 in 6000 to 10,000 live births [29, 30].

**Inheritance: Autosomal Dominant.**

**Genetic Pathways Involved:** Mutations in either the TSC1 gene (locus 9q34) or the TSC2 gene (locus 16p13.3). TSC1 and TSC2 encode the heterodimerizing tumor suppressor proteins hamartin and tuberin, respectively. The heterodimerization of hamartin with tuberin plays a role in the inhibition of the mTOR pathway. The mTOR pathway is important in regulating protein translation, cell cycle progression, and response to hypoxia [31].

**Associated Brain Tumors:** The characteristic brain tumor in TSC is subependymal giant cell astrocytoma (SEGA), a low-grade slow-growing tumor arising in the periventricular area and comprising glioneuronal lineage mixed cells that can be found in approximately 5–20% patients. Tubers (cortical or subcortical) and subependymal nodules are regarded as hamartomas. They are present in approximately 90% of children with TSC [32].

**Other Features:** Pleomorphic features involving many organ systems, including benign hamartomas of the brain, eyes, heart, lung, liver, kidney, and skin, characterize TSC.

### 16.1.12 Von-Hippel Lindau (VHL)

**Incidence: 1 in 36,000 individuals** [32].

**Inheritance: Autosomal Dominant.**

**Genetic pathways involved:** The gene for VHL, pVHL is located on chromosome 3p25 and encodes the tumor suppressor protein pVHL. Hypoxia-inducible factor 1 a (HIF1a) and hypoxia-inducible factor 2 a (HIF2a) are two of the major proteins regulated by pVHL, and pVHL is thus involved in a critical pathway for the adaptation of cells to hypoxia by downregulating hypoxia-inducible transcription factors. In VHL, loss of the sole functioning pVHL allele causes a condition analogous to hypoxia [33].

**Associated Brain Tumors:** Patients with VHL are prone to developing hemangioblastomas at a younger age. Hemangioblastomas are WHO grade I tumors, well-circumscribed, capillary vessel-rich benign neoplasms causing symptoms through pressure on adjacent structures and hemorrhage. Hemangioblastomas occur in about 60%–80% of VHL patients and may be multiple, scattered across the brain and spinal cord. The cerebellum is the most common site (44%–72%) followed by the spinal cord, brainstem, and, less commonly, supratentorial structures. Endolymphatic sac tumors of the middle ear are large highly vascular masses in the temporal bone located posterior to the internal auditory canal, near the vestibular aqueduct. Incidence is around 14% in patients with VHL and presents at a younger age and more frequently B/L. [34, 35]

**Other Features:** Renal angiomas, clear cell renal cell carcinomas (RCCs), pheochromocytomas, endolymphatic sac tumors of the temporal bone, serous cystadenomas and neuroendocrine tumors of the pancreas, and papillary cystadenomas of the epididymis and broad ligament.

## 16.2 Less Common Syndromes

### 16.2.1 Carney Complex

**Inheritance:** Autosomal dominant.

**Genetic Pathways Involved:** Mutations in the tumor suppressor gene PRKAR1 at locus 17q24, a mediator in cyclic adenosine monophosphate (cAMP) signaling pathways.

**Associated Brain Tumors**: It is characterized by psammomatous melanotic schwannoma (PMS) in 10% of patients, a rare nerve sheath tumor that can involve the CNS and is characterized by high melanin pigmentation and psammoma bodies at histologic examination. PMS can have an aggressive nature with distant metastatic disease.

### 16.2.2 Rubinstein Tayabi Syndrome (RTS)

**Inheritance**: Autosomal dominant disorder.

**Incidence:** one in 100,000 to 125,000 individuals.

**Genetic Pathways Involved**: mutations in the CREBBP gene encoding CREB-binding protein, which is involved in the regulation of SHH and cell division implicated in carcinogenesis.

**Associated Brain Tumors**: RTS is characterized by an increased incidence of medulloblastomas, meningiomas, and oligodendrogliomas.

### 16.2.3 Melanoma-Astrocytoma Syndrome

Melanoma-astrocytoma syndrome is an uncommon entity that was first described in 1993 and subsequently linked to mutations in CDKN2A and CDKN2B at locus 9p21. This syndrome is characterized by the presence of cutaneous malignant melanoma and CNS tumors including astrocytoma, neurofibroma, schwannoma, and meningioma.

| Genetic syndrome | Chromosome/ Gene involved | Protein product | Major pathways involved | CNS tumors | Other tumors |
|---|---|---|---|---|---|
| Ataxia telangiectasia | 11q22/ATM | Ataxia telangiectasia mutated | DNA repair, CHK2, p53 | Meningioma, glioblastoma, pilocytic astrocytoma, Medulloblastoma | Leukemia lymphoma, breast, and gastric cancers |
| Cowden syndrome | 10q23/PTEN | Phosphatase and tensin homologous protein | PI3K/ mTOR | Dysplastic cerebellar gangliocytoma, glial tumors | Follicular thyroid, breast, endometrial carcinoma |

(continued)

| Genetic syndrome | Chromosome/ Gene involved | Protein product | Major pathways involved | CNS tumors | Other tumors |
|---|---|---|---|---|---|
| FAP | 5q21/APC | Adenomatous polyposis coli, β-catenin | WNT | Medulloblastoma, astrocytoma, ependymoma | Colorectal carcinoma |
| HNPCC | MLH1<br>PMS2<br>MSH2<br>MSH6 | MutLα (MLH1 and PMS2 dimer)<br>MutSα (MSH2 and MSH6 complex) | DNA repair | Glioblastoma and other glial tumors | Colorectal carcinoma |
| Gorlin syndrome | 9q/PTCH<br>10q24/SUFU | Transmembrane glycoprotein | SHH | Desmoplastic medulloblastoma, meningioma, oligodendroglioma, craniopharyngioma | Basal cell carcinoma, odontogenic keratocyst, cardiac/ ovarian fibromas |
| Li-Fraumeni syndrome | 17p13/TP53 | p53 | Cell cycle, apoptosis | Astrocytoma, choroid plexus carcinoma, medulloblastoma, PNET | Breast cancer, adrenocortical carcinoma, bone/ soft-tissue sarcoma |
| Multiple endocrine neoplasia (MEN1) | 11q13/MEN1 | Menin | Cell cycle | Pituitary micro and macroadenoma | Parathyroid adenoma, pancreatic and duodenal neuroendocrine tumors |
| Neurofibromatosis type 1 | 17q11/NF1 | Neurofibromin | Ras | Optic/chiasmatic gliomas, plexiform neurofibromas, Pilocytic astrocytoma, glioblastomas | Leukemia, pheochromocytoma, rhabdomyosarcoma |
| Neurofibromatosis type 2 | 22q12/NF2 | Merlin | Cell cycle | Vestibular schwannoma, meningioma, Ependymoma | None |
| Von-Hippel Lindau syndrome (VHL) | 3p25/VHL | pVHL | Hypoxia HIF1a, HIF2a | Hemangioblastoma, endolymphatic sac tumors | Clear cell RCC, renal angiomas, pancreatic cystadenoma, Pheochromocytoma |
| Tuberous sclerosis | 9q34/TSC1<br>16q13/TSC2 | Hamartin<br>Tuberin | mTOR | Subependymal giant cell astrocytoma | Cardiac Rhabdomyoma, Renal Angiomyolipoma |

## References


1. Swift M, Reitnauer PJ, Morrell D, Chase CL. Breast and other cancers in families with ataxia-telangiectasia. N Engl J Med. 1987;316(21):1289–94.
2. Nissenkorn A, Ben-Zeev B. Ataxia telangiectasia. Handb Clin Neurol. 2015;132:199–214.
3. Savitsky K, Bar-Shira A, Gilad S, et al. A single ataxia telangiectasia gene with a product similar to PI-3 kinase. Science. 1995;268(5218):1749–53.
4. Wallis LI, Griffiths PD, Ritchie SJ, Romanowski CA, Darwent G, Wilkinson ID. Proton spectroscopy and imaging at 3T in ataxia-telangiectasia. AJNR Am J Neuroradiol. 2007;28(1):79–83.
5. Habeckbek M, Brinar VV, Rados M, Zadro I, Zarković K. Brain MRI abnormalities in ataxia-telangiectasia. Neurologist. 2008;14(3):192–5.
6. Zhou XP, Marsh DJ, Morrison CD, et al. Germline inactivation of PTEN and dysregulation of the phosphoinositol3-kinase/Akt pathway cause human Lhermitte-Duclos disease in adults. Am J Hum Genet. 2003;73(5):1191–8.
7. Huang S, Zhang G, Zhang J. Similar MR imaging characteristics but different pathological changes: a misdiagnosis for Lhermitte-Duclos disease and review of the literature. Int J Clin Exp Pathol. 2015;8(6):7583–7.
8. Treister D, Kingston S, Hoque KE, Law M, Shiroishi MS. Multimodal magnetic resonance imaging evaluation of primary brain tumors. Semin Oncol. 2014;41(4):478–95.
9. Therkildsen C, Ladelund S, Rambech E, Persson A, Petersen A, Gilbert M. Glioblastomas, astrocytomas and oligodendrogliomas linked to Lynch syndrome. Eur J Neurol. 2015;22(4):717–24.
10. Deming DA, Lystra AA, Nettekoven L, et al. PIK3CA and APC mutations are synergistic in the development of intestinal cancers. Oncogene. 2014;33(17):2245–54.
11. Attard TM, Giglio P, Koppula S, Snyder C, Lynch HT. Brain tumors in individuals with familial adenomatous polyposis: a cancer registry experience and pooled case report analysis. Cancer. 2007;109(4):761–6.
12. Hahn H, Wicking C, Zaphiropoulous PG, et al. Mutations of the human homolog of Drosophila patched in the nevoid basal cell carcinoma syndrome. Cell. 1996;85(6):841–51.
13. Lo Muzio L, Nocini PF, Savoia A, et al. Nevoid basal cell carcinoma syndrome: clinical findings in 37 Italian affected individuals. Clin Genet. 1999;55(1):34 40.
14. Nikolaou V, Stratigos AJ, Tsao H. Hereditary nonmelanoma skin cancer. Semin Cutan Med Surg. 2012;31(4):204–10.
15. Smith MJ, Beetz C, Williams SG, et al. Germline mutations in SUFU cause Gorlin syndrome-associated childhood medulloblastoma and redefine the risk associated with PTCH1 mutations. J Clin Oncol. 2014;32(36):4155–61.
16. Thalakoti S, Geller T. Basal cell nevus syndrome or Gorlin syndrome. Handb Clin Neurol. 2015;132:119–28.
17. Sartip K, Kaplan A, Obeid G, Kadom N. Neuroimaging of nevoid basal cell carcinoma syndrome (NBCCS) in children. Pediatr Radiol. 2013;43(5):620–7.
18. Lalloo F, Varley J, Ellis D, et al. Prediction of pathogenic mutations in patients with early-onset breast cancer by family history. Lancet. 2003;361(9363):1101–2.
19. Ranger AM, Patel YK, Chaudhary N, Anantha RV. Familial syndromes associated with intracranial tumors: a review. Childs Nerv Syst. 2014;30(1):47–64.
20. Brandi ML, Gagel RF, Angeli A, et al. Guidelines for diagnosis and therapy of MEN type 1 and type 2. J Clin Endocrinol Metab. 2001;86(12):5658–71.
21. Chandrasekharappa SC, Guru SC, Manickam P, et al. Positional cloning of the gene for multiple endocrine neoplasia type 1. Science. 1997;276(5311):404–7.
22. Burgess JR, Shepherd JJ, Parameswaran V, Hoffman L, Greenaway TM. The spectrum of pituitary disease in multiple endocrine neoplasia type 1 (MEN 1): clinical, biochemical, and radiological features of the pituitary disease in a large MEN 1 kindred. J Clin Endocrinol Metab. 1996;81(7):2642–6.
23. Hirbe AC, Gutmann DH. Neurofibromatosis type 1: a multidisciplinary approach to care. Lancet Neurol. 2014;13(8):834–43.

24. Huson SM, Harper PS, Compston DA. Von Recklinghausen neurofibromatosis: a clinical and population study in south-east Wales. Brain. 1988;
25. Gutmann DH, Parada LF, Silva AJ, Ratner N. Neurofibromatosis type 1: modeling CNS dysfunction. J Neurosci. 2012;32(41):14087–93.
26. Nguyen R, Kluwe L, Fuensterer C, Kentsch M, Friedrich RE, Mautner VF. Plexiform neurofibromas in children with neurofibromatosis type 1: frequency and associated clinical deficits. J Pediatr. 2011;159(4):652–655.e2.
27. Trofatter JA, MacCollin MM, Rutter JL, et al. A novel moesin-, ezrin-, radixin-like gene is a candidate for the neurofibromatosis 2 tumor suppressor. Cell. 1993;72(5):791–800.
28. Mautner VF, Lindenau M, Baser ME, et al. The neuroimaging and clinical spectrum of neurofibromatosis 2. Neurosurgery 1996;38(5):880–885; discussion 885–886.
29. Curatolo P, Bombardieri R, Jozwiak S. Tuberous sclerosis. Lancet. 2008;372(9639):657–68.
30. Kwiatkowski DJ, Manning BD. Molecular basis of giant cells in tuberous sclerosis complex. N Engl J Med. 2014;371(8):778–80.
31. Goh S, Butler W, Thiele EA. Subependymal giant cell tumors in tuberous sclerosis complex. Neurology. 2004;63(8):1457–61.
32. Lonser RR, Glenn GM, Walther M, et al. von Hippel-Lindau disease. Lancet. 2003;361(9374):2059–67.
33. Latif F, Tory K, Gnarra J, et al. Identification of the von Hippel-Lindau disease tumor suppressor gene. Science. 1993;260(5112):1317–20.
34. Bausch B, Wellner U, Peyre M, et al. Characterization of endolymphatic sac tumors and von Hippel-Lindau disease in the International Endolymphatic Sac Tumor Registry. Head Neck. 2016;38(suppl 1):E673–9.
35. Slater A, Moore NR, Huson SM. The natural history of cerebellar hemangioblastomas in von Hippel-Lindau disease. AJNR Am J Neuroradiol. 2003;24(8):1570–4.

# Particle Therapy in Paediatric Oncology 17

Rakesh Kapoor, Devangana Bora, and Divya Khosla

## 17.1 Introduction

Ionising radiation is classified into electromagnetic radiation (X rays and gamma rays) or particular radiation (electrons, protons, α-particles, neutrons, deuterons and heavy charged particles).

As of now, the most commonly used energy for radiotherapy (RT) is photon or x-ray based. Robert Wilson first proposed the use of heavy particles in radiotherapy in 1940s.Various charged particles currently used in radiation oncology are:

(i) Neutrons
(ii) Proton heavy particles
(iii) Carbon and neon ions
(iv) Mesons
(v) Neon ions

Amongst charged particles, neutrons were the first to enter in widespread clinical trials. Despite initial promise, neutrons have not been able to show widespread applicability except in the treatment of some radio-resistant tumours such a salivary gland malignancies, bone and soft tissue sarcoma and non-hormone responsive prostatic cancer. The therapeutic prospects of protons were initially reported in 1946 by Wilson [1], and the first patient was treated with protons in 1954 at the University of California [2]. In this chapter, we will mainly focus on protons and their implications in paediatric oncology.

R. Kapoor (✉) · D. Bora · D. Khosla
Department of Radiotherapy and Oncology, PGIMER, Chandigarh, India


R. Madan et al. (eds.), *Evidence Based Practice in Pediatric Radiation Oncology*, https://doi.org/10.1007/978-981-96-4872-6_17

## 17.2 Principles of Particle Therapy

Due to their size, charged particles have differing depth dosage characteristics from photons. When their velocity slows down in the final millimetres of their journey, they deposit the majority of their energy, creating the abrupt and localised peak of dose deposition known as the Bragg peak. Hence, the tissues proximal and distal to the Bragg peak receive minimal radiation dose. The energy of the proton beam affects how deep the Bragg peak forms. The dosage that will be deposited in the tissues depends on the beam's intensity. One can give pre-specified dosages with more accuracy and conformity by altering the energy of the charged particles and the intensity of the beam.

To get the optimal target coverage, multiple Bragg peaks of different energies and intensities are combined, which forms the Spread-Out Bragg Peaks (SOBP). Unlike protons, carbon ions deposit the energy distally due to nuclear fragmentation [3]. Additionally, carbon ions have sharper lateral dose penumbra at larger depths as compared to photon or protons. The ratio of the dose needed to create a particular biological effect with $Co^{60}$ photons to the dose needed to produce the same biologic effect with charged particles is known as the relative biologic effectiveness (RBE). Table 17.1 shows the comparison between proton, photon and carbon-based radiotherapy [4].

## 17.3 Radiotherapy in Paediatric Oncology

Given that practically all therapies have late effects that are sometimes severe and lasting, decision-making in the field of paediatrics is excruciatingly difficult. Around 1050 children are anticipated to die of cancer in the United States in 2022, when there will likely be 10,470 new cases of cancer diagnosed in children between the ages of 1 and 14 [11]. As the survival in childhood cancer patients is increasing, a greater number of childhood cancer survivors translate to a greater number of adults living with long term treatment toxicities, many of which are attributed to RT. Children are more prone to the radiation toxicities and radiation-induced secondary neoplasms (RISM) as their organs are still in the developmental phase [12].

**Table 17.1** Comparison between proton, photon and carbon-based radiotherapy

| | Carbon ions | Protons | Photons |
|---|---|---|---|
| Year of first treatment | 1994[a] | 1954 | Late 1800 & early 1900s[b] |
| Number of sites treating as of June 2019 | 12[c] | 83[d] | Routine |
| Bragg-Peak | Present | Present | Absent |
| Estimated RBE[a] | 2.5–5 | 1.1 | Low |
| Relative LET | Highest | High | Low |
| Relative risk of second malignancy[e,f] | Low | Low | High |

[a]Mohamad et al. [5], [b]Gianfaldoni et al. [6], [c]Lazar et al. [7], [d]Particle Therapy Co-operative Group [8], [e]Eley et al. [9], [f]Mohamad et al. [10]

In one study, it was seen that radiation exposure to breast in lymphoma patients increases the risk of breast cancer particularly when breast tissue was exposed to radiation at a younger age [13].

The Childhood Cancer Survivor Study (CCSS) reported that the mortality rate due to primary disease in children is declining while morbidity and mortality due to secondary cancers and long-term treatment toxicities is on the rises [14]. Thus, it is important to employ effective ways of delivering radiation while minimising toxicities and late effects.

## 17.4 Proton Therapy for the Paediatric Population

While considering the proton beam radiotherapy for clinical application, it has to be agreed upon that the paediatric population as compared to adults will reap its greatest benefits. There is a host of other wide-ranging issues such as its cost, complexity and availability of such centres. Peter Johnstone et al. disputed whether all paediatric patients should receive treatment at the sparsely spaced proton facilities, which are not always located closer to homes, or if they could instead receive treatment using other cutting-edge photon technologies closer to their homes [15]. When comparing protons with photons utilising intensity-modulated radiotherapy (IMRT), volumetric modulated arc therapy (VMAT), or tomotherapy, some researchers have debated if reduction in the overall dosage to the tumour will have a clinically relevant impact on the long-term effects of radiation and disease control as studies are scarce and long term outcomes need to be monitored closely. Literature at hand points that not only protons are comparable to photons in terms of local control but are also a way forward in minimising late effects of radiation.

## 17.5 Medulloblastoma

The most frequent malignant brain tumour in children, accounting for roughly 20% of all paediatric brain tumours, is Medulloblastoma [16]. Cranio-spinal irradiation (CSI) is one of the most important components of multi-modality treatment in MB. Dr. Edith Paterson advanced the concept of CSI and reported that irradiation of entire neuraxis improves the 3-year survival to 65% [17]. However, addition of CSI is associated with a considerable risk of neurocognitive and endocrinological impairment and second malignancies in survivors because substantial doses are absorbed by the structures anterior to the spinal cord, including the bilateral lungs, hearts, bowels, breast tissue and gonads, given the high exit doses in photon therapy.

Zhang R and colleagues predicted the risk of radiation-induced second malignancies in proton versus photon CSI and found that the total lifetime attributable risk of the incidence of second cancer was significantly lower after proton CSI with a lifetime risk ratio of 0.18 [18]. Proton CSI has been shown to decrease cardiac morbidity and haematological side effects as compared to photon CSI [18]. However, some authors have hypothesised that the biologic uncertainties connected to proton therapy may increase the likelihood of disease recurrence in medulloblastoma patients. A meta-analysis and a systematic review done to compare proton versus photon radiotherapy in paediatric CNS malignancies showed that proton therapy offered significant dosimetric advantage over photon [19].

## 17.6 Skull Base Tumours

Skull base tumours are heterogeneous group of tumours comprising of chordomas, chondrosarcomas, meningiomas, pituitary adenomas, acoustic neuromas, craniopharyngiomas, Ewing sarcoma, esthesioneuroblastomas and glomus jugulare. Although the majority of cases are typically seen in the fifth or sixth decades of life, they are known to affect all age people [20].

Maximum safe surgical resection followed by adjuvant radiation or radiotherapy alone for unresectable tumours is the current standard of care. Irradiation of these tumours is often difficult because of their proximity to important organs and high recurrence rates. For these tumours, proton therapy not only delivers highly conformal radiation but also helps in dose escalation. Earlier studies have shown that adjuvant radiation to a total dose exceeding 70 Gy improves outcome in chordoma. However, due to the nearby essential organs' inherent radiobiological sensitivity, this dose cannot be delivered by photons. The five-year recurrence-free survival rate for cranial base chordomas varies between 59% and 73% with the use of proton therapy [21].

The standard of care for meningiomas is surgery; however, incomplete excision results in higher recurrences. Good local control rates have been achieved with cutting-edge radiotherapy methods as 3D-CRT, IMRT, and stereotactic radiation [22]. The outcomes with proton have been encouraging with local control rates and OS of 90% at 5 years [23–25]. In one study, a hypofractionated stereotactic (HSP) or single-session stereotactic (SSSP) technique was also used to provide proton therapy [26]. The 3- and 5-year LC rates for HSP with three or more fractions were 100% and 91%, respectively. Regardless of the fractionation, the documented toxicities have been minimal and the 3-year tumour control rate was 94%.

Olfactory neuroblastomas or esthesioneuroblastomas develop near the base of the frontal cranium from olfactory stem cells that come from neural crest cells. Surgery followed by adjuvant RT is the standard of care for these tumours [27]. However, the treatment guidelines for paediatric and adolescent patients have been extrapolated from adult patients. Nishimura et al. reported a series of 14 patients, who received proton therapy to a total dose of 65 Gy (RBE) in 2.5 Gy per fraction [28]. The OS and PFS at 5 years have been reported as 93% and 84%, respectively.

Combs et al. [29] documented a range of negative consequences in around 150 individuals treated by proton therapy. Alopecia (37%), visual impairment (28%), motor dysfunction (27%), headaches (27%) and light fatigue (27%) were the most often reported early effects. Nonetheless, it is important to emphasise that these remain equivalent to photon-based toxicities.

## 17.7 Mediastinal Hodgkin's Lymphoma

With a bimodal age distribution, mediastinal lymphomas constitute 12% of all lymphoma cases. A study by Simpson et al. [30] showed that lymphomas form a major burden (50%) of all mediastinal tumours in the paediatric population. Also due to various advancements in the treatment, survival rates today are as high as 80% across all stages. Hence, throughout the past 10 years, attention has been focused on reducing radiotherapy target volumes to lessen treatment-related adverse effects. Radiation for mediastinal lymphoma increases the risk of ischemic heart disease, hypothyroidism, pulmonary fibrosis and second cancers. Despite the major advancements in highly conformal radiation delivery techniques like IMRT along with reduction in radiation dose and volume, proton therapy is under the clinical radar with hopes to significantly decrease the dose to the heart, spinal cord, lungs and breast. Since the risks of geographical misses are substantial, extreme attention is required to prevent an increase in the probability of recurrences.

Lautenschlaeger et al. [31] compared the dose received by the thoracic structures and breast tissues by various photon and proton plans. The authors concluded that PTV coverage was comparable for both IMRT and IMPT with proton plans being slightly more superior in terms of its conformity index. The comparison of the mean doses received by the organs at risks showed higher dose sparing by protons. In addition, the mean doses received by the breast tissues had reduced by 3.1 and 3.2 Gy, respectively, for protons and photons, both delivered via intensity modulation. Also, the mean doses received by the cardia was increased by more than 3 Gy in photon plans than that of proton plans. The dose sparing was evident across all cardiac substructures, the lungs, oesophagus and the cord. Even though newer techniques like the "Butterfly" technique with photons have resulted in better target coverage and organ sparing, the superiority of protons remain to be unchallenged. Though data is still in the early stages, use of protons for such malignancies looks promising in not only decreasing toxicities, but improving survival.

## 17.8 Neuroblastoma and Nephroblastoma

Radiation therapy is employed in neuroblastomas and nephroblastomas, in accordance to the risk stratification. Around one-third of those who receive radiation have long-term consequences, such as stunted growth and development, nephrotoxicity and secondary cancers. Proton therapy in these patients helps to reduce radiation doses to organs at risk (OARs). When irradiated with photons, this would ensure a higher dose to organs mainly spinal cord and bowel. A study by Vogel et al. [32] found that with photon therapy, the mean and median dose to 50% or more to the contralateral kidney (D50) were 135 cGy and 139 cGy, while with proton therapy, these were 52 cGy RBE and 5 cGy RBE, respectively.

## 17.9 Sarcomas

Sarcomas are a diverse group of cancers of soft tissues and bones, commonly seen in children. Proton therapy has shown clinical benefit in these patients [33].

**Rhabdomyosarcoma (RMS)** It is the most common soft-tissue sarcoma in children. Embryonal and alveolar are the two most prevalent histological categories that differ in age, tumour site, tendency for distant spread and long-term outcome [34]. Treatment comprises of combination of surgery, chemotherapy and RT depending on the age of the child, tumour site and stage. With relapse rates ranging from 15% to 37%, local recurrence is the most common pattern of failure [35]. Proton beam therapy has the dosimetric advantage and reduces doses to OARs as compared to photon-based IMRT plans, reducing acute and late side effects [36, 37]. In one study, 55 children who received proton beam therapy (median RT dose: 50.4 GyE) for various site RMS were retrospectively analysed [38]. A total of 153 adverse events of grade 3 were observed including 141 haematological toxicities in 48 patients. The authors mentioned that the acute effects were similar to photon therapy and observed 1 and 2 years survival of 92% and 85%, respectively. Leiser et al. [39] did not observe acute Grade >3 toxicity or treatment interruption in 83 RMS patients treated with proton beam therapy. In one study, 17 patients with parameningeal RMS were treated with proton therapy to a median dose of 50.4 GyE [40]. The authors observed a 5-years failure free and overall survival of 59% and 64%, respectively. Late sequelae in disease free patients included failure to maintain height, hormonal imbalance, slight facial dysmorphisms, delayed eruption of adult dentition, dental caries, and persistent nose and sinus congestion.

**Ewing sarcomas** Ewing sarcoma family of tumours are aggressive, solid malignant tumours that most commonly affect children and adolescents. A typical multimodal treatment plan includes induction chemotherapy, local therapy that includes surgery and/or RT [41]. Proton therapy is especially beneficial in limiting dose to the nearby organs/structures when the tumour is juxtaposed to a joint and joint space.

In one study, 15 paediatric Ewing sarcoma patients were treated with proton therapy to a median dose of 55.8GyE [42]. In this study, 4-year OS and EFS rates were 94.6% and 84.8%, respectively [42]. Another study reported 5-year local control and metastasis-free survival rates of 81.5% and 76.4%, respectively, with median RT dosage of 54.9GyE [43].

Despite the current literature showing advantage of proton therapy, availability and cost of particle therapy are the liming factors particularly in low middle-income countries (LMIC). At present, there is only one proton centre in India, while in the USA, 41 regional proton therapy centres are available. In Europe, more than 20 clinical centres offering some form of heavy particle radiotherapy has opened up in the last decade. Proton therapy cost ranges from about $30,000 to $120,000, as compared to photon IMRT, which costs around $15,000. The construction cost of a proton centre can go up to $200 million.To date, the results of proton therapy are promising due to its unique physical and biological properties resulting in lower integral dose and reduced late effects. Owing to cost and limited availability of proton facilities in LMIC, careful patient selection is very important.

## References


1. Wilson RR. Radiological use of fast protons. Radiology. 1946;47(5):487–91.
2. Lawrence JH, Tobias CA, Born JL, McCOMBS RK, Roberts JE, Anger HO, et al. Pituitary irradiation with high-energy proton beams: a preliminary report. Cancer Res. 1958;18(2):121–34.
3. Durante M, Debus J. Heavy charged particles: does improved precision and higher biological effectiveness translate to better outcome in patients? Semin Radiat Oncol. 2018;28(2):160–7.
4. Malouff TD, Mahajan A, Krishnan S, Beltran C, Seneviratne DS, Trifiletti DM. Carbon ion therapy: a modern review of an emerging technology. Front Oncologia. 2020;10:82.
5. Md S, et al. Carbon Ion Radiotherapy: A Review of Clinical Experiences and Preclinical Research, with an emphasis on DNA damage/repair. Cancers [Internet] 2017 [cited 2022 Nov 28];9(6). Available from: https://pubmed.ncbi.nlm.nih.gov/28598362/
6. An overview on radiotherapy: from its history to its current applications in dermatology. Open Access Maced J Med Sci [Internet] 2017 [cited 2022 Nov 28];5(4). Available from: https://pubmed.ncbi.nlm.nih.gov/28785349/
7. Lazar AA, Schulte R, Faddegon B, Blakely EA, Roach M. Clinical trials involving carbon-ion radiation therapy and the path forward. Cancer. 2018;124(23):4467–76.
8. PTCOG - PTCOG [Internet]. [cited 2022 Nov 28]. Available from: https://www.ptcog.ch/index.php/component/users/?view=login&Itemid=435
9. Eley JG, Friedrich T, Homann KL, Howell RM, Scholz M, Durante M, et al. Comparative risk predictions of second Cancers after carbon-ion therapy versus proton therapy. Int J Radiat Oncol Biol Phys. 2016;95(1):279–86.
10. Risk of subsequent primary cancers after carbon ion radiotherapy, photon radiotherapy, or surgery for localised prostate cancer: a propensity score-weighted, retrospective, cohort study. Lancet Oncol [Internet]. 2019 [cited 2022 Nov 28];20(5). Available from: https://pubmed.ncbi.nlm.nih.gov/30885458/
11. Childhood Cancers - NCI [Internet]. 2015 [cited 2022 Nov 28]. Available from: https://www.cancer.gov/types/childhood-cancers
12. Paulino AC, Constine LS, Rubin P, Williams JP. Normal tissue development, homeostasis, senescence, and the sensitivity to radiation injury across the age spectrum. Semin Radiat Oncol. 2010;20(1):12–20.
13. Bhatia S, Robison LL, Oberlin O, Greenberg M, Bunin G, Fossati-Bellani F, et al. Breast cancer and other second neoplasms after childhood Hodgkin's disease. N Engl J Med. 1996;334(12):745–51.
14. Armstrong GT, Liu Q, Yasui Y, Neglia JP, Leisenring W, Robison LL, et al. Late mortality among 5-year survivors of childhood cancer: a summary from the childhood cancer survivor study. J Clin Oncol. 2009;27(14):2328–38.
15. Johnstone PAS, McMullen KP, Buchsbaum JC, Douglas JG, Helft P. Pediatric CSI: are protons the only ethical approach? Int J Radiat Oncol. 2013;87(2):228–30.
16. Mahapatra S, Amsbaugh MJ. Medulloblastoma [Internet]. StatPearls [Internet]. StatPearls Publishing; 2022 [Cited 2023 Mar 6]. Available from: https://www.ncbi.nlm.nih.gov/books/NBK431069/
17. Paterson E, Farr RF. Cerebellar Medulloblastoma: treatment by irradiation of the whole central nervous system. Acta Radiol. 1953;39(4):323–36.
18. Zhang R, Howell RM, Giebeler A, Taddei PJ, Mahajan A, Newhauser WD. Comparison of risk of radiogenic second cancer following photon and proton craniospinal irradiation for a pediatric medulloblastoma patient. Phys Med Biol. 2013;58(4):807–23.

19. Carbonara R, Di Rito A, Monti A, Rubini G, Sardaro A. Proton versus Photon Radiotherapy for Pediatric Central Nervous System Malignancies: A systematic review and meta-analysis of Dosimetric comparison studies. J Oncol 2019;2019:5879723.
20. McMaster ML, Goldstein AM, Bromley CM, Ishibe N, Parry DM. Chordoma: incidence and survival patterns in the United States, 1973-1995. Cancer Causes Control CCC. 2001;12(1):1–11.
21. Hug EB, Loredo LN, Slater JD, DeVries A, Grove RI, Schaefer RA, et al. Proton radiation therapy for chordomas and chondrosarcomas of the skull base. J Neurosurg. 1999;91(3):432–9.
22. Noël G, Bollet MA, Calugaru V, Feuvret L, Haie-Meder C, Dhermain F, et al. Functional outcome of patients with benign meningioma treated by 3D conformal irradiation with a combination of photons and protons. Int J Radiat Oncol Biol Phys. 2005;62(5):1412–22.
23. Weber DC, Schneider R, Goitein G, Koch T, Ares C, Geismar JH, et al. Spot scanning based proton therapy for intracranial meningioma: long-term results from the Paul Scherrer Institute. Int J Radiat Oncol Biol Phys. 2012;83(3):865–71.
24. Slater JD, Loredo LN, Chung A, Bush DA, Patyal B, Johnson WD, et al. Fractionated proton radiotherapy for benign cavernous sinus meningiomas. Int J Radiat Oncol Biol Phys. 2012;83(5):e633–7.
25. Wenkel E, Thornton AF, Finkelstein D, Adams J, Lyons S, De La Monte S, et al. Benign meningioma: partially resected, biopsied, and recurrent intracranial tumors treated with combined proton and photon radiotherapy. Int J Radiat Oncol Biol Phys. 2000;48(5):1363–70.
26. Vernimmen FJ, Harris JK, Wilson JA, Melvill R, Smit BJ, Slabbert JP. Stereotactic proton beam therapy of skull base meningiomas. Int J Radiat Oncol Biol Phys. 2001;49(1):99–105.
27. Dulguerov P, Allal AS, Calcaterra TC. Esthesioneuroblastoma: a meta-analysis and review. Lancet Oncol. 2001;2(11):683–90.
28. Nishimura H, Ogino T, Kawashima M, Nihei K, Arahira S, Onozawa M, et al. Proton-beam therapy for olfactory neuroblastoma. Int J Radiat Oncol Biol Phys. 2007;68(3):758–62.
29. Combs SE, Kessel K, Habermehl D, Haberer T, Jäkel O, Debus J. Proton and carbon ion radiotherapy for primary brain tumors and tumors of the skull base. Acta Oncol Stockh Swed. 2013;52(7):1504–9.
30. Simpson I, Campbell PE. Mediastinal masses in childhood: a review from a paediatric pathologist's point of view. Prog Pediatr Surg. 1991;27:92–126.
31. Lautenschlaeger S, Iancu G, Flatten V, Baumann K, Thiemer M, Dumke C, et al. Advantage of proton-radiotherapy for pediatric patients and adolescents with Hodgkin's disease. Radiat Oncol 2019;14(1):157.
32. Pencil beam scanning proton therapy for treatment of the retroperitoneum after nephrectomy for Wilms tumor: A dosimetric comparison study. Pediatr Blood Cancer [Internet]. 2017 [cited 2023 Mar 6];64(1). Available from: https://pubmed.ncbi.nlm.nih.gov/27565764/
33. Frisch S, Timmermann B. The evolving role of proton beam therapy for sarcomas. Clin Oncol R Coll Radiol G B. 2017;29(8):500–6.
34. Malempati S, Hawkins DS. Rhabdomyosarcoma: review of the children's oncology group (COG) soft-tissue sarcoma committee experience and rationale for current COG studies. Pediatr Blood Cancer. 2012;59(1):5.
35. Patterns of failure in pediatric rhabdomyosarcoma after proton therapy. Int J Radiat Oncol Biol Phys [Internet]. 2016. [cited 2023 Mar 6];96(5). Available from: https://pubmed.ncbi.nlm.nih.gov/27742542/
36. Ladra MM, Edgington SK, Mahajan A, Grosshans D, Szymonifka J, Khan F, et al. A Dosimetric comparison of proton and intensity modulated radiation therapy in pediatric rhabdomyosarcoma patients enrolled on a prospective phase II proton study. Radiother Oncol J Eur Soc Ther Radiol Oncol. 2014;113(1):77–83.
37. Cotter SE, Herrup DA, Friedmann A, Macdonald SM, Pieretti RV, Robinson G, et al. Proton radiotherapy for pediatric bladder/prostate rhabdomyosarcoma: clinical outcomes and dosimetry compared to intensity-modulated radiation therapy. Int J Radiat Oncol Biol Phys. 2011;81(5):1367–73.

38. Mizumoto M, Murayama S, Akimoto T, Demizu Y, Fukushima T, Ishida Y, et al. Preliminary results of proton radiotherapy for pediatric rhabdomyosarcoma: a multiinstitutional study in Japan. Cancer Med. 2018;7(5):1870.
39. Tumour control and Quality of Life in children with rhabdomyosarcoma treated with pencil beam scanning proton therapy. Radiother Oncol J Eur Soc Ther Radiol Oncol [Internet]. 2016 [cited 2023 Mar 6];120(1). Available from: https://pubmed.ncbi.nlm.nih.gov/27247053/
40. Childs SK, Kozak KR, Friedmann AM, Yeap BY, Adams J, MacDonald SM, et al. Proton radiotherapy for parameningeal rhabdomyosarcoma: clinical outcomes and late effects. Int J Radiat Oncol Biol Phys. 2012;82(2):635–42.
41. Proton radiotherapy for pediatric Ewing's sarcoma: initial clinical outcomes. Int J Radiat Oncol Biol Phys [Internet] 2012. [cited 2023 Mar 6];82(3). Available from: https://pubmed.ncbi.nlm.nih.gov/21856094/
42. Nakao T, Fukushima H, Fukushima T, Suzuki R, Hosaka S, Yamaki Y, et al. Interinstitutional patient transfers between rapid chemotherapy cycles were feasible to utilize proton beam therapy for pediatric Ewing sarcoma family of tumors. Rep Pract Oncol Radiother 2018;23(5):442–450.
43. Weber DC, Murray FR, Correia D, Bolsi A, Frei-Welte M, Pica A, et al. Pencil beam scanned protons for the treatment of patients with Ewing sarcoma. Pediatr Blood Cancer. 2017;64(12)

# High Grade Glioma in Children

# 18

Supriya Mallick

## 18.1 Introduction

In pediatric age group, CNS tumors are the second commonest malignant tumor, of which nearly 10% are considered high grade glioma [1]. Despite improvement in diagnostics modalities and available therapeutic options, prognosis of these patients is poor with 40% mortality [1].

In the 2014 International Society of Neuropathology (ISN) at Haarlem consensus meeting came up with a multilayered diagnostic approach for gliomas and is considered a landmark change as it was aimed to address inter- and intra-observer variation and heterogeneous behavior of tumor in the same class or group [2]. These layers comprise of molecular data (layer 4), WHO grade (Layer 3), histological classification (Layer 2), and Integrated diagnosis (layer 1). These systems were later adopted by WHO in 2016. However, to add on to the existing knowledge and disseminate, it quickly a Consortium to Inform Molecular and Practical Approaches to CNS Tumor Taxonomy (cIMPACT-NOW) was formed. The cIMPACT-NOW data highlights that pediatric high-grade gliomas are not a single entity rather theses are a mix of tumors widely variable based of their molecular characteristic (Image 18.1).

### 18.1.1 H 3.3 Mutant

WHO in the 2016 classification introduced the terminology of diffuse midline glioma. In most of the cases, these tumors arise from pons resulting in diffuse enlargement of pons and are characterized by H3.3K27 M mutation [3]. A lysine-to-methionine mutation happens in position 27 in histone 3.1, 3.2 (rarely), or 3.3

S. Mallick (✉)
Department of Radiation Oncology, National Cancer Institute, Jhajjar, Haryana, India

2nd Campus AIIMS, New Delhi, Delhi, India



R. Madan et al. (eds.), *Evidence Based Practice in Pediatric Radiation Oncology*,
https://doi.org/10.1007/978-981-96-4872-6_18

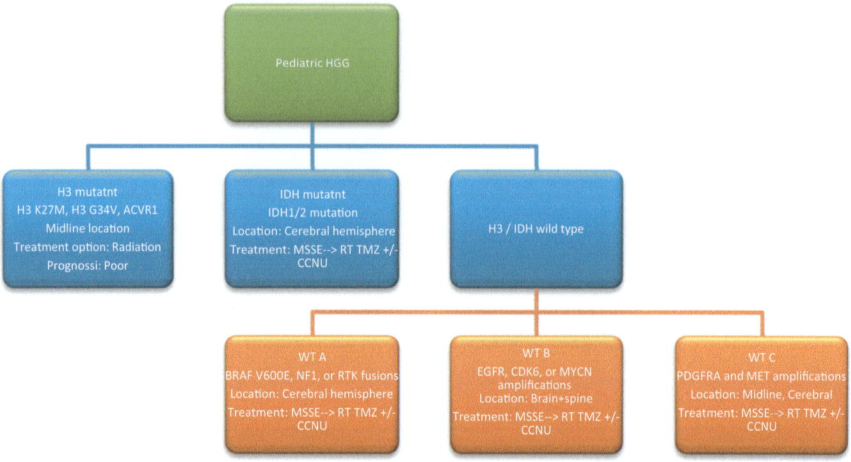


**Image 18.1** Molecular classification of pediatric HGG

(H3K27M). Midline gliomas are mostly reported in pediatric population with median age of 6–7 years. Nearly half of the patients present with rapidly progressing variety of neurological symptoms and cranial nerve VI and VII are most commonly involved. Cranial nerve palsies (facial asymmetry and diplopia), long tract signs (clonus, hyperreflexia, weakness, positive Babinski reflex, and increased tone), and cerebellar signs (ataxia, dysmetria) are considered “classic triad” and indicated necessity of immediate imaging. Cranial nerves VI and VII are the most commonly affected and specific dysfunction of these is characteristic of DIPG. Obstructive hydrocephalus can also be a presenting compliant in nearly 10–30% of the patients.

Magnetic resonance imaging (MRI) brain is the standard imaging, which shows an infiltrative mass with its epicenter in the pons. The mass appears hypointense in T1 weighted image without contrast enhancement in most of the cases and hyperintense in T2 weighted image/FLAIR. The characteristic presentation and imaging finding are considered diagnostic of these tumors. In the recent years, many centers have reported stereotactic biopsy as a safe intervention, particularly helpful for characterizing the tumors and enabling a tailored therapeutic approach.

Because of diffuse involvement of pons, most of the time surgery is not possible and radiation therapy is considered the only effective treatment. However, prognosis of these patients is dismal [4]. Radiotherapy alone is considered the standard of care with median survival less than a year. A conformal radiation of 54–60 Gy is delivered in 5.5–6 weeks @2 Gy per fraction. Children’s Cancer Group (CCG) and Pediatric Oncology Group (POG) advocated hyper-fractionated radiation up to 78 Gy or 75.6 Gy but reported no additional benefit beyond 54 Gy [5]. Two small phase II trials reported hypofractionated radiation (39 Gy in 13 fraction) to be an effective treatment option with similar survival outcome compared to conventional radiation [6, 7]. A target delineation is based on CT-T2W/FLAIR image fusion which forms the gross tumor volume. An additional 1.5–2 cm margin forms the clinical target volume. Role of chemotherapy has been extensively evaluated for DIPG patients. CCSG randomized 74 patients to receive radiation alone or radiation followed by PCV chemotherapy. But the additional chemotherapy did not alter the outcome. In another trial, CCG randomized patients to receive either carboplatin, etoposide, and vincristine ($n$ = 32) or cisplatin, etoposide, cyclophosphamide, and vincristine ($n$ = 31) followed by radiation. But this approach also reported similar results. ACNS0126 randomized DIPG patients to receive radiation with concurrent Temozolomide (90 mg/m$^2$/day for 42 days), followed by maintenance with 10 cycles TMZ (200 mg/m$^2$/day for 5 days). However, compared to CCG 9941 trial, Temozolomide did not alter survival outcome and was found similar in other trials also [8, 9].

### 18.1.2 IDH Mutant

Isocitrate dehydrogenase (IDH) gene mutations have been recognized as most important mutation in the glioma genesis. IDH exists in two forms: NADP dependent (IDH 1 and IDH2) and NADP independent IDH3. IDH 1 is present in cytoplasm and peroxisome and located in long arm of chromosome (2q32). Its important role is antioxidation in eukaryotes, whereas IDH 2 is present in mitochondria (long arm of chromosome 15 15q21). In normal circumstance, IDH1 catalyzes the oxidative decarboxylation of isocitrate to alpha ketoglutarate in the TCA cycle. But when IDH 1/IDH 2 is mutated, it produces 2-hydroxy gluterate, which subsequently produces VEGF and HIF alpha, and both lead to the development of tumor microenvironment and invasion and ultimately glioma genesis [10]. A heterozygous missense mutation of amino acid residue of 132, arginine [R] replaced by histidine [H] R132H, is the commonest IDG mutation followed by 172. IDH mutations are more common in lower grade gliomas and secondary gliomas. IDH mutations have been reported to be common in older children with malignant glioma and are associated with MGMT methylation and better efficacy of Temozolomide [11]. Retrospective studies have reported variable rate of MGMT methylation, and it was reported to be as high as 50% [12]. Surgery has been considered the cornerstone of therapy with an aim to achieve maximal safe surgical excision. After surgery patients are treated with radiation to a dose of 60 Gy in 30 fractions over 6 weeks. A planning CT scan with delayed contrast is taken and is fused with postoperative T1/FLAIR weighted MRI image. The low-risk clinical target volume (CTV 50) included MRI abnormality visible on the T2 sequences of the postoperative MRI with isotropic 2–2.5 cm margin. The high-risk CTV (CTV60) includes a1.5–2 cm margin around the T1 contrast enhancing tumor and post-operative cavity. Alternatively, a T1 abnormality, along with post-operative cavity with 1.5–2 cm expansion, forms the CTV, which is treated with full 60 Gy dose [13]. Role of chemotherapy has also been extensively studied in such patients. Wolff et al. randomized patients with high-grade glioma to receive maintenance chemotherapy with lomustine, vincristine, and cisplatin or sandwich chemotherapy with ifosfamide, etoposide, methotrexate, cisplatin, and cytosine arabinoside [14]. The authors reported favorable results for patients treated with sandwich approach and female patients with grade III histology, and those who received radiation more than 54 Gy had better outcome [Wolff]. Several retrospective single institute studies reported radiation with concurrent chemotherapy followed by maintenance chemotherapy to be favorable regimen [15, 16]. Gupta et al. reported median overall survival of 17.4 months and median progression-free survival (PFS) of 15.1 months for the entire cohort. The authors reported 1- and 3-year PFS to be 54.4% and 24.6%, respectively. A phase II HERBY trial tested bevacizumab along with radiation and Temozlomide for the treatment of pediatric high-grade glioma [18]. However, addition of bevacizumab failed to improve both EFS and OS. A joint ITCC and SIOPE-brain tumor study evaluated Irinotecan along with Temozolomide followed by standard treatment but failed to achieve any benefit of this approach [19]. Children's Oncology Group trial ACNS0423 subjected patients with pediatric high-grade glioma to receive radiation with concurrent temozolomide followed by six cycles of adjuvant chemotherapy with lomustine 90 mg/m(2) on day 1 and temozolomide 160 mg/m(2)/day ×5 every 6 weeks. The authors reported addition significantly better EFS and OS in participants without gross-total resection when treated with combination regimen [19].

### 18.1.3 H3/IDH Wild Type

Tumors lacking either H3.3 or IDH mutation are further subdivided into three groups: WTA, WT B, and WT C, which is due to characteristic mutation they harbor. As of now the cornerstone of therapy remains maximal safe surgical resection followed by radiation along with concurrent Temozolomide (75 mg/m$^2$) followed by six cycles of maintenance Temozolomide (150–200 mg/m$^2$). Target volume for radiation is similar to IDH mutants. WT-A tumors harbor BRAF V600E, NF1 mutations, or RTK fusions, which are often found in pediatric low-grade gliomas and are found to have better survival outcome. Vemurafenib, a BRAF V600E inhibitor, and selumetinib, a MEK inhibitor, have shown promising results in low grade gliomas and may show better outcome in high grade gliomas as well. WT-B tumors mostly harbor EGFR amplification. A spectrum of EGFR inhibitors has been used in high-grade gliomas but has not been effective. Newer EGFR inhibitors, osimertinib have with higher BBB penetration has shown promising results in preclinical studies. PDGFRA and MET amplification are hallmark of WT-C type tumors, and Dasatinib, which targets PDGFRA, has shown promising results.

## References

1. Ostrom QT, de Blank PM, Kruchko C, Petersen CM, Liao P, Finlay JL, Stearns DS, Wolff JE, Wolinsky Y, Letterio JJ, Barnholtz-Sloan JS. Alex's Lemonade Stand Foundation Infant and Childhood Primary Brain and Central Nervous System Tumors Diagnosed in the United States in 2007-2011. Neuro Oncol. 2015;16 Suppl 10(Suppl 10):x1–x36.

2. Louis DN, Perry A, Burger P, Ellison DW, Reifenberger G, von Deimling A et al (2014) International Society of Neuropathology-Haarlem consensus guidelines for nervous system tumor classification and grading. Brain Pathol 24:429–435.
3. Haag D, Mack N, Benites Goncalves da Silva P, Statz B, Clark J, Tanabe K et al. H3.3-K27M drives neural stem cell-specific gliomagenesis in a human iPSC-derived model. Cancer Cell. 2021 Mar 8;39(3):407-422.e13.
4. Dagar A, Ghosh A, Aashita, Kumar A, N YIK, Kamboj K, Sharma A, Raj J, Sharma D, Mallick S. Survival and toxicity outcomes of hypofractionated conformal radiotherapy compared to conventionally fractionated radiotherapy in the treatment of diffuse intrinsic pontine gliomas. Childs Nerv Syst. 2025;41(1):85.
5. Packer RJ, Boyett JM, Zimmerman RA, Albright AL, Kaplan AM, Rorke LB, Selch MT, Cherlow JM, Finlay JL, Wara WM. Outcome of children with brain stem gliomas after treatment with 7800 cGy of hyperfractionated radiotherapy. A Childrens Cancer Group Phase I/II Trial. Cancer. 1994;74(6):1827–34.
6. Izzuddeen Y, Gupta S, Haresh KP, Sharma D, Giridhar P, Rath GK. Hypofractionated radiotherapy with temozolomide in diffuse intrinsic pontine gliomas: a randomized controlled trial. J Neurooncol. 2020;146(1):91–95.
7. Zaghloul MS, Eldebawy E, Ahmed S, Mousa AG, Amin A, Refaat A, Zaky I, Elkhateeb N, Sabry M. Hypofractionated conformal radiotherapy for pediatric diffuse intrinsic pontine glioma (DIPG): a randomized controlled trial. Radiother Oncol. 2014;111(1):35–40.
8. Jalali R, Raut N, Arora B, Gupta T, Dutta D, Munshi A, Sarin R, Kurkure P. Prospective evaluation of radiotherapy with concurrent and adjuvant temozolomide in children with newly diagnosed diffuse intrinsic pontine glioma. Int J Radiat Oncol Biol Phys. 2010;77(1):113–8.
9. Cohen KJ, Heideman RL, Zhou T, Holmes EJ, Lavey RS, Bouffet E, Pollack IF. Temozolomide in the treatment of children with newly diagnosed diffuse intrinsic pontine gliomas: a report from the Children's Oncology Group. Neuro Oncol. 2011;13(4):410–6.
10. Huang J, Yu J, Tu L, Huang N, Li H, Luo Y. Isocitrate Dehydrogenase Mutations in Glioma: From Basic Discovery to Therapeutics Development. Front Oncol. 2019;9:506.
11. Pollack IF, Hamilton RL, Sobol RW, Nikiforova MN, Lyons-Weiler MA, LaFramboise WA, Burger PC, Brat DJ, Rosenblum MK, Holmes EJ, Zhou T, Jakacki RI; Children's Oncology Group. IDH1 mutations are common in malignant gliomas arising in adolescents: a report from the Children's Oncology Group. Childs Nerv Syst. 2011;27(1):87–94.
12. Srivastava A, Jain A, Jha P, Suri V, Sharma MC, Mallick S, Puri T, Gupta DK, Gupta A, Sarkar C. MGMT gene promoter methylation in pediatric glioblastomas. Childs Nerv Syst. 2010;26(11):1613–8.
13. Mallick S, Gandhi AK, Joshi NP, Kumar A, Puri T, Sharma DN, Haresh KP, Gupta S, Julka PK, Rath GK, Sarkar C. Outcomes of pediatric glioblastoma treated with adjuvant chemoradiation with temozolomide and correlation with prognostic factors. Indian J Med Paediatr Oncol. 2015;36(2):99–104.
14. Wolff JE, Gnekow AK, Kortmann RD, Pietsch T, Urban C, Graf N, Kühl J. Preradiation chemotherapy for pediatric patients with high-grade glioma. Cancer. 2002 Jan 1;94(1):264-71.
15. Gupta S, Mallick S, Benson R, Haresh KP, Julka PK, Rath GK. Extent of surgical resection and adjuvant temozolomide improves survival in pediatric GBM: a single center experience. Childs Nerv Syst. 2017;33(6):951–956.
16. Jung TY, Lee JY, Kim DS, Park HJ, Kim CY, Ra YS, Lee MJ, Kim SH, Baek HJ, Kim IH, Park KD, Kim SK. Pediatric supratentorial high-grade glioma: multicenter retrospective observational study of the Korean Society for Pediatric Neuro-Oncology. J Neurooncol. 2015;121(2):413–9.
17. Grill J, Massimino M, Bouffet E, Azizi AA, McCowage G, Cañete A, Saran F, Le Deley MC, Varlet P, Morgan PS, Jaspan T, Jones C, Giangaspero F, Smith H, Garcia J, Elze MC, Rousseau RF, Abrey L, Hargrave D, Vassal G. Phase II, Open-Label, Randomized, Multicenter Trial (HERBY) of Bevacizumab in Pediatric Patients With Newly Diagnosed High-Grade Glioma. J Clin Oncol. 2018;36(10):951–958.

18. Hargrave D, Geoerger B, Frappaz D, Pietsch T, Gesner L, Cisar L, Breazna A, Dorman A, Cruz-Martinez O, Fuster JL, Rialland X, Icher C, Leblond P, Ashley D, Perilongo G, Elliott M, English M, Clausen N, Grill J. A phase II single-arm study of irinotecan in combination with temozolomide (TEMIRI) in children with newly diagnosed high grade glioma: a joint ITCC and SIOPE-brain tumour study. J Neurooncol. 2013;113(1):127–34.
19. Jakacki RI, Cohen KJ, Buxton A, Krailo MD, Burger PC, Rosenblum MK, Brat DJ, Hamilton RL, Eckel SP, Zhou T, Lavey RS, Pollack IF. Phase 2 study of concurrent radiotherapy and temozolomide followed by temozolomide and lomustine in the treatment of children with high-grade glioma: a report of the Children's Oncology Group ACNS0423 study. Neuro Oncol. 2016;18(10):1442–50.

# Medulloblastoma and Other Embryonal Tumors in Children

# 19

Shikha Goyal, Renu Madan, and Sandeep Mohindra

## 19.1 Introduction

Embryonal tumors comprise 9.4% of all brain tumors in children <19 years; 6.5% of these are medulloblastomas and 1.5% ATRT [1]. Below 9 years, embryonal tumors are the second most common brain tumor type after gliomas. Median age at presentation for medulloblastomas is 7 years. Non-WNT/non-SHH medulloblastomas represent 50%, while SHH-activated and TP53 wildtype represent 33% of medulloblastoma subtypes. Five-year survival improves with increasing age at diagnosis, being ~70% above 10 years.

WHO CNS 2021 classification lists four molecular subtypes of medulloblastoma, while histologic defined medulloblastoma is limited to just one category. Other CNS embryonal tumors are divided into six types: atypical teratoid/rhabdoid tumor, cribriform neuroepithelial tumor, embryonal tumor with multilayered rosettes, CNS neuroblastoma, *FOXR2*-activated, CNS tumor with *BCOR* internal tandem duplication, and CNS embryonal tumor [2]. While all embryonal tumors were deemed grade 4 earlier, the current classification does not make that assumption for all tumors—some CNS embryonal tumors are deemed grade 3 as well although the knowledge of their clinical behavior is less well known.

Medulloblastomas are the most common malignant tumors in childhood and second most common brain or cerebellar tumors after pilocytic astrocytoma. Although

S. Goyal (✉) · R. Madan
Department of Radiotherapy and Oncology, Postgraduate Institute of Medical Education and Research, Chandigarh, India

S. Mohindra
Department of Radiotherapy & Oncology, Post Graduate Institute of Medical Education and Research, Chandigarh, India

Department of Neurosurgery, PGIMER, Chandigarh, India


R. Madan et al. (eds.), *Evidence Based Practice in Pediatric Radiation Oncology*, https://doi.org/10.1007/978-981-96-4872-6_19

they may occur in adults, diagnosis after 40 years is rare, similar to other embryonal tumors. Although most are sporadic, 5–6% may have syndromic association (nevoid basal cell carcinoma syndrome, familial adenomatous polyposis, or Li-Fraumeni syndrome).

## 19.2 Clinical Presentation

Symptoms are either due to mass effect or involvement of adjacent structures. Most common presentation is due to obstructive hydrocephalus leading to high intracranial pressure, with a 2–3 month history of headache (morning), projectile vomiting, and altered mentation. Midline tumors may cause gait or truncal ataxia, while lateralized tumors cause incoordination. With the involvement of brainstem, cranial nerves, or cerebellum, there may be double vision, swallowing difficulty or dizziness.

Neurologic examination may reveal ataxia, broad-based gait, abnormal heel-to-toe-walk or finger-to-nose test, titubation of head, nystagmus, or intention tremor. With prolonged intracranial hypertension, abducens nerve palsy is the most common finding, but papilledema or vision loss may also happen.

## 19.3 Imaging

CT head may reveal dilated ventricles and a hyperdense mass in posterior fossa that may enhance with contrast. MRI is the preferred modality and shows hydrocephalus with periventricular ooze, a heterogeneously enhancing cerebellar mass with fourth ventricular compression. Lesions are iso- or hypointense on T1 and heterogeneous on T2. Some lesions may show necrosis, bleed, or cysts. As the disease has propensity for leptomeningeal spread, a contrast screening study of the spine should also be obtained in addition to cranial imaging. Ideally, spine imaging should be performed preoperatively but if not done, it should be delayed for 2 weeks to avoid confusion due to surgical debris. Leptomeningeal disease may be evident as nodular or linear enhancement along the ventricles, cerebral convexities, brainstem, spinal canal, or within cauda equina. Metastases to cerebral parenchyma or outside CNS have been rarely noted.

The location of the tumor has some relation to molecular subtype. Tumors in CP angle may represent Wnt, lateralized cerebellar lesions are more often seen with SHH, while non-Wnt/non-SHH tumors commonly have a midline vermian location [3].

## 19.4 Cerebrospinal Fluid Evaluation

Nearly 30% of medulloblastomas may have CSF dissemination at diagnosis, which may be evident on imaging. A CSF examination is mandatory even in an image-negative spine—biochemistry may show mild pleocytosis and raised protein, while cytology may reveal malignant cells. In patients with obstructive hydrocephalus, lumbar puncture and CSF analysis may have to be delayed for ~2 weeks after surgical resection.

Systemic imaging: CT of chest/abdomen to rule out extra-CNS metastases is rarely indicated only in patients with indicative symptoms.

## 19.5 Histopathology and Molecular Subtypes

Medulloblastomas are seen as soft, friable, and often necrotic masses on gross pathology. Microscopically, they have high cellularity, round to oval nuclei, frequent mitoses, and Homer Wright rosettes. On IHC, synaptophysin, neuron-specific enolase, and nestin are positive. Nuclear beta-catenin is positive in WNT tumors, and p53 is absent in those with TP53 mutations.

Detailed histopathology information is available in a separate chapter.

WHO 2021 CNS classification for embryonal tumors focuses on a molecular classification, although the earlier histology categories also exist [2].

Medulloblastomas are categorized into four molecular groups based on gene expression profiling: WNT-activated, SHH-activated and TP53-wildtype, SHH-activated and TP53-mutant, or non-WNT/non-SHH. Through methylation and transcriptome profiling, subgroups having distinct clinical profile, prognosis, and treatment needs are also being identified. Non-molecularly defined medulloblastoma was earlier classified into four types morphologically (classic, desmoplastic/nodular, medulloblastoma with extensive nodularity (MBEN), and large cell/anaplastic) in WHO 2016 classification but now identified with only one entity: medulloblastomas, histologically defined. Individual morphologic types may be associated with a particular molecular category, for example, WNT with classic morphology, desmoplastic/nodular and MBEN with SHH, and large cell/anaplastic with groups other than WNT [4].

The histopathologic as well as molecular subtypes are prognostic; they may also dictate treatment regimes in future studies. Histologic desmoplastic/nodular or MBEN, or molecular WNT tumors have a better prognosis, while histologic large cell/anaplastic or molecular non-WNT/non-SHH (especially erstwhile group 3 with MYC amplification) or SHH with TP53 mutations have a worse prognosis [4]. Classic histology or molecular SHH without TP53 mutation and erstwhile group 4 have an intermediate prognosis. Nearly 30% medulloblastomas have SHH pathway alterations. Nearly 10–20% of these may have somatic TP53 mutations. While TP53 mutant SHH altered medulloblastomas are seen in adolescence with a 5-year survival of 40%, TP53 wild type are seen in infants as well as adults and have a better 5-year survival of 80%. Nearly 10% medulloblastomas have Wnt pathway alterations; these may be seen in children as well as adults. Presentation in infancy is rare. This small subgroup has the least potential for dissemination and the best outcome, with survival exceeding 95% in children. Non-Wnt/non-SHH tumors were earlier classified as group 3 and group 4 tumors. Group 3 comprise 25% of medulloblastomas and occur in children. Many anaplastic/large cell tumors are part of this group and have a high propensity for metastases at presentation. Five-year survival is 50%. Group 4 tumors comprise 35% medulloblastomas; most have classic histology and occur in adolescent males. In children, nearly 40% may have metastases at presentation and 5-year survival is 75%, while survival in adults is inferior.

## 19.6 Genetics of Origin and Metastases

All molecular subgroups have different cellular origin. SHH tumors arise from cerebellar granule cell progenitor cells in the upper rhombic lip, Wnt from lower rhombic lip multipotential progenitors of the dorsal brainstem, and non-SHH/non-Wnt from cells in the rhombic lip germinal zone, which give rise to glutamatergic neurons including photoreceptor cells and unipolar brush cells of the cerebellum. When these progenitor cells undergo repeated stimulation or fail to exit the cell cycle, they may give rise to medulloblastoma.

Recurrences and metastases also retain the molecular signature. SHH tumors have a higher propensity of local recurrence, while non-SHH/non-Wnt have a higher tendency for distant spread.

## 19.7 Genetic Testing and Counselling

Due to higher predisposition to germline mutations, it is recommended that patients with SHH and Wnt (with absent somatic CTNNB1 mutation) tumors and some with non-Wnt/non-SHH tumors (family history of BRCA tumors, HRR deficient) should undergo genetic testing and counselling [5].

## 19.8 Differential Diagnosis

Other possibilities that need to be ruled out for posterior fossa masses in children on imaging include pilocytic astrocytoma (single cyst with enhancing cyst wall and a solid enhancing mural nodule), posterior fossa ependymoma (arise from roof of fourth ventricle and may extend inferiorly through foramina of Magendie and Luschka), and atypical teratoid/rhabdoid tumor (commonly lateralized in cerebellar hemispheres, hemorrhage may be present). Although radiology is indicative, definite distinction can be made only on histopathology.

Diffusion imaging may show low ADC values in medulloblastoma or ATRT.

## 19.9 Risk Stratification

This is traditionally performed using modified Chang criteria, which include the child's age, amount of residual disease in postoperative bed, and the spread of disease. Children older than 3 years with residual disease <1.5 $cm^2$ and no CSF or extraneural spread are categorized as standard risk, while those with any of these three characteristics: younger than 3 years, a larger residual ($\geq$1.5 $cm^2$), or CSF/extraneural spread are categorized as high risk [6]. Whether each of the high risk factors confers poor prognosis of their own merit or is more commonly associated with a more aggressive molecular tumor subtype is a matter of debate and is being evaluated. Future risk strata may include molecular subtype in addition to the traditional criteria.

## 19.10 Prognostic Factors

Apart from the three factors used for risk stratification noted above (age < 3 years, disseminated disease at presentation, and large postop residual >1.5 $cm^2$), other adverse prognostic factors include

- Large cell/anaplastic histology
- MYC amplification
- Genetic predisposition/germline mutations (*PTCH1*, *PALB2*, *BRCA2*, *SUFU*)
- TP53 mutation
- GL12 mutation
- Loss of chromosome 17p

## 19.11 Treatment

Treatment strategy consists of two initial steps: interventions to relieve high intracranial pressure and specific tumor-directed therapy based on risk category.

**Ventriculoperitoneal shunt** Obstructive hydrocephalus due to compression of fourth ventricle by the tumor may be relieved placing VP shunt if definitive surgery is delayed or the child is too sick to undergo an upfront surgical resection. Some children may need steroids to manage the vasogenic edema around the tumor that may be contributing to hydrocephalus.

**Maximal safe resection** Definitive surgery with removal of maximum tumor without causing severe neurologic deficits such as cranial nerve damage, for the posterior fossa tumor instantly relieves obstructive symptoms, provides tissue diagnosis, and is an essential component for disease control. It is possible to perform a near total resection (with >90% of tumor excised) in 80% patients. Nearly 25% of patients operated for vermian lesions may develop cerebellar mutism or posterior fossa syndrome. Extent of resection determines the traditional risk category especially in non-metastatic patients, but it may become less relevant in the era of molecular classification [7].

**Adjuvant radiation therapy** Irrespective of risk category/disease extent, radiation therapy is essential for cure in all patients. The entire subarachnoid space or craniospinal axis is the target due to the high propensity of the tumor for CSF dissemination. Patterns of relapse and survival patterns observed when treating limited volumes (posterior fossa, posterior fossa and spine, craniospinal axis) have led to establishment of CSI as the minimum standard for adjuvant RT [8]. It may be difficult to deliver large volume irradiation in very young children, especially those younger than 3 years; hence, the outcome is less favorable in these patients and they may need systemic therapy to delay or omit radiotherapy. Broadly, the child receives radiotherapy to whole brain and spine for phase 1, while phase 2 involves irradiation to the site of gross disease (posterior fossa tumor as well as any other gross nodular lesions in brain or spine) (Fig. 19.1).

Conventional radiotherapy technique consists of 3D conformal radiotherapy. Since CSI entails irradiation of long segments and complex fields, one field is not

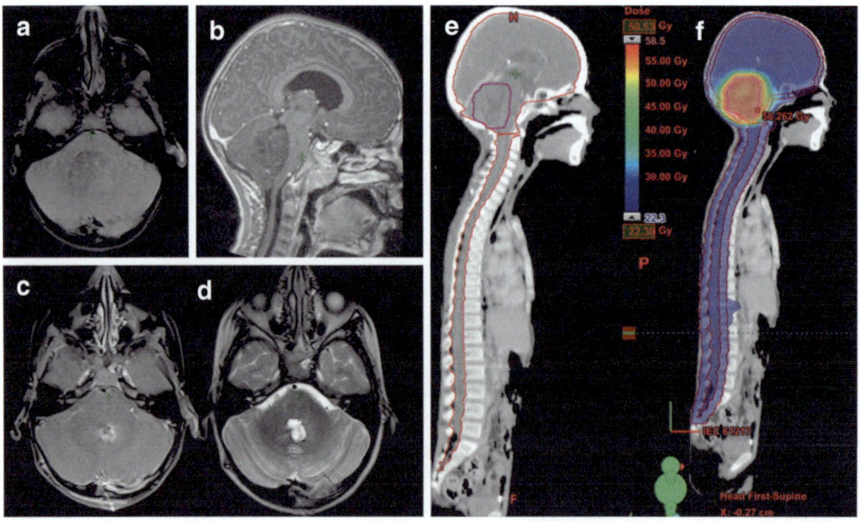


**Fig. 19.1** Preoperative T1 contrast MRI (**a**) axial and (**b**) sagittal sections showing an heterogeneously enhancing midline tumor in posterior fossa with brainstem compression and obstructive hydrocephalus. Postoperative MRI of the same patient with minimal residual tumor<1.5 $cm^2$ on axial (**c**) T1 contrast and (**d**) T2 weighted images. (**e**) Radiotherapy planning CT (sagittal view) of this patient showing the clinical target volumes for whole brain and whole spine (red) and tumor bed boost (magenta). (**f**) Dose color wash of the RT plan with 23.4 Gy to craniospinal axis and 54 Gy to tumor bed

sufficient to treat the entire target and several fields (usually two parallel opposed portals for brain and 1–2 fields for spine with junction matching) are used. Although initial treatments were planned with patient in prone position with hands by sides with easy visualization of spinal fields, use of simulations (X-ray or CT-based) has made treatment in a more comfortable supine position feasible. Supine position is also preferred if the child needs anesthesia. These days, many modern technological advancements such as IMRT and VMAT have enabled better dose distribution (with avoidance of regions of unacceptably high or low doses) at junctions, as well as reduction of dose to critical organs such as eyes, thyroid, heart, bowel, etc. Tomotherapy has obviated the need for junction placement or matching. These techniques conform high dose to targets but deliver a much larger volume of low dose to entire body due to multiple or rotational beams, thus increasing the integral dose as well as increasing the risk of hematologic toxicity [9]. Proton therapy is able to mitigate these adverse effects with a much better beam profile, thus considerably reducing the exit dose to several organs outside the target volume. However, its availability is limited in India and the cost of therapy is prohibitive for most.

When using conventional simulation, the field borders use bony references as landmarks. When treating whole brain, care is taken to include cribriform plate, posterior third of orbit, temporal lobes, and pituitary fossa to avoid missing the meninges in these regions (German helmet technique). The fields flash into air on cranial and posterior aspect. The brain-spine junction is kept in lower part of cervical spine to avoid exit of the spinal field into the oral cavity and mandible in children. 1–2 spinal fields are used with width encompassing the transverse processes of vertebrae (to include neural foramina) and depth of prescription such that the spinal cord with margin receives the prescription dose. The lower edge of the spinal field should include the entire thecal sac with 1 cm margin—this may be assessed using the spinal MRI and is usually kept at S2-S3 junction.

When using CT-based planning, the entire subarachnoid space needs to be delineated as target for craniospinal RT. SIOPE guidelines may be used to delineate clinical target volume, and same areas as mentioned in conventional simulation need to be delineated, including meningeal reflections over various cranial nerves including entire length of optic nerve, internal auditory canal, superior orbital fissure, foramen rotundum, foramen ovale, jugular foramen, hypoglossal canal, and exiting nerve roots at all intervertebral junctions [10]. Additional PTV margin (depending on expected motion and setup error depending on the cranial and spinal segment) is given—this margin may be lesser in cranial region (4–6 mm) but higher in lumbar spine (8–10 mm) due to larger chances of motion; the immobilization technique—single vs dual—may also impact the margin needed [11].

SFOP guidelines were conventionally used to plan the posterior fossa boost, with the borders placed 5 mm anterior to clivus (anterior), parallel to anterior margin, but extending into air behind occiput (posterior), cranial margin kept 1 cm superior to the midpoint of a horizontal line bisecting the skull into top and bottom halves, and caudal margin kept a cm below the foramen magnum [12].

In CT-based planning as per SIOPE, the entire posterior fossa (MRI may aid visualization) including brainstem and prepontine cistern constitutes the boost CTV

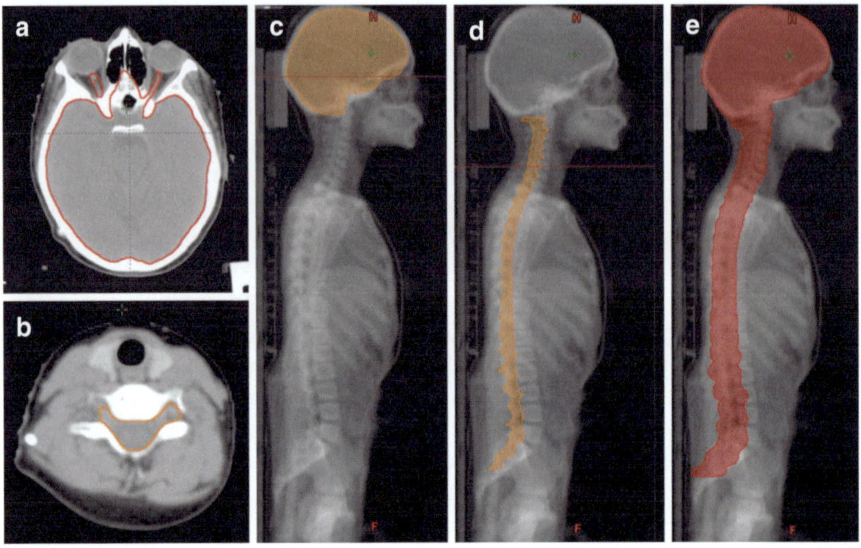


**Fig. 19.2** CT-based delineation of CSI targets as per SIOPE guidelines. (**a**) Whole brain, (**b**) spinal cord including neural foramina. Lateral digitally reconstructed radiograph projections of (**c**) CTV brain, (**d**) CTV spine, and (**e**) PTV CSI

in high risk cases, and a PTV margin of 3–5 mm may be given [13]. When treating standard risk medulloblastoma, the tumor bed and any residual tumor on co-registered T1 contrast MRI is delineated as the GTV, CTV boost consists of 1–1.5 cm expansion around GTV, constrained at natural barriers such as bone, and PTV boost is given an additional 3–5 mm margin. (Fig. 19.2).

During CT-based planning, all normal tissues and organs from vertex till obturator foramen are delineated individually as organs at risk. Constraints for these organs may be given using QUANTEC or PENTEC guidelines.

## 19.12 Infants and Young Children

Radiotherapy is challenging in this category due to its potential to cause long-term severe neurologic sequelae due to impediment with brain growth, and treatment may consist of systemic therapy (chemotherapy) with or without autologous hematopoietic stem cell rescue.

Infants with SHH medulloblastoma were treated in HIT-2000 trial with systemic chemotherapy and intraventricular methotrexate [14]. After 2006, focal RT (54 Gy) was added for classic or large cell/anaplastic histologic types. SHH group showed excellent outcomes (93% 5y PFS and 100% 5y OS), suggesting a role of intraventricular Mtx in SHH-I category for improving outcomes. Although all patients had suboptimal IQ scores compared to normal children, the IQ decline was much more pronounced after RT. With the St Jude's risk adapted consolidation therapy, focal

RT did not seem to benefit in any category, while SHH-II group did not seem to need intraventricular methotrexate either to maintain similar control [15].

Non-Wnt/non-SHH medulloblastoma had a survival rate of under 20% at 5 years despite risk adapted therapy in St Jude study [15].

## 19.13 Children ≥3 Years (High Risk)

These children are at high risk of relapse and have poor survival despite aggressive adjuvant therapy.

The conventional dose of CSI in this group is 36–39.6 gray (Gy) at 1.5–1.8 Gy per fractions, followed by a boost to entire posterior fossa till 54–55.8 Gy at 1.8 Gy per fraction. Additional sites of intracranial or spinal metastases are given boost based on tolerance of that region (total 45–50.4 Gy in spinal cord and 54 Gy in intracranial or cauda region). Reduction of boost volume may be feasible in some high risk cases but prospective data is lacking [16]. Earlier studies used concurrent vincristine during RT but the current trend is to omit vincristine due to minimal impact on survival while adding to toxicity. This practice has yielded 5y survival of 58.7% in high risk patients [17]. For patients with metastatic group 3 medulloblastoma, concurrent carboplatin has shown promise and may be considered in patients with very good nutritional status as long as craniospinal RT delivery is not compromised due to hematologic toxicity and poor tolerance [18, 19]. A study from TMH Mumbai has shown that benefit of carboplatin may be maintained even when administered only for first 15 days of CSI [20]. Prophylactic G-CSF given on weekends may help reduce hematologic toxicity with CSI and reduce treatment interruptions [21].

Following RT, all children receive multiagent chemotherapy, starting 6 weeks after completion of radiotherapy.

Attempts have been made to improve outcomes in high risk patients with use of autologous stem cell transplant or more intensive chemotherapy regimens following CSI dose reduction, with encouraging event free survival approaching 70% at 5 years [22, 23]. Hyperfractionated RT-CSI dose up to 39 Gy in 30 fractions (2 daily fractions of 1.3 Gy each) and posterior fossa boost till 60 Gy (2 daily fractions of 1.5 Gy each) has also shown encouraging survival [24].

Figure 19.3 shows the postoperative MRI in a child with high risk medulloblastoma.

## 19.14 Children ≥3 Years (Standard Risk)

In children with standard risk disease, craniospinal RT dose is 23.4 Gy in 13 fractions, followed by boost till 54 Gy to the site of gross disease (involved field radiotherapy). In these children, there is now data to suggest that boost volume can be limited to tumor bed and not the entire posterior fossa, which reduces the dose to cochlea, temporal lobes, optic structures, as well as pituitary, without compromising

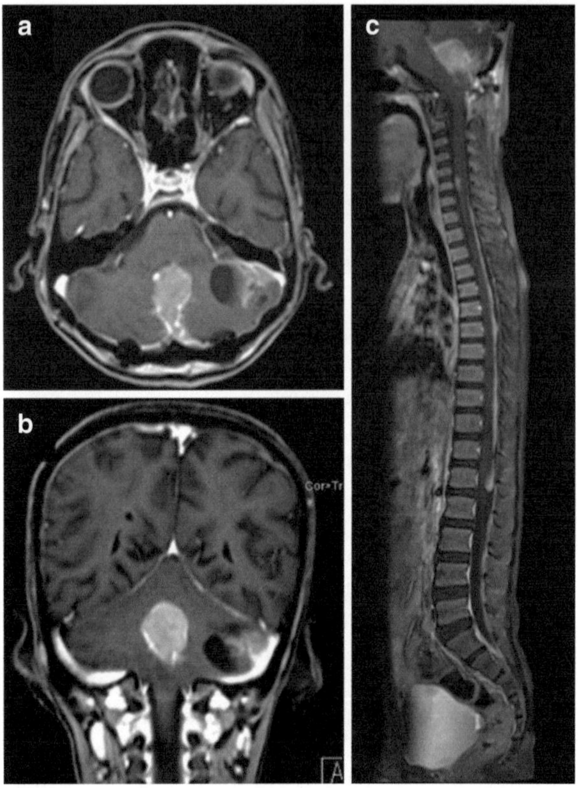


**Fig. 19.3** A 5 year old child had undergone subtotal resection of a midline posterior fossa lesion, which revealed group 3 medulloblastoma on histopathology. Postoperative T1 contrast MRI in (**a**) axial (brain), (**b**) coronal (brain), and (**c**) sagittal (spine) orientations demonstrate a large enhancing residual tumor in postoperative bed, another left cerebellar lesion with solid-cystic components, multiple areas of leptomeningeal enhancement along the spinal cord and cauda equina. The child was treated with craniospinal irradiation (36 Gy in 20 fractions), boost to posterior fossa (19.8 Gy in 11 fractions) and to enhancing region in spine (9 Gy in 5 fractions) (Plan not shown)

on outcome. This approach of reduced CSI dose and reduced boost volumes yields 5-year survival approaching 85% [13]. Although reduction in boost volumes should yield lower morbidity in terms of neurocognitive and hearing functions, this has not been observed in the follow-up reported so far. Weekly vincristine that was earlier considered standard is no longer recommended. Further attempts to reduce CSI dose to 18 Gy resulted in higher results in poorer event free survival, confined to group 4 (5y EFS 77.2% vs 97.1%, $p = 0.047$). It was also observed that SHH group had lesser failures when given IFRT instead of posterior fossa boost. Ongoing trials are exploring CSI dose reduction to 15–18 Gy in Wnt tumors. Efforts to omit CSI in Wnt tumors have yielded higher failures; hence, CSI remains standard even in this favorable subgroup [25].

Hyperfractionation has been explored in these patients with the intent to reduce neuro- and ototoxicity but has not yielded better therapeutic ratio in one study while in a small Indian study, both neurocognitive function and hearing were better [26–28].

When adjuvant chemotherapy is not given in these patients, reduced dose CSI (23.4 Gy) results in higher spinal failures and poorer event free survival compared to standard dose CSI (36 Gy); hence, standard dose CSI may be preferred in some standard risk patients when chemotherapy administration is not feasible for any reason [29].

## 19.15 Adjuvant Chemotherapy

Adjuvant chemotherapy is integral to the treatment regime in high risk category as well as with reduced dose CSI in standard risk category. Treatment is typically started 6 weeks after RT. Various regimes have been explored historically incorporating combinations of vincristine, lomustine, cisplatin, and cyclophosphamide. In standard risk, pre-radiotherapy chemotherapy worsens outcomes while it may have some use in high risk or metastatic disease.

The ACNS0331 trial that established the role of IFRT for boost used 9 cycles of chemotherapy—cycles 1–2, 4–5, 7–8 used vincristine, lomustine, and cisplatin, while cycles 3, 6, 9 used vincristine and cyclophosphamide [13]. Randomized comparisons of chemotherapy regimes combining vincristine and cisplatin with either lomustine or cyclophosphamide demonstrate similar outcomes but different toxicity profiles [30]. This combination of vincristine (1.4 mg/m$^2$ D1 and 8), cisplatin 75 mg/m$^2$ D1, and lomustine75 mg/m$^2$ orally, given 6 weekly for 8 cycles, is now popular as Packer's regime. In low and middle income countries, alternative regime replacing lomustine with cyclophosphamide (1000 mg/m$^2$ Day 1 and 2) and given 3–4 weekly for 6–8 cycles is used due to lower myelosuppression and thus lower need for supportive care. In India, a modified regime delivering 6 cycles of this schedule but limiting cisplatin to cycles 2, 4 and 6 results in lesser ototoxicity but similar control rates [31, 32]. Selection and duration of the regime is similar irrespective of the risk category.

Chemotherapy is also used as a strategy to delay radiotherapy in very young children <3 years after surgery. Although various drug combinations including high dose or intravenous methotrexate have been used with encouraging outcomes, the regime carboplatin 600 mg/m$^2$ D1, cyclophosphamide 1000 mg/m$^2$ D1, and etoposide 100 mg/m$^2$ D1–3 every 4 weeks is recommended for 12 cycles or till the child turns 3 years [32]. Following chemotherapy, RT is delivered if feasible after the child turns 3—decisions are made on individual case parameters—standard risk may be offered conformal RT to tumor bed or CSI with boost, while high risk is offered CSI with boost.

## 19.16 Complications of Therapy

Surgery: Posterior fossa syndrome and persistent or worsened cranial nerve palsies and ataxia may happen [33]. Children who have VP shunts may have repetitive blockage or infections if appropriate care is not taken.

Radiotherapy: Craniospinal RT in young children may lead to severe IQ impairment due to interference with nervous system maturation. Even in older children, neurocognitive decline may be expected in long term [34]. Irradiation of hypothalamic-pituitary axis may lead to several hormonal deficiencies with resultant precocious puberty, hypogonadism, hypothyroidism, adrenal insufficiency, and reduced skeletal growth due to growth hormone deficiency [35]. Irradiation of cochlea, lens, larynx, mandible, spine, thyroid, lungs, heart, kidneys, bowel, and genitalia may result in long-term deficits in these organs. Radiation-induced vasculopathy may cause a higher risk of stroke in survivors.

Chemotherapy: It may result in repeated myelosuppression and risks of bleeding and infection that may need hospitalization and supportive management. Lomustine may cause delayed thrombocytopenia, while cisplatin may cause ototoxicity.

Infertility is contributed both by radiation therapy and chemotherapy. Patients may also need hormone replacement therapy to overcome gonadal insufficiency.

Second malignancies: The incidence is estimated around 4.2% at 10 years in standard risk patients; the most common sites include brain and thyroid [36].

COG has released long-term survivor guidelines that may aid in meticulous follow-up in these patients [37].

## 19.17 Post-Treatment Follow-Up

Patients are recommended for follow-up 3-monthly for first 2 years, then 6–12 monthly for the next 5–10 years, then every 1–2 years. Clinical history and physical examination along with MRI of brain and, if indicated, spine imaging (especially in patients with spine disease) should be undertaken on each visit.

## 19.18 Recurrences After Curative Therapy

Nearly 20–30% medulloblastomas may recur during follow-up. Recurrence patterns are divided equally between local disseminated and both together. Children have earlier relapses compared to adults; most occur within first 3 years. There is no standard approach to management of recurrences. Localized recurrences may benefit from resection, followed by systemic chemotherapy and possibly reirradiation, depending to the disease-free interval. Some patients with favorable response post-surgery and chemotherapy may benefit from high dose chemotherapy (including thiotepa-based regimes) with autologous stem cell rescue with 10-year survival of 24%; additional radiotherapy improved event free survival [38]. Phase 2 studies have shown benefit of vismodegib, an SHH pathway inhibitor in recurrent SHH tumors [39].

Infants who were not exposed to RT earlier may receive CSI as part of salvage regime after crossing the age of 3 years. Children who were older at first diagnosis and have SHH tumors, localized recurrence, and salvage CSI were prognostic for better survival [40].

## 19.19 Other Embryonal Tumors

### 19.19.1 Atypical Teratoid/Rhabdoid Tumor

These tumors are highly aggressive tumors characterized by the loss of INI1 (SMARCB1, chromosome 22) or SMARCA4. They occur in very young children, with the cerebellum (particularly cerebellopontine angle) being the most common site. Tumors may occasionally be multifocal. Symptoms may be related to raised intracranial pressure or adjacent structure invasion (cranial nerve palsies). MRI may demonstrate T1 hypo- and T2 iso- to hypointense lesions with cysts or hemorrhage; leptomeningeal enhancement may be present at diagnosis. Definite distinction from medulloblastoma can be made only on histology which demonstrates rhabdoid cells, necrosis, and increased mitoses. INI1 nuclear staining is lost and is pathognomonic. A third of patients may have germline mutations. For ATRT as well, molecular analysis has demonstrated three subtypes: ATRT-TYR, ATRT-SHH, and ATRT-MYC, which may have differences in age at presentation and prognosis.

Treatment is based on the same principles as medulloblastoma, including surgery, radiotherapy, and chemotherapy. Unlike medulloblastoma, where radiotherapy is delayed in young children, RT is offered even in young children due to aggressive nature of disease; however, focal radiotherapy to tumor bed may be opted instead of craniospinal radiation in young children. Targeted therapies (e.g., aurora kinase inhibitors) are being investigated. Despite aggressive therapy, prognosis is poor with 5-year survival 30–40% [41]. Children with germline mutations tend to be younger and have poorer outcomes than those with sporadic mutations.

Figure 19.4 shows the images of a patient with posterior fossa ATRT.

**Embryonal tumor with multilayered rosettes** ETMRs are tumors with genetic alterations C19MC on FISH and usually positive for LIN28A on IHC. Germline DICER1 mutations may be seen rarely, but these tumors may lack C19MC amplification. They have a tendency to present at the age of 2–3 years, mainly in females, are supratentorial (frontal > parietotemporal), and may have leptomeningeal disease at diagnosis in 25%. Clinical presentation may be related to the site of disease and may range from focal neurogic deficits to raised intracranial pressure. MRI may show large circumscribed enhancing lesions with cystic change or calcification; no features are specific to ETMR. Treatment is similar to other embryonal tumors, including radiotherapy according to age. PARP inhibitors may have a therapeutic role. Prognosis is dismal with median survival less than a year.

**CNS neuroblastoma, FOXR2-activated** This entity was introduced in 2021 classification and accounts for 10% of CNS embryonal tumors. Tumors are supratentorial. IHC may show OLIG2 positivity. NGS may help identify FOXR2alterations.

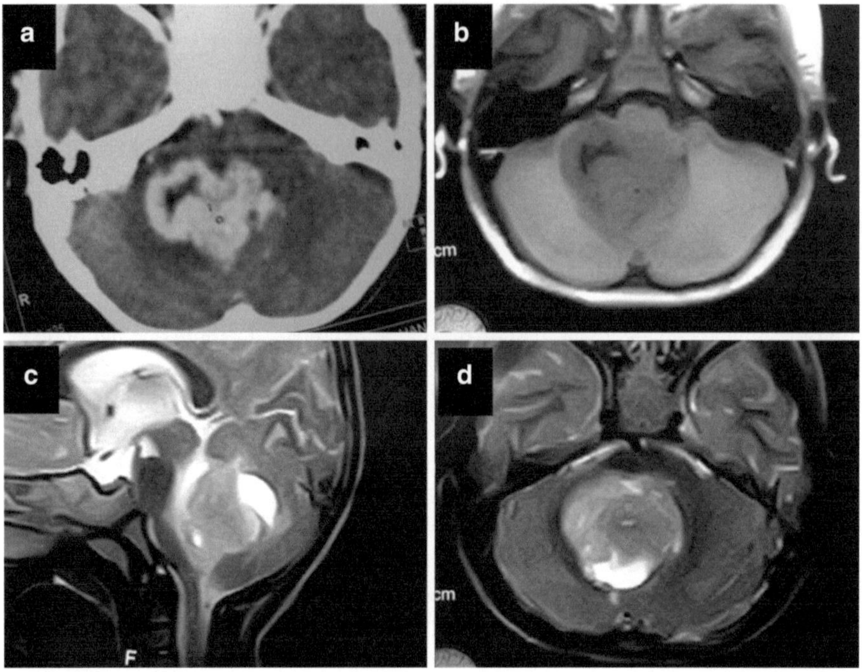


**Fig. 19.4** (**a**) CT head shows a hyperdense fourth ventricular mass with internal necrosis. Corresponding MR images in (**b**) T1 axial, (**c**) T2 sagittal, and (**d**) T2 axial orientations demonstrate the T1 hypointense and T2 hetereointense lesion with internal necrosis and cystic change causing obstructive hydrocephalus. After craniotomy and resection, postoperative histopathology was revealed as atypical teratoid rhabdoid tumor

**CNS tumor with BCOR internal tandem duplication** This entity was also introduced in 2021 classification. These tumors present in children under 5 years and have extensive multilobar involvement at diagnosis.

**CNS embryonal tumor NEC/NOS** This category includes tumors that have embryonal histology but do not have a distinct molecular profile for inclusion in above groups. These are rare and occur more commonly in infants and young children.

## References

1. Ostrom QT, Price M, Ryan K, Edelson J, Neff C, Cioffi G, Waite KA, Kruchko C, Barnholtz-Sloan JS. CBTRUS statistical report: Pediatric Brain Tumor Foundation childhood and adolescent primary brain and other central nervous system tumors diagnosed in the United States in 2014-2018. Neuro-Oncology. 2022;24(Suppl 3):iii1–iii38.

2. Louis DN, Perry A, Wesseling P, Brat DJ, Cree IA, Figarella-Branger D, Hawkins C, Ng HK, Pfister SM, Reifenberger G, Soffietti R, von Deimling A, Ellison DW. The 2021 WHO classification of tumors of the central nervous system: a summary. Neuro Oncol. 2021;23(8):1231–51.
3. Perreault S, Ramaswamy V, Achrol AS, Chao K, Liu TT, Shih D, Remke M, Schubert S, Bouffet E, Fisher PG, Partap S, Vogel H, Taylor MD, Cho YJ, Yeom KW. MRI surrogates for molecular subgroups of medulloblastoma. AJNR Am J Neuroradiol. 2014;35(7):1263–9.
4. Ellison DW, Dalton J, Kocak M, Nicholson SL, Fraga C, Neale G, Kenney AM, Brat DJ, Perry A, Yong WH, Taylor RE, Bailey S, Clifford SC, Gilbertson RJ. Medulloblastoma: clinicopathological correlates of SHH, WNT, and non-SHH/WNT molecular subgroups. Acta Neuropathol. 2011;121(3):381–96.
5. Waszak SM, Northcott PA, Buchhalter I, Robinson GW, Sutter C, Groebner S, et al. Spectrum and prevalence of genetic predisposition in medulloblastoma: a retrospective genetic study and prospective validation in a clinical trial cohort. Lancet Oncol. 2018;19(6):785–98.
6. Chang CH, Housepian EM, Herbert C Jr. An operative staging systemand a megavoltage radiotherapeutictechnicforcerebellarmedulloblastomas. Radiology. 1969;93(6):1351–9.
7. Thompson EM, Bramall A, Herndon JE 2nd, Taylor MD, Ramaswamy V. The clinical importance of medulloblastoma extent of resection: a systematic review. J Neuro-Oncol. 2018;139(3):523–39.
8. Landberg TG, Lindgren ML, Cavallin-Ståhl EK, Svahn-Tapper GO, Sundbärg G, Garwicz S, Lagergren JA, Gunnesson VL, Brun AE, Cronqvist SE. Improvements in the radiotherapy of medulloblastoma, 1946-1975. Cancer. 1980;45(4):670–8.
9. Petersson K, Gebre-Medhin M, Ceberg C, Nilsson P, Engström P, Knöös T, Kjellén E. Haematological toxicity in adult patients receiving craniospinal irradiation--indication of a dose-bath effect. Radiother Oncol 2014;111(1):47–51.
10. Ajithkumar T, Horan G, Padovani L, Thorp N, Timmermann B, Alapetite C, Gandola L, Ramos M, Van Beek K, Christiaens M, Lassen-Ramshad Y, Magelssen H, Nilsson K, Saran F, Rombi B, Kortmann R, Janssens GO, SIOPE BTG Radiotherapy Group. SIOPE—brain tumor group consensus guideline on craniospinal target volume delineation for high-precision radiotherapy. Radiother Oncol. 2018;128(2):192–7.
11. Krishnatry R, Gudi S, Siwach A, Patil A, Rajesh RK, Shekhar HK, Sutar V, Chatterjee A, Goda JS, Jalali R, Gupta T. Impact of immobilisation and image guidance protocol on planning target volume margins for supine craniospinal irradiation. Rep Pract Oncol Radiother. 2022;27(2):250–9.
12. Carrie C, Hoffstetter S, Gomez F, Moncho V, Doz F, Alapetite C, Murraciole X, Maire JP, Benhassel M, Chapet S, Quetin P, Kolodie H, Lagrange JL, Cuillere JC, Habrand JL. Impact of targeting deviations on outcome in medulloblastoma: study of the French Society of Pediatric Oncology (SFOP). Int J Radiat Oncol Biol Phys. 1999;45(2):435–9.
13. Michalski JM, Janss AJ, Vezina LG, Smith KS, Billups CA, Burger PC, et al. Children's oncology group phase III trial of reduced-dose and reduced-volume radiotherapy with chemotherapy for newly diagnosed average-risk medulloblastoma. J Clin Oncol. 2021;39(24):2685–97.
14. Mynarek M, von Hoff K, Pietsch T, et al. Nonmetastatic medulloblastoma of early childhood: results from the Prospective Clinical Trial HIT-2000 and an extended validation cohort. J Clin Oncol. 2020;38(18):2028–40.
15. Robinson GW, Rudneva VA, Buchhalter I, et al. Risk-adapted therapy for young children with medulloblastoma (SJYC07): therapeutic and molecular outcomes from a multicentre, phase 2 trial. Lancet Oncol. 2018;19(6):768–84.
16. Tian S, Sudmeier LJ, Zhang C, Madden NA, Buchwald ZS, Shu HG, Curran WJ, Eaton BR, Esiashvili N. Reduced-volume tumor-bed boost is not associated with inferior local control and survival outcomes in high-risk medulloblastoma. Pediatr Blood Cancer. 2020;67(1):e28027.
17. Gajjar A, Robinson GW, Smith KS, et al. Outcomes by clinical and molecular features in children with medulloblastoma treated with risk-adapted therapy: results of an International Phase III Trial (SJMB03). J Clin Oncol. 2021;39(7):822–35.

18. Jakacki RI, Burger PC, Zhou T, et al. Outcome of children with metastatic medulloblastoma treated with carboplatin during craniospinal radiotherapy: a Children's Oncology Group Phase I/II study. J Clin Oncol. 2012;30(21):2648–53.
19. Leary SES, Packer RJ, Li Y, Billups CA, Smith KS, Jaju A, Heier L, Burger P, Walsh K, Han Y, Embry L, Hadley J, Kumar R, Michalski J, Hwang E, Gajjar A, Pollack IF, Fouladi M, Northcott PA, Olson JM. Efficacy of carboplatin and isotretinoin in children with high-risk medulloblastoma: a randomized clinical trial from the Children's Oncology Group. JAMA Oncol. 2021;7(9):1313–21.
20. Gupta T, Sinha S, Chinnaswamy G, Vora T, Prasad M, Bhat V, Goda JS, Krishnatry R, Chatterjee A, Epari S, Sahay A, Moiyadi A, Shetty P, Patil V, Khatua S, Jalali R, Kurkure P. Safety and efficacy of concurrent carboplatin during full-dose craniospinal irradiation for high-risk/metastatic medulloblastoma in a resource-limited setting. Pediatr Blood Cancer. 2021;68(5):e28925.
21. Madan R, Kumar N, Gupta A, Gupta K, Salunke P, Khosla D, Yadav BS, Kapoor R. Effect of prophylactic granulocyte-colony stimulating factor (G-CSF) on acute hematological toxicity in medulloblastoma patients during craniospinal irradiation (CSI). Clin Neurol Neurosurg. 2020;196:105975.
22. Gajjar A, Chintagumpala M, Ashley D, Kellie S, Kun LE, Merchant TE, Woo S, Wheeler G, Ahern V, Krasin MJ, Fouladi M, Broniscer A, Krance R, Hale GA, Stewart CF, Dauser R, Sanford RA, Fuller C, Lau C, Boyett JM, Wallace D, Gilbertson RJ. Risk-adapted craniospinal radiotherapy followed by high-dose chemotherapy and stem-cell rescue in children with newly diagnosed medulloblastoma (St Jude Medulloblastoma-96): long-term results from a prospective, multicentre trial. Lancet Oncol. 2006;7(10):813–20.
23. Sung KW, Lim DH, Son MH, Lee SH, Yoo KH, Koo HH, Kim JH, Suh YL, Joung YS, Shin HJ. Reduced-dose craniospinal radiotherapy followed by tandem high-dose chemotherapy and autologous stem cell transplantation in patients with high-risk medulloblastoma. Neuro-Oncology. 2013;15(3):352–9.
24. Gandola L, Massimino M, Cefalo G, Solero C, Spreafico F, Pecori E, Riva D, Collini P, Pignoli E, Giangaspero F, Luksch R, Berretta S, Poggi G, Biassoni V, Ferrari A, Pollo B, Favre C, Sardi I, Terenziani M, Fossati-Bellani F. Hyperfractionated accelerated radiotherapy in the Milan strategy for metastatic medulloblastoma. J Clin Oncol. 2009;27(4):566–71.
25. Gupta T, Pervez S, Dasgupta A, Chatterjee A, Epari S, Chinnaswamy G, Jalali R. Omission of upfront craniospinal irradiation in patients with low-risk WNT-pathway medulloblastoma is associated with unacceptably high risk of Neuraxial failure. Clin Cancer Res. 2022;28(19):4180–5.
26. Lannering B, Rutkowski S, Doz F, Pizer B, Gustafsson G, Navajas A, et al. Hyperfractionated versus conventional radiotherapy followed by chemotherapy in standard-risk medulloblastoma: results from the randomized multicenter HIT-SIOP PNET 4 trial. J Clin Oncol. 2012;30(26):3187–93.
27. Gupta T, Jalali R, Goswami S, Nair V, Moiyadi A, Epari S, Sarin R. Early clinical outcomes demonstrate preserved cognitive function in children with average-risk medulloblastoma when treated with hyperfractionated radiation therapy. Int J Radiat Oncol Biol Phys. 2012;83(5):1534–40.
28. Gupta T, Mohanty S, Kannan S, Jalali R. Prospective longitudinal assessment of sensorineural hearing loss with hyperfractionated radiation therapy alone in patients with average-risk medulloblastoma. Neurooncol Pract. 2014;1(3):86–93.
29. Thomas PR, Deutsch M, Kepner JL, Boyett JM, Krischer J, Aronin P, et al. Low-stage medulloblastoma: final analysis of trial comparing standard-dose with reduced-dose neuraxis irradiation. J Clin Oncol. 2000;18(16):3004–11.
30. Packer RJ, Gajjar A, Vezina G, Rorke-Adams L, Burger PC, Robertson PL, Bayer L, LaFond D, Donahue BR, Marymont MH, Muraszko K, Langston J, Sposto R. Phase III study of craniospinal radiation therapy followed by adjuvant chemotherapy for newly diagnosed average-risk medulloblastoma. J Clin Oncol. 2006;24(25):4202–8.

31. Nageswara Rao AA, Wallace DJ, Billups C, Boyett JM, Gajjar A, Packer RJ. Cumulative cisplatin dose is not associated with event-free or overall survival in children with newly diagnosed average-risk medulloblastoma treated with cisplatin based adjuvant chemotherapy: report from the Children's Oncology Group. Pediatr Blood Cancer. 2014;61(1):102–6.
32. Gupta T, Sarkar C, Rajshekhar V, Chatterjee S, Shirsat N, Muzumdar D, Pungavkar S, Chinnaswamy G, Jalali R. Indian Society of Neuro-Oncology consensus guidelines for the contemporary management of medulloblastoma. Neurol India.;65(2):315–332.
33. Robertson PL, Muraszko KM, Holmes EJ, Sposto R, Packer RJ, Gajjar A, Dias MS, Allen JC, Children's Oncology Group. Incidence and severity of postoperative cerebellar mutism syndrome in children with medulloblastoma: a prospective study by the Children's Oncology Group. J Neurosurg. 2006;105(6 Suppl):444–51.
34. Palmer SL, Armstrong C, Onar-Thomas A, Wu S, Wallace D, Bonner MJ, Schreiber J, Swain M, Chapieski L, Mabbott D, Knight S, Boyle R, Gajjar A. Processing speed, attention, and working memory after treatment for medulloblastoma: an international, prospective, and longitudinal study. J Clin Oncol. 2013;31(28):3494–500.
35. Laughton SJ, Merchant TE, Sklar CA, Kun LE, Fouladi M, Broniscer A, Morris EB, Sanders RP, Krasin MJ, Shelso J, Xiong Z, Wallace D, Gajjar A. Endocrine outcomes for children with embryonal brain tumors after risk-adapted craniospinal and conformal primary-site irradiation and high-dose chemotherapy with stem-cell rescue on the SJMB-96 trial. J Clin Oncol. 2008;26(7):1112–8.
36. Packer RJ, Zhou T, Holmes E, Vezina G, Gajjar A. Survival and secondary tumors in children with medulloblastoma receiving radiotherapy and adjuvant chemotherapy: results of Children's Oncology Group trial A9961. Neuro Oncol. 2013;15(1):97–103.
37. Landier W, Bhatia S, Eshelman DA, Forte KJ, Sweeney T, Hester AL, et al. Development of risk-based guidelines for pediatric cancer survivors: the Children's Oncology Group long-term follow-up guidelines from the Children's Oncology Group late effects committee and nursing discipline. J Clin Oncol. 2004;22(24):4979–90.
38. Dunkel IJ, Gardner SL, Garvin JH Jr, Goldman S, Shi W, Finlay JL. High-dose carboplatin, thiotepa, and etoposide with autologous stem cell rescue for patients with previously irradiated recurrent medulloblastoma. Neuro-Oncology. 2010;12(3):297–303.
39. Robinson GW, Orr BA, Wu G, Gururangan S, Lin T, Qaddoumi I, et al. Vismodegib exerts targeted efficacy against recurrent sonic hedgehog-subgroup medulloblastoma: results from phase II Pediatric Brain Tumor Consortium Studies PBTC-025B and PBTC-032. J Clin Oncol. 2015;33(24):2646–54.
40. Erker C, Mynarek M, Bailey S, Mazewski CM, Baroni L, Massimino M, et al. Outcomes of infants and young children with relapsed medulloblastoma after initial craniospinal irradiation-sparing approaches: an international Cohort Study. J Clin Oncol. 2023;41(10):1921–32.
41. Reddy AT, Strother DR, Judkins AR, Burger PC, Pollack IF, Krailo MD, Buxton AB, Williams-Hughes C, Fouladi M, Mahajan A, Merchant TE, Ho B, Mazewski CM, Lewis VA, Gajjar A, Vezina LG, Booth TN, Parsons KW, Poss VL, Zhou T, Biegel JA, Huang A. Efficacy of high-dose chemotherapy and three-dimensional conformal radiation for atypical teratoid/rhabdoid tumor: a report from the Children's Oncology Group Trial ACNS0333. J Clin Oncol. 2020;38(11):1175–85.

# 20 Pediatric Ependymoma

Arnav Tiwari, M. Karthigeyan, Renu Madan, and Narendra Kumar

## 20.1 Introduction

Ependymomas are glial neoplasms arising from the ependymal lining of the ventricle or central canal of spinal cord. These tumors account for 8–10% of central nervous system tumors in children. Although the pediatric ependymomas can occur both in brain and spine, the latter is less frequently seen; approximately 90% of childhood ependymomas are present in the intracranial compartment. The World Health Organization (WHO) 2021 recently classifies the ependymal tumors, depending on their site of origin into supratentorial, posterior fossa, and spinal types which are further characterized according to their molecular profile [1]. Based on histological grade, the ependymomas have been conventionally categorized into grade 1 (subependymoma), grade II (classic), and grade III (anaplastic) variety, albeit the tumor determined outcomes with regard to their histological grade alone have been inconsistent.

## 20.2 Intracranial Ependymomas

Intracranial ependymomas (IE) are the third most common brain neoplasm in children and constitute about 6–10% of intracranial tumors in this age group [2]. Over 50% of IE are reported to occur in children <3 years of age [3]. Of the IE, 70% are

A. Tiwari · N. Kumar
Department of Radiotherapy and Oncology, PGIMER, Chandigarh, India

M. Karthigeyan
Department of Neurosurgery, PGIMER, Chandigarh, India

R. Madan (✉)
Department of Radiotherapy and Oncology, Postgraduate Institute of Medical Education and Research, Chandigarh, India



R. Madan et al. (eds.), *Evidence Based Practice in Pediatric Radiation Oncology*, https://doi.org/10.1007/978-981-96-4872-6_20

infratentorially located arising from the fourth ventricular floor, while 30% manifest in the supratentorial portion [4]. Mostly, the supratentorial ependymomas (50–60%) are extra-ventricular in origin and, however, are found adjacent to the ventricular wall particularly lateral ventricle, while a few originate from remote brain parenchyma ependymal cell rests.

Traditionally, ependymomas are classified as WHO grades 1, 2, and 3. However, according to the latest WHO classification, these are now categorized into the following groups [1]:

1. Supratentorial ependymoma (ST-EP).
   (a) ST-EP, *ZFTA* fusion-positive.
   (b) ST-EP, *YAP1* fusion-positive.
   (c) ST-EP, grade 2/3.
2. Posterior fossa ependymoma (PF-EP).
   (a) PF-EP, group A.
   (b) PF-EP, group B.
   (c) PF-EP, grade 2/3.
3. Spinal ependymomas.
   (a) Spinal ependymoma, *MYCN*-amplified.
   (b) Myxopapillary ependymoma, grade 2.
   (c) Spinal ependymoma, grade 2/3.
4. Subependymoma, grade 1.

Detailed pathology has been discussed in a separate chapter.

### 20.2.1 Initial Work-Up/Evaluation

#### 20.2.1.1 Clinical Presentation

The clinical presentation of IE depends on the tumor location, their size, and extent. The infratentorial lesions, by virtue of their location in the floor of fourth ventricle, can manifest with nausea and vomiting due to the area postrema involvement and other features like ataxia, cranial nerve involvement, and cerebellar signs. The supratentorial ependymomas generally tend to present with raised intracranial pressure symptoms, focal deficits, seizures, and cognitive involvement [5].

#### 20.2.1.2 Imaging

The preferred imaging modality in the initial evaluation of IE is a contrast enhanced magnetic resonance imaging (CEMRI). Apart from aiding the diagnosis, it better delineates the lesion and helps planning the degree of surgical excision. IE usually present as a mass occupying the fourth ventricle with secondary obstructive hydrocephalus. They typically show spread into the foramen of Magendie to extend into cervico-medullary junction and spinal cord (60%) and up to the cerebellopontine angle (CPA) through the foramen of Luschka (15%) [4]. This growth characteristic (plastic appearance) highly aids to differentiate ependymoma from other common pediatric tumors such as medulloblastomas and choroid plexus papilloma; the tumors usually insinuate and encase the adjacent neurovascular structures. At times, the posterior fossa ependymomas can be seen to arise from a non-midline location such as CP angle. These non-midline tumors originate from the ependymal cell rests in the foramen of Luschka, extend laterally into the CPA, and have been reported to carry relatively poor prognosis because of their tendency to encase lower cranial nerves and major brainstem vasculature [4, 6]. On MRI, the ependymomas are generally T1 hypo- to isointense and T2 hyperintense and often exhibit avid heterogeneous contrast enhancement, along with areas of necrosis and calcification. However, it is not infrequent to find few non-enhancing portions admixed with the enhancing tumor. A computed tomography delineates calcifications better that has been reported in up to 50% of the ependymal tumors, and the lesion is usually isointense in appearance [4].

The supratentorial ependymomas that usually are of higher grade (anaplastic type) are aggressive and present as heterogeneous contrast-enhancing intraparenchymal mass with both solid and cystic components (Fig. 20.2). These tumors when compared with infratentorial ependymomas have a higher tendency for cystic changes, calcification, and hemorrhages and thus show heterogeneous T1 and T2 signal intensities [4].

#### 20.2.1.3 Cerebrospinal Fluid Dissemination

A cerebrospinal fluid (CSF) seeding in ependymomas although a less common feature compared with medulloblastomas can occur in about 5–12% of patients and is an important factor determining the disease staging and patient prognosis. The CSF spinal seeding is more likely with infratentorial ependymomas, especially the high-grade tumors. A younger age, incomplete resection, and higher proliferative index are also observed to be predisposing factors [4, 7]. Considering this risk of CSF dissemination, the European Association of Neuro-Oncology (EANO) recommends mandatory craniospinal imaging and CSF cytology (which is performed not earlier than 2–3 weeks to minimize the risk of a false positive result) following surgery [3]. On MRI, the leptomeningeal tumor spread may appear as smooth enhancement along the spinal cord surface, focal enhancement along intradural space or as nodularity, thickening, and clumping of nerve roots.

### 20.2.2 Surgical Aspects and Related Outcomes

Many children, when presenting with raised intracranial pressure symptoms, may require a CSF diversion procedure (ventriculoperitoneal shunt or ventriculostomy) before proceeding with the definitive oncologic resection. However, an upward brain herniation post CSF release can be a concern especially with large posterior fossa tumors. Hence, a controlled CSF release during this surgical procedure is necessary.

Ependymoma resection of the fourth ventricle/posterior fossa poses unique challenges because of their location. Complete tumor resection should be the aim as it provides a greater likelihood of cure. Nevertheless, the radicality of tumor excision has to be often balanced with potential damage to the cranial nerves at the floor of brain stem. Though the positioning deployed in our institution is prone or concorde, other positions such as lateral oblique and semi-sitting has also been practiced. Craniotomy over craniectomy is preferred because the former lessens the chance of pseudomeningocele, CSF leak, and chronic postoperative pain and also eases wound reopening with better soft tissue planes in redo surgeries; an additional C1 laminectomy may be needed for tumors extending into the cervical canal. One should be cautious during dural opening as young children often have large dural venous lakes which can lead to sudden blood loss and hemodynamic instability. In large tumors extending through the Foramen of Magendie, the lesion can be readily seen in the cistern magna once the dura is opened. Surgical corridors such as transvermian and telovelar routes have been described for the tumor access. Because the fourth ventricular ependymomas receive its main vascularity from the distal segments of posterior inferior cerebellar arteries, identification and coagulation of these feeders can help reduce intraoperative bleeding. Gentle tumor debulking has to be performed using suction and tumor forceps and cavitron ultrasonic surgical aspirator (CUSA), avoiding undue traction on the brainstem. Any change in cardiac rate and blood pressure during tumor removal heralds brainstem manipulation and should be considered a warning sign. Utilizing intraoperative neuromonitoring (IONM) techniques such as brainstem auditory evoked potentials, motor/sensory evoked potentials, and electromyography with direct cranial nerves stimulation greatly assist tumor excision and avoid potential operative deficits. Visualization of the cerebral aqueduct with free CSF flow marks the limit of decompression at the superior pole of the tumor. The inferior pole of the tumor at the medulla/cervicomedullary junction has to be meticulously dissected off the floor of the fourth ventricle which is the usual site of the origin of these tumors. At surgery, if the tumor is found to be adherent to the fourth ventricular floor, it is prudent to leave a thin layer of tumor tissue to avoid iatrogenic brainstem and cranial nerve injuries. Because the ependymomas insinuate along the lateral cisternal space, a thorough inspection along the lateral aspect of brain stem and Foramen of Luschka is necessary to avoid overlooking of residual tumor. In the CPA ependymomas, the encasement of cranial nerves is frequent and adds to the operative morbidity in these children [6]. In comparison, supratentorial ependymomas usually exhibit better interface with the surrounding brain making their removal relatively easy.

Published literature provides convincing evidence that maximal resection is the main stay and offers the chance of best possible outcomes in pediatric IE (class II evidence, level of recommendation B, EANO) [2, 3, 6]. The extent of tumor resection has been demonstrated to be the single most important factor concerning the prognosis and survival in these children [2]. Hence, in pediatric IE, a gross total resection (GTR) must be rigorously attempted when feasible. However, the frequent location of IE in the posterior fossa in children may limit resection due to the cranial nerve encasement and brain stem adherence. Although earlier studies have shown GTR could be achieved only in about 50% of cases, the advent of modern surgical techniques have of late increased the resection rates close to 80–95% [6, 8]. Even in the event of a postoperative MRI showing residual lesion, a relook surgery should be considered, when GTR still appears to be the realistic goal. This is because GTR has been demonstrated to produce the best overall survival (OS) and progression-free survival (PFS) in pediatric ependymomas; it provides 5-year OS of at-least 70–80% and progression-free survival of 51–75% when compared with subtotal resection (STR) with corresponding rates of 22–47% and 0–26% [6]. It has been noted that children <3 years show relatively poor survival than older children, which is partly attributed to a difficulty in achieving GTR at a younger age (particularly infants) with small posterior fossa and decreased blood volume. These children may quickly become unstable even with relatively less blood loss, precluding complete resection.

## 20.3 Spinal Ependymomas

In contrast to IE, spinal ependymomas are relatively less common in children and account for only <13% of CNS ependymomas but have better prognosis as compared to IE [9]. Median age at diagnosis is 13 years which is higher than that of IE (7 years) [10, 11]. They, however, are documented to be the second most common pediatric intramedullary tumor. In the pediatric spine, the classic (grade II) and myxopapillary ependymomas are the frequent subtypes. Spinal ependymomas in children are usually seen in association with neurofibromatosis (NF) type 2 and are often multiple in this setting.

### 20.3.1 Initial Work-Up/Evaluation

#### 20.3.1.1 Clinical Presentation

Pediatric ependymomas can present anywhere along the spinal column. Classic grade II ependymomas exhibit indolent course and most commonly arise from the cervical spine [12]. In a pediatric series, about half of these were distributed between the cervicomedullary, cervical, and thoracic region, while the other half were present in the lower spinal cord [11]. On the other hand, the myxopapillary ependymomas almost always originate in the conus medullaris, cauda equina, and filum terminale. Although the initial WHO classifications regarded them as grade I tumors, they have been fairly shown to exhibit clinically aggressive behavior, and considering this fact the latest WHO 2021 version has moved them into grade 2 category. Their prognosis, compared to that of the adults, differs with a high propensity for recurrence and neural-axis and extra neural dissemination. Because of the slow growing nature of spinal ependymomas, their presentation may be non-specific and can be easily overlooked, causing a delay in diagnosis. Some common manifestations such as pain, gait imbalance, motor milestone regression, motor weakness, scoliosis and torticollis, and bladder disturbance have been observed. Occasionally, hydrocephalus attributed to an altered CSF dynamics has been seen. In a pediatric cohort, a usual presentation noted was back pain followed by lower extremity pain and numbness [11].

#### 20.3.1.2 Imaging

On imaging, spinal ependymomas are centrally located, well-circumscribed lesions that symmetrically enlarge the spinal canal. These are usually T1 hypo-isointense with variable T2 hyperintensities; the heterogeneous appearance owes to the presence of intralesional hemorrhage and calcifications. Polar cysts rather than intratumoral cysts are common. It can show both homogenous and heterogenous enhancement after contrast administration; however, occasionally a rim enhancement is also observed. Hemosiderin caps (cap sign), which are rim of low signal intensity along the tumor margin, may be seen in 20–60% of ependymomas. The spinal astrocytomas that are frequently occurring pediatric intramedullary tumors are differentiated from the ependymomas by their infiltrative nature with ill-demarcated margins, eccentric cord expansion, varying degrees of cord edema, and T2 hyperintensities. A screening MRI of the entire cranio-spinal axis is suggested especially in large tumors (>4 spinal segments) or in recurrent cases.

Pediatric MPE are characteristically located as intradural extramedullary tumors in the lumbosacral region arising from the filum terminale and can show foraminal extension and vertebral body scalloping. On T1 MRI, they show T1 iso- to hyperintense and T2 heterogenously hyperintense signals and demonstrate heterogeneous contrast enhancement. MPE can show high vascularity with intratumoral hemorrhage, explaining their T1 hyper-intensity. The T2 intensity may be variable due to the presence of intratumoral hemorrhage, cyst formation, and mineralization.

### 20.3.2 Surgical Considerations

Spinal ependymomas are operated by a posterior approach with midline myelotomy. In children, for tumors spanning over multiple segments, a laminoplasty may be preferred over laminectomy in view of risk of post laminectomy kyphosis over long term in a growing spine. An ultrasonography if available can be used to localize the tumor extent before dural opening. It is suggested that these children be operated under neuromonitoring assistance. The ependymomas, compared to astrocytomas, display a clear plane interface with the spinal cord parenchyma, and the principle is to dissect between these two planes. Ideally, GTR should be the goal in all cases albeit with the concern of neurological preservation, and the best possibility lies in the first attempt at tumor removal. Subtotal resection may be opted if there is an absent clear plane or in the event of any change in the IONM potentials. An in toto tumor excision has been generally suggested unless its size, adherence to the cauda equina or conus region necessitates initial debulking, in order to minimize the chance of subarachnoid spilling. It is prudent to stay within the capsule during tumor retrieval to prevent neoplastic dissemination. After tumor removal, the filum can be identified and divided to ensure gross tumor removal.

In general, smaller tumors (up to three segments) are well defined and display capsule at surgery that increases the chance of complete resection. Larger tumors usually lack a capsule suggesting the possibility that an increasing tumor size slowly breaks the capsule with infiltration of the surrounding nerve roots and subarachnoid dissemination [13].

Similar to the cranial counterpart, the extent of resection and tumor location are the main factors determining the outcomes. In pediatric cohorts, GTR when compared with subtotal resection plus adjuvant radiotherapy has been related to a better OS and PFS [10, 11]. Tumors located in the lower half tend to behave more aggressive with early and more frequent recurrence [12]. Encapsulation of tumor and GTR are the strongest determinant of PFS.

In children, studies have documented a relatively aggressively behavior of MPE when compared with adults. In a systematic review, the overall recurrence rate of MPE in children was significantly higher as compared to adults (40.5% vs. 23.4%), along with a shorter time to recurrence (median time; 20.6 vs. 75.1 months) [14].

**Postoperative Investigations** Postoperative MRI should be performed in all cases to look for the extent of residual disease (ideally within 72 h of surgery). In cases where MRI is not done within 3 days of surgery, it should be suspended for 3 weeks. A second look surgery should be considered when the residual disease in present and GTR is a realistic goal. As mentioned above, lumbar puncture should be done (no sooner than 14 days after surgery) to look for CSF dissemination. The presence of M0 disease is confirmed by a negative lumbar puncture within 2 weeks following surgery, although a positive result within this time frame necessitates a repeat sample.

**Post-operative Management** Postoperative radiotherapy (RT) and chemotherapy are the main component of adjuvant treatment depending upon patient's age, location, CSF dissemination, and extent of the residual disease irrespective of the molecular subtype [3].

## 20.4 Post-operative Radiotherapy (PORT)

**Adjuvant Therapy After GTR** Several studies have shown that addition of PORT improves survival in IE [15].

All patients of age >12 months should receive PORT for grade 2 and 3 ependymoma with the exception of completely resected grade 2 supratentorial ependymoma. This subgroup constitutes a favorable prognostic group and can be kept on observation rather than immediate PORT. A phase 2 trial (COG ACNS0121) showed that 61% of patients with grade 2 supratentorial ependymoma had no progression and all patients were alive after 5 years of observation after gross total resection. This approach was evaluated in ACNS0831 trial; however, the final results of this trial are awaited.

**Adjuvant Therapy After STR** Patients after STR tend to have poor prognosis as compared to those after GTR. In these patients, a course of chemotherapy is suggested post-operatively followed by second look surgery if feasible and then PORT. Combination of vincristine, etoposide, cyclophosphamide, and platinum are considered as the most active agents [16].

**Focal RT Versus Craniospinal Irradiation (CSI)** All grade 2–3 IE patients should receive focal RT unless there is CSF dissemination. Focal RT dose for patients above 3 years of age is 59.4 Gy at 1.8 Gy fraction. However, for younger children, as young as 12–18 months, radiation dose is limited to 54 Gy to avoid neurocognitive deficits [17].

In case of CSF dissemination, CSI with a boost to focal lesions (to a total dose of 54–59.4 Gy) should be considered in patients >3 years of the age.

**Children Less Than 12 Months** In very young children (<12 months), PORT is constrained due to concern about potential developmental complications [18].

In order to delay the need of adjuvant RT, adjuvant chemotherapy is indicated after surgery. However; none of the randomized trials compare immediate PORT versus chemotherapy after surgery in this group of patients. Various combinations of chemotherapy including vincristine, etoposide, cyclophosphamide, platinum-based chemotherapy, and high dose methotrexate have shown a response rate of 40–50% [19].

## 20.5 Target Volume Delineation

For focal RT, gross target volume (GTV) includes tumor bed and any residual disease on post-operative MRI. Older standards (COG ACNS0121) advised 1 cm expansion from GTV to clinical target volume (CTV), whereas more recent protocols employ a 0.5 cm margin to GTV (ACNS0831). A set-up margin is added to CTV according to institutional protocols. Figure 20.1 shows target volume delineation and dose color wash for posterior fossa ependymoma.

**Maintenance Chemotherapy** Role of post-RT chemotherapy is unclear. Preliminary results from children oncology group (ACNS0831) suggested that maintenance chemotherapy (four cycles of VCR, cyclophosphamide, cisplatin, and etoposide) after focal radiotherapy is effective in few patients [20]. However, the final results from this trial are awaited. Another ongoing phase III trial by international society of pediatric oncology (SIOP-EP-II) is also randomizing patients to adjuvant chemotherapy versus observation after surgery and PORT [21].

**Recurrent Intracranial Ependymoma** Although slow growing, ependymomas carry risk of recurrence in spite of maximum resection, and therefore, a periodic clinico-radiologic surveillance is necessary. Long-term prognosis for recurrent disease remains dismal, and there is no consensus on treatment for recurrent disease. However, even in recurrent tumors that are amenable for excision, surgery and/or re-irradiation should be offered. In children with recurrent tumors who underwent surgery and GTR, a 5-year event free survival of 19% has been reported, while with

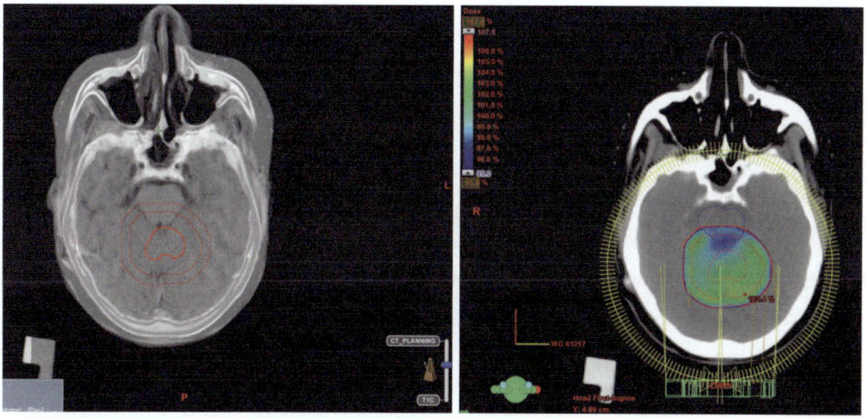

**Fig. 20.1** Figure 20.1 is showing target volume delineation using CT/MRI fusion (left) and dose colour wash for posterior fossa ependymoma treated with Volumetric Modulated Arc Technique (Right)

incomplete resection and no surgery, it was 14% and 8%, respectively [22]. Re-irradiation may achieve durable response in carefully selected patients [23]. Re-irradiation options include focal RT, CSI, or hypo-fractionated stereotactic RT depending on the age, location, extent of recurrence, and time to previous radiation. Patients who receive focal Re-irradiation remain at risk for the development of disseminated disease. In one study, outcomes were most favorable in patients who experienced distant only failure without anaplasia and received CSI at recurrence [24]. Recently completed phase II trial (RERTEP) has explored the treatment options for recurrent ependymoma with results pending.

Role of chemotherapy in recurrent ependymoma remains unclear and conventional chemotherapy can provide palliation in some patients [25].

**Molecular Targets** The potential molecular target in IE includes epidermal growth factor receptor (EGFR) and vascular growth factor receptor (VGFR). However, till date, all these approaches remain investigational.

**Prognosis** Long-term prognosis in IE remains poor despite aggressive treatment with a 10-year survival of approximately 50–70% [26].

**Radiotherapy in Spinal Ependymoma** A post-operative contrast enhanced MRI be done 2–3 weeks after surgery to look for extent of resection. As there is the risk of leptomeningeal dissemination, a screening MRI of entire cranio-spinal axis and CSF cytology should be done after 2–3 weeks of surgery [3]. Complete resection is the goal of the treatment, and there are no standardized adjuvant treatment protocols

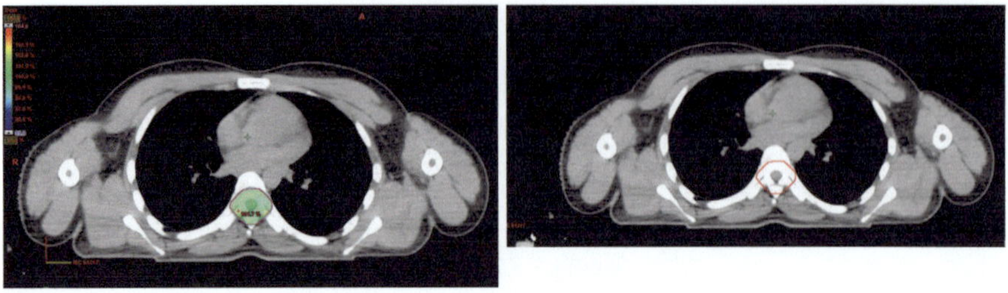

**Fig. 20.2** Figure 20.2 is showing planning target volume on CT (left) and dose colour wash for spinal ependymoma, treated with Volumetric Modulated Arc Technique (Right)

for pediatric spinal ependymoma. Nonetheless, focal postoperative irradiation is advised by the European Association of NeuroOncology (EANO) for all anaplastic (WHO grade III) tumors and incompletely resected classic (WHO grade II) tumors to a dose of 45–54 Gy [3]. For myxopapillary ependymomas, which have a higher probability of local recurrence than conventional grade II tumors, post-op RT improves local control and PFS even after complete resection [27]. There are no separate guidelines for radiotherapy target volume delineation in spinal EPN, which are often extrapolated from that of IE. Figure 20.2 shows target volume delineation and dose color wash for spinal ependymoma.

Radiation consequences have been discussed in a separate chapter.

To summarize, recognition of clinical features along with initiation of appropriate treatment is essential in pediatric ependymomas. Gross total resection should be the intent for a favorable clinical outcome; nevertheless, this has to be weighed against the potential for additional surgical morbidity. Post-operative radiotherapy improves survival and is recommended for all grade 2 and grade 3 intracranial ependymoma with some exceptions mentioned above. Regular clinical and imaging surveillance is essential to detect early recurrence.

## References

1. Louis DN, Perry A, Wesseling P, Brat DJ, Cree IA, Figarella-Branger D, et al. The 2021 WHO classification of tumors of the central nervous system: a summary. Neuro Oncol. 2021;23(8):1231–51.
2. Cage TA, Clark AJ, Aranda D, Gupta N, Sun PP, Parsa AT, et al. A systematic review of treatment outcomes in pediatric patients with intracranial ependymomas: a review. J Neurosurg Pediatr. 2013;11(6):673–81.
3. Rudà R, Reifenberger G, Frappaz D, Pfister SM, Laprie A, Santarius T, et al. EANO guidelines for the diagnosis and treatment of ependymal tumors. Neuro Oncol. 2018;20(4):445–56.
4. Yuh EL, Barkovich AJ, Gupta N. Imaging of ependymomas: MRI and CT. Childs Nerv Syst. 2009;25(10):1203–13.
5. Childhood Ependymoma Treatment (PDQ®)–Health Professional Version—NCI. 2023 [cited 2023 May 8]. https://www.cancer.gov/types/brain/hp/child-ependymoma-treatment-pdq.

6. Sanford RA, Merchant TE, Zwienenberg-Lee M, Kun LE, Boop FA. Advances in surgical techniques for resection of childhood cerebellopontine angle ependymomas are key to survival. Childs Nerv Syst. 2009;25(10):1229–40.
7. Maksoud YA, Hahn YS, Engelhard HH. Intracranial ependymoma. Neurosurg Focus. 2002;13(3):e4.
8. Lillard JC, Venable GT, Khan NR, Tatevossian RG, Dalton J, Vaughn BN, et al. Pediatric supratentorial ependymoma: surgical, clinical, and molecular analysis. Neurosurgery. 2019;85(1):41–9.
9. McGuire CS, Sainani KL, Fisher PG. Incidence patterns for ependymoma: a surveillance, epidemiology, and end results study. J Neurosurg. 2009;110(4):725–9.
10. Lin Y, Jea A, Melkonian SC, Lam S. Treatment of pediatric Grade II spinal ependymomas: a population-based study. J Neurosurg Pediatr. 2015;15(3):243–9.
11. Safaee M, Oh MC, Mummaneni PV, Weinstein PR, Ames CP, Chou D, et al. Surgical outcomes in spinal cord ependymomas and the importance of extent of resection in children and young adults. J Neurosurg Pediatr. 2014;13(4):393–9.
12. Oh MC, Sayegh ET, Safaee M, Sun MZ, Kaur G, Kim JM, et al. Prognosis by tumor location for pediatric spinal cord ependymomas. J Neurosurg Pediatr. 2013;11(3):282–8.
13. Klekamp J. Spinal ependymomas. Part 2: ependymomas of the filum terminale. Neurosurg Focus. 2015;39(2):E7.
14. Feldman WB, Clark AJ, Safaee M, Ames CP, Parsa AT. Tumor control after surgery for spinal myxopapillary ependymomas: distinct outcomes in adults versus children: a systematic review. J Neurosurg Spine. 2013;19(4):471–6.
15. Merchant TE, Li C, Xiong X, Kun LE, Boop FA, Sanford RA. Conformal radiotherapy after surgery for paediatric ependymoma: a prospective study. Lancet Oncol. 2009;10(3):258–66.
16. Van Poppel M, Klimo P, Dewire M, Sanford RA, Boop F, Broniscer A, et al. Resection of infantile brain tumors after neoadjuvant chemotherapy: the St. Jude experience. J Neurosurg Pediatr. 2011;8(3):251–6.
17. Koshy M, Rich S, Merchant TE, Mahmood U, Regine WF, Kwok Y. Post-operative radiation improves survival in children younger than 3 years with intracranial ependymoma. J Neurooncol. 2011;105(3):583–90.
18. Zapotocky M, Beera K, Adamski J, Laperierre N, Guger S, Janzen L, et al. Survival and functional outcomes of molecularly defined childhood posterior fossa ependymoma: cure at a cost. Cancer. 2019;125(11):1867–76.
19. Garvin JH, Selch MT, Holmes E, Berger MS, Finlay JL, Flannery A, et al. Phase II study of pre-irradiation chemotherapy for childhood intracranial ependymoma. Children's Cancer Group protocol 9942: a report from the Children's Oncology Group. Pediatr Blood Cancer. 2012;59(7):1183–9.
20. Smith A, Onar-Thomas A, Ellison D, Owens-Pickle E, Wu S, Leary SES, et al. EPEN-54. ACNS0831, phase III randomized trial of post-radiation chemotherapy in patients with newly diagnosed ependymoma ages 1 to 21 years. Neuro Oncol. 2020;22(Suppl 3):iii318–9.
21. Leblond P, Massimino M, English M, Ritzmann TA, Gandola L, Calaminus G, et al. Toward improved diagnosis accuracy and treatment of children, adolescents, and young adults with ependymoma: the international SIOP ependymoma II protocol. Front Neurol. 2022;13:887544.
22. Zacharoulis S, Ashley S, Moreno L, Gentet JC, Massimino M, Frappaz D. Treatment and outcome of children with relapsed ependymoma: a multi-institutional retrospective analysis. Childs Nerv Syst. 2010;26(7):905–11.
23. Bouffet E, Hawkins CE, Ballourah W, Taylor MD, Bartels UK, Schoenhoff N, et al. Survival benefit for pediatric patients with recurrent ependymoma treated with reirradiation. Int J Radiat Oncol Biol Phys. 2012;83(5):1541–8.
24. Tsang DS, Burghen E, Klimo P, Boop FA, Ellison DW, Merchant TE. Outcomes after reirradiation for recurrent pediatric intracranial ependymoma. Int J Radiat Oncol Biol Phys. 2018;100(2):507–15.

25. Brandes AA, Cavallo G, Reni M, Tosoni A, Nicolardi L, Scopece L, et al. A multicenter retrospective study of chemotherapy for recurrent intracranial ependymal tumors in adults by the Gruppo Italiano Cooperativo di Neuro-Oncologia. Cancer. 2005;104(1):143–8.
26. Ritzmann TA, Chapman RJ, Kilday JP, Thorp N, Modena P, Dineen RA, et al. SIOP ependymoma I: final results, long-term follow-up, and molecular analysis of the trial cohort—a BIOMECA Consortium Study. Neuro Oncol. 2022;24(6):936–48.
27. Schild SE, Nisi K, Scheithauer BW, Wong WW, Lyons MK, Schomberg PJ, Shaw EG. The results of radiotherapy for ependymomas: the Mayo Clinic experience. Int J Radiat Oncol Biol Phys. 1998;42(5):953–8.

# 21 Pediatric Low-Grade Glioma

Kavindra Singh, Sushanta Kumar Sahoo, and Shikha Goyal

## 21.1 Introduction

Central nervous system (CNS) tumors are the most common pediatric solid tumors, the most prevalent tumor type being pediatric low-grade glioma (pLGG, 45%), and the most common histology being pilocytic astrocytoma (15.3%) [1]. The current classification of pediatric gliomas relies heavily on molecular diagnostics.

The WHO 2021 classification categorizes these as either (a) pediatric type diffuse low-grade gliomas, (b) circumscribed astrocytic tumors, and (c) glioneuronal and neuronal tumors [2]. These may encompass a spectrum of pathologies seen throughout the neuraxis. Unlike adult low-grade glioma (LGG) that are predominantly located in the cerebral hemispheres and may undergo transformation to high grade gliomas, pLGG may occur anywhere in CNS and rarely undergo high-grade transformation. With the recent advancement of molecular and genetic research in diagnosis and therapy, our understanding of the diagnostic and risk categorization of these tumors has also expanded, which has therapeutic relevance as well.

The presentation of these tumors depends on their location within CNS. Owing to their slow growing nature, these are often detected at a stage when they have achieved a large size leading to raised intracranial pressure (ICP) except in few locations where they present early. Standard workup includes imaging of neuraxis to look for the extent of disease. Surgery is the preferred treatment for most tumors, with only a few exceptions like deep seated location, tumors occupying eloquent areas of brain, tumors in the vicinity of brainstem, and some factors which

K. Singh · S. K. Sahoo
Neurosurgery, PGIMER, Chandigarh, India

S. Goyal (✉)
Department of Radiotherapy and Oncology, Postgraduate Institute of Medical Education and Research, Chandigarh, India



R. Madan et al. (eds.), *Evidence Based Practice in Pediatric Radiation Oncology*,
https://doi.org/10.1007/978-981-96-4872-6_21

sometimes prohibit gross total tumor removal (GTR). Overall, their prognosis depends on the tumor type and location and extent of resection. In patients undergoing GTR, overall 10-year progression-free survival (PFS) exceeds 85% compared to 50% only in those undergoing subtotal resection (STR) [3]. The latter (with STR) often need adjuvant therapy but may still have unsatisfactory disease control with long-term morbidity.

## 21.2 Classification

Pediatric low-grade gliomas are a heterogeneous group of tumors with predominantly glial or mixed glioneuronal histology. Unlike their malignant counterparts, these tumors lack necrosis, mitosis, and microvascular proliferation on histopathology. WHO 2021 classification has supplemented the earlier histologic classification with molecular markers for more robust categorization of clinical behavior and prognosis. Pediatric type diffuse LGG now include three new tumor types: diffuse astrocytoma-*MYB* or *MYBL1*-altered, polymorphous low grade neuroepithelial tumor of the young (PLNTY), and diffuse low-grade glioma-MAPK altered. Glioneuronal and neuronal tumor group also has three new types: diffuse glioneuronal tumor with oligodendroglioma-like features and nuclear clusters (DGONC), myxoid glioneuronal tumor (MGT), and multinodular and vacuolating tumor (MVNT) [2, 4]. A list of tumors in the category of pLGG are summarized in Table 21.1.

**Table 21.1** Tumors comprising pLGG as per WHO CNS 2021 classification

| Pediatric type diffuse LGG | Circumscribed astrocytic gliomas | Glioneuronal and neuronal tumor |
|---|---|---|
| • Diffuse astrocytoma, MYB- or MYBL1-altered<br>• Angiocentric glioma<br>• Polymorphous low grade neuroepithelial tumor of the young (PLNTY)<br>• Diffuse low-geade glioma, MAPK pathway-altered | • Pilocytic astrocytoma<br>• Pleomorphic xanthoastrocytoma<br>• SEGA<br>• Chordoid glioma<br>• High-grade astrocytoma with piloid features<br>• Astroblastoma, MN1-altered | • Ganglioglioma<br>• Desmoplastic infantile astrocytoma and ganglioglioma<br>• Dysembryoplastic neuroepithelial tumor<br>• Diffuse glioneuronal tumor with oligodendroglioma-like features and nuclear clusters<br>• Gangliocytoma<br>• Papillary glioneuronal tumor<br>• Rosette-forming glioneuronal tumor<br>• Multinodular and vacuolating neuronal tumor (MVNT)<br>• Dysplastic cerebellar gangliocytoma (Lhermitte-Duclos disease)<br>• Central neurocytoma<br>• Extraventricular neurocytoma<br>• Cerebellar liponeurocytoma |

## 21.3 Diagnostic Imaging

Neuroimaging constitutes the first investigation to confirm the suspicion of a low grade glioma. Most patients would get a computed tomography (CT) scan initially, but magnetic resonance imaging (MRI) is preferred. Imaging studies are discussed in a separate chapter in detail. MRI of most LGGs shows a lesion in hemispheric location with no or minimal mass effect, T1 hypointensity, and variable enhancement. Pilocytic astrocytomas are usually well defined and T1 hypointense and show brilliant enhancement. Cerebellar lesions typically demonstrate a cyst with enhancing wall and a solid enhancing mural nodule. Other low-grade gliomas may be less well defined and may not enhance with contrast.

Spinal pilocytic astrocytomas are usually eccentric, well defined, with displacement rather than infiltration of spinal cord. The dorsal cord is most often affected. Syringomyelia and cysts may be associated, but edema is uncommon. Lesions are T1 iso-/hypointense and T2 hyperintense; enhancement is variable but less common than intracranial lesions.

## 21.4 Genetics and Molecular Makers

Despite a morphology similar to adult LGG, the common alterations seen in adult gliomas such as chromosome 1p and 19q codeletions, TP53 mutations, or IDH1 and IDH2 mutations are almost never encountered in pLGG. In the last decade, we have gained unparalleled insight into the underlying biology of pLGG. The single most important genetic event in the pathophysiology of pLGG is the upregulation of RAS/MAPK pathway. Below is the list of commonly seen molecular alterations in different pLGG patients. Most pilocytic astrocytomas have MAPK pathway alterations. Sporadic infratentorial/cerebellar pilocytic astrocytomas commonly show BRAF alterations, while these are rare in supratentorial lesions, the most common being 7q34 gain via duplication and fusion between BRAF oncogenes and KIAA1549 [5]. BRAF v600E point mutations may occur occasionally in supratentorial tumors; these may also occur in pleomorphic xanthoastrocytoma (PXA), pilomyxoid astrocytoma (PMA), ganglioglioma, and diffuse astrocytoma, conferring a higher risk of malignant transformation and worse outcome than BRAF fusion. These changes are utilized as targets in recurrent or progressive disease with promising results. Other somatic mutations seen in low-grade gliomas, especially in pilocytic astrocytoma, may be related to FGFR1, PTPN11, and NTRK2.

Genetic syndromes are linked to pLGG include neurofibromatosis type-1 (NF1), tuberous Sclerosis Complex (TSC), Noonan syndrome, and Constitutional Mismatch Repair Syndrome (CMMRD). Germline mutation in chromosome 17q is linked with development of optic pathway or hypothalamic pilocytic astrocytoma.

Testing with IHC or sequencing for histone mutations may also help categorize otherwise morphologically grade 2 gliomas into high-grade gliomas, with a poorer prognosis (Table 21.2).

**Table 21.2** Molecular markers in pLGG

| Molecular alteration | Common associates |
|---|---|
| BRAF V600 | Pilocytic astrocytoma, pleomorphic xanthoastrocytoma, ganglioglioma, PLNTY |
| KIAA1549BRAF and other BRAF fusion | Pilocytic astrocytoma |
| FGFR fusions and point mutations | Pilocytic astrocytoma, PLNTY, DNET, extraventricular neurocytoma, glioneuronal tumor, rosette forming glioneuronal tumor |
| NF1 | Pilocytic astrocytoma, diffuse astrocytoma |
| KRAS mutations | Pilocytic astrocytoma |
| CRAF fusions | Pilocytic astrocytoma |
| MAP2K1 activating mutation | Multinodular vacuolating neuronal tumor |
| MYB fusion/amplification | Angiocentric glioma |
| MYB/MYBL1 abnormalities | Diffuse astrocytoma and isomorphic diffuse astrocytoma |

## 21.5 General Management Principles

The role of multidisciplinary decision-making cannot be more emphasized than in this disease where the long-term survival, functional preservation, and long-term morbidity from therapy all need a fine balance. One cannot compromise survival and function by reserving necessary interventions while overenthusiastic treatments may introduce long-term disabilities in terms of sensorimotor deficits, intelligence and memory effects, and endocrine dysfunction, leading to poor societal adjustment.

### 21.5.1 Surgical Treatment

Surgery is the treatment of choice for most pLGGs and its timing guided by the clinical condition of the child at presentation and specific radiographic features. Most children present with insidious onset of symptoms. Children with severe symptoms from mass effect need emergent resection. Many LGGs are part of long-term epilepsy-associated tumors (LEAT), e.g., angiocentric glioma, ganglioglioma, and DNET, where gross total resection also affords freedom from epilepsy.

In children harboring supratentorial tumors, anti-epileptic drugs (AED) are started in preoperative period. Our preferred AED is levetiracetam, because of its minimal interaction with other drugs. In children with a history of seizures, and who are already on AEDs, same drugs are continued in perioperative period. Another important addition is a corticosteroid such as dexamethasone, especially in tumors with surrounding perilesional edema. It is given as bolus dose followed by a tapering maintenance dose which is continued post-operatively.

Surgery aims to remove the maximum possible tumor without causing neurological deficits and to obtain tissue for histopathology. PFS benefit of GTR over STR has been mentioned earlier. GTR may, however, not be feasible in poorly circumscribed, non-pilocytic LGGs with infiltration of deep nuclei or other eloquent areas, or those crossing midline. Stereotactic biopsy remains an option for deep located, small tumors where diagnosis is in doubt.

Owing to their slow growth, these tumors may pose an intraoperative challenge of differentiation from normal brain parenchyma. When available, intraoperative tools such as neuronavigation, intraoperative ultrasound, or MRI may help achieve maximal safe resection. Neuromonitoring including somatosensory evoked potentials (SSEP), motor evoked potentials (MEP), and direct stimulation, etc., has proven useful, especially when working in or near critical structures like brainstem, motor cortex, and insular region, etc.

### 21.5.2 Adjuvant Therapy

The need for adjuvant therapy in pediatric LGG is somewhat controversial for the following reasons:

(a) Long-term risk of malignant transformation is not exactly known because of small volume of cases.
(b) They behave differently compared to their adult counterparts; hence, extrapolation of adult data is not appropriate.
(c) Many of these tumors which are sub-totally resected may not demonstrate growth on follow-up imaging and remain quiescent for a long time.
(d) Effect of radiotherapy or other adjuvant treatment in small children is of particular concern, and the pros and cons of individual modalities need to be considered.

Adjuvant therapy is considered only in children where GTR is not achieved (STR or biopsy only), and the tumor shows considerable growth over periodic imaging as the progression-free period may be long even after STR [6]. Even in these situations, repeat surgery, if feasible, is preferred over adjuvant therapy. Modalities for adjuvant therapy include radiotherapy (RT) or systemic therapy (chemotherapy and targeted therapy) based on tumor type and molecular profile. Among the modalities available, RT is perhaps the most utilized. Concerns pertaining to the use of RT include risk of malignant transformation, cognitive delay, endocrinopathy, and vasculopathy which need to be considered before planning the same.

#### 21.5.2.1 Adjuvant Radiotherapy

Cranial RT for pLGG has been criticized and withheld in favor of follow-up or systemic therapies (chemotherapy and targeted therapy) owing to concerns regarding long-term toxicity. However, it must be understood that despite the overall good prognosis, a subset (10–15%) will progress early and have compromised survival despite systemic therapy. Identification of this poor prognostic group (diffuse astrocytoma, thalamic, or midbrain location) may help reduce the disability from multiple surgical failures and systemic therapy effects by early institution of RT [7]. A 20-year retrospective study from St Jude's on children with unresectable LGG or glioneuronal tumors (biopsy-proven) treated with RT included 150 patients, with a median follow-up exceeding 11 years [8]. Diffuse astrocytoma or tumors in thalamic/midbrain location were deemed high risk and had worse 10-year overall survival (OS) than pilocytic astrocytoma or ganglioglioma located outside the thalamus or midbrain (deemed low risk), 76.4% vs. 95.6% ($p = 0.003$). Delay in RT (after at least one course of systemic therapy) in high-risk group led to further OS detriment.

The expected late morbidity in this subset of patients who may gain in survival from adjuvant RT may be managed with using more conformal techniques such as intensity modulated RT (IMRT) or volumetric modulated arc therapy (VMAT). Proton therapy, when available, may potentially reduce the incidence of second neoplasms, which is a major concern when opting to omit RT in these patients. In the St Jude's cohort, tumor bed was given a 5 mm margin for clinical target volume (CTV) and a 3–5 mm margin for planning target volume (PTV); this volume was planned for a dose of 54 gray (Gy) over 6 weeks (5 fractions per week).

#### 21.5.2.2 Chemotherapy

The role of chemotherapy in pLGG is limited and aims to avoid or delay RT in very young children. The most popular combination of carboplatin/vincristine may induce partial response or stable disease with a 68% PFS at 3 years; responses are independent of NF1 status but better in children younger than 5 years [9]. A 4-drug combination TPCV (thioguanine, procarbazine, lomustine, and vincristine) shows better 5-year event free survival (EFS) but no OS gain in grade 1–2 gliomas with <95% resection or residual >1.5 $cm^2$ (newly diagnosed or progressed following resection) in children under 10 years (except pontine tumors or optic nerve gliomas not involving chiasm). Children younger than 1 year and those with residual tumors larger than 3 cm or located in thalamus had poorer OS [10].

#### 21.5.2.3 Targeted Therapy

Newer molecules that target the MAPK pathway are effective in recurrent/chemo-refractory disease (50% tumors progress on chemotherapy) and may be considered especially in pilocytic astrocytomas. Although no long-term randomized phase 3 data exist, phase 2 studies have been promising to introduce these drugs in case of need. MEK1/2 inhibitors (trametinib, selumetinib, cobimetinib, binimetinib) have shown encouraging outcomes. BRAF inhibitors such as dabrafenib and vemurafenib in BRAF mutant lesions are also under investigation. Combinations of MEK inhibitors with drugs inhibiting mTOR (everolimus), VEGF (bevacizumab),

**Table 21.3** Adjuvant therapy for select group of p-LGG

| Type of tumor | Adjuvant therapy |
|---|---|
| Diffuse astrocytoma | Chemo + radiotherapy |
| Pilocytic astrocytoma | MEK1/2 inhibitor |
| Pleomorphic xanthoastrocytoma | BRAF targeted therapies |
| SEGA | mTOR pathway inhibitor |

or FGFR (erdafitinib, zoligratinib) pathways are being evaluated in recurrent pLGGs [11].

Table 21.3 shows the approach (available/investigational) for adjuvant therapy.

Herein we discuss some of the most commonly seen tumors in clinical practice.

## 21.6 Circumscribed Astrocytic Tumors

### 21.6.1 Pilocytic Astrocytoma

#### 21.6.1.1 Epidemiology

It is the most common brain tumor and low-grade glioma and the second most common brain tumor (after embryonal tumors) seen in pediatric population aged 0–19 years, with a higher male preponderance. Incidence of pilocytic astrocytoma has steadily increased from 2004 to 2018 (annual percentage change = 1.2%) [1]. The term pilocytic is used to describe cells with hair-like, bipolar processes. Tumors can arise both in supratentorial and infratentorial compartment. Cerebellum is the most location, followed by supratentorial, optic pathway, hypothalamus, brainstem, and rarely, spinal cord [12]. Nearly 70% of optic pathway or hypothalamic gliomas are associated with NF-1, and nearly 15–20% of children with NF-1 may develop optic pathway glioma, half of which may develop symptoms worthy of therapy before the child turns 5 years [13].

#### 21.6.1.2 Clinical presentation

Tumor location determines clinical presentation. Being slow growing tumors, they usually achieve a significant size by the time they are detected. Cerebellar pilocytic astrocytomas may present with ataxia, signs of increased ICP, and in late cases, cranial nerve palsies. Optic pathway and hypothalamic tumors present with decreased visual acuity and/or field defect, nystagmus, endocrine disturbance in form of diabetes insipidus and short stature, precocious puberty, electrolyte disturbances, proptosis, and in some cases, obstruction of cerebrospinal fluid (CSF) pathway with hydrocephalus (causing headache, vomiting, enlargement of the head, missed developmental milestones, or behavioral abnormalities). The diencephalic syndrome, which includes extreme weight loss, failure to thrive despite normal or accelerated development, hyperkinesis, hyperalertness, and mood elation, can be brought on by tumors that affect both the optic chiasm and the hypothalamus. Sporadic optic pathway tumors are usually more symptomatic and worsen earlier than NF-1-associated tumors, warranting earlier intervention. NF-1 associated tumors are often multifocal and involve bilateral optic nerves. Tectal plate tumors are invariably believed to be pilocytic and are typically treated without biopsy confirmation. On examination, these individuals may show signs of Parinaud's syndrome or papilledema.

#### 21.6.1.3 Natural course

Even though the tumor is close to the ventricles, the likelihood of CSF spread is low; reports of it mostly occur in aggressive and recurring tumors (3–5%). Median survival may exceed 5 years even with leptomeningeal spread [14].

These tumors can occasionally experience spontaneous regression. GTR is curative. In a multicenter trial of grade 1 gliomas, resection to a higher degree showed a better PFS at 5 years in pilocytic astrocytomas but not in gangliogliomas or dysembryoplastic neuroepithelial tumors (DNET) [15].

Occipital/parietal lobe tumors have a worse PFS than temporal lobe tumors. Intraoperative MRI may improve resectability but not necessarily affect survival. Optic pathway gliomas, however, cannot be removed surgically, and even a biopsy may result in visual loss. They are usually asymptomatic and may not warrant treatment if linked to NF-1. In the absence of NF-1, sporadic optic pathway gliomas may be more aggressive and require therapy.

#### 21.6.1.4 Imaging

On CT imaging, these lesions are well-defined iso- or hypodense round or oval lesions and exhibit marked contrast enhancement. On MRI, they are typically T1 hypo- or isointense and T2 hyperintense when solid and T1 and T2 hyperintense in cystic variants (Fig. 21.1). On post-contrast sequences, they show strong and diffuse contrast enhancement and in cases of cystic PA, intense and heterogeneous enhancement of a characteristic mural nodule is seen. The cyst wall also reveals T2 hyperintensity with minimal edema, if present. The cyst fluid is T1 iso- to hypointense but T2/FLAIR hyperintense and more proteinaceous than CSF. The skull bone may occasionally be thin in peripheral lesions. Typically, these tumors are monofocal. Tumors in hypothalamus and optic pathway have less well-defined borders; T1 iso- or hypointense optic pathway tumors have a T2 hyperintense signal and show variable enhancement (from none to striking, only 50% enhance). There may be varying degrees of optic pathway involvement; spontaneous lesions often develop from the chiasm, whereas NF-1-related lesions more frequently develop from the optic nerve. Magnetic resonance spectroscopy (MRS) may show elevated choline and lactate peaks and low *N*-acetylaspartate (NAA). On DWI sequences, there is no diffusion restriction. Differential diagnosis depends on the location—in posterior fossa, differentials include medulloblastoma, ependymoma, and hemangioblastoma, and in supratentorial compartment, differentials are PMA, PXA, ganglioglioma, and demyelinating disease.

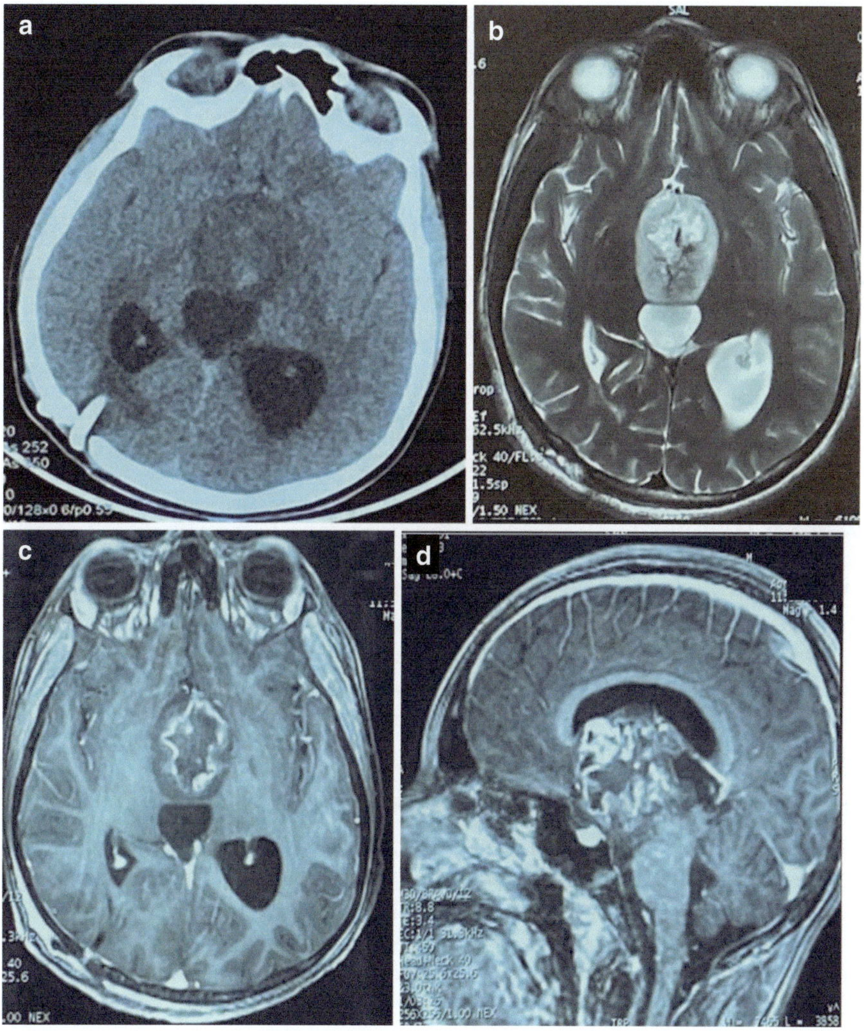


**Fig. 21.1** (**a**) NCCT head in a patient with hypothalamic glioma showing a hypodense lesion in the hypothalamic area. The lesion is hyperintense on T2W MRI (**b**) and shows irregular enhancement on contrast MRI (**c**, **d**)

#### 21.6.1.5 Pathology

These are considered WHO grade 1. On macroscopic examination, they are soft to firm and greyish in color. Cysts are commonly seen within the tumor as well as surrounding the tumor tissue. On microscopic examination, they are sparse to moderately cellular with fibrillated areas and Rosenthal fibers. The granular bodies are periodic acid-Schiff (PAS), alpha1-antitrypsin, and alpha1-antichymotrypsin positive, whereas the piloid cells are glial fibrillary acid protein (GFAP) positive. They have relatively low Ki-67/MIB-1 index of up to 3%.

Genetics: Nearly 15–20% of children with NF-1 under 7 years are predisposed to developing optic pathway gliomas [16]. Nearly 2% brainstem lesions are associated with NF-1; individuals who exhibit additional NF-1 stigmata should be recognized. Numerous genetic pathways are linked to the development and cause of illness. Causes of MAPK/Erk pathway upregulation include inactivation of NF1 gene in NF-1 and BRAF gene changes (mutation, fusion, or overexpression) in sporadic tumors. In contrast to BRAFV600E point mutation in supratentorial and diencephalic lesions, KIAA1549-BRAF fusions are more frequent in lesions of the optic pathway and cerebellum [17]. Tumors with *BRAFV600E* mutation and CDKN2A deletion have poorer PFS and OS, while those with *KIAA1549-BRAF* fusions have better outcomes.

Deregulation of the phosphoinositol 3 kinase (PI3K) pathway, Matrilin 2 overexpression, and other molecular changes can result in the development of aggressive or recurring disease. High CD133 and MDR1 expression in recurrent tumors treated with many courses of chemotherapy may function via the PI3K-Akt-NF-B signaling pathway and result in drug resistance [18].

#### 21.6.1.6 Treatment

Surgery remains the primary treatment, with no adjuvant therapy needed after GTR. Patients with small residual disease may be followed up for progression. Tumors in brainstem or optic pathway may preclude complete resection, sometimes amenable to biopsy only, and these may need adjuvant or salvage therapy more commonly than cerebellar or hemispheric lesions. Recurrence rates following GTR are less than 5%, but after partial resection are close to 50%. Non-critical site tumors may be followed up even after partial resection and re-excision may be considered if increasing in extent.

Brainstem or spinal lesions may benefit from adjuvant RT after incomplete resection or biopsy. RT may also be used for symptomatic sporadic visual pathway tumors, cancers resistant to chemotherapy, or recurring tumors that cannot be surgically removed again. Gross tumor volume (GTV) is defined as residual tumor seen on a recent T1 contrast MRI. Additional margins of 5–10 mm are applied to generate CTV, with a further margin of 3–5 mm to generate the PTV, and this final volume is planned to receive a dose of 50.4 Gy in 28 fractions using conformal approaches. Depending on how close the tumor is to vital normal structures, other treatments including IMRT, VMAT (with or without imaging guidance), and proton therapy may be used.

Adjuvant RT results in long-term survival exceeding 95% and EFS rates of 70–90% [19]. Not every patient with an optic pathway pilocytic astrocytoma will restore their eyesight. RT should not be used in children with NF-1 because they may become more susceptible to second malignancies and vasculopathies. Vincristine-carboplatin chemotherapy, however, may hinder progression and postpone RT in unresectable or residual tumors in young children [9].

Adjuvant RT is not recommended for these tumors since they afflict young children and have a good prognosis unless mass effect from residual disease in locations like brainstem is causing neurological damage. Before administering RT to adolescents and young adults with any low-grade tumors, the possibility of malignant transformation should be discussed. Chemotherapy may help unresectable tumors in very young children by delaying disease progression. In recurrent/unresectable/disseminated conditions, adult pilocytic astrocytomas may respond to antiangiogenic therapy such as bevacizumab due to their high vascularity and high VEGF expression, but such data are sparse in children. Farnesyl transferase inhibitors, MEK inhibitors, and mTOR inhibitors may all be used therapeutically. Through the suppression of the MAPK pathway, systemic drugs like dabrafenib and trametinib are being researched for the management of aggressive tumors. Age and tumor location both affect survival. Compared to unresectable tumors (brainstem, spine), tumors with GTR have a higher likelihood of survival.

Spinal pilocytic astrocytomas: Although overall prognosis is good and extent of resection does not impact OS, GTR is feasible in only 70–80%. Nearly one-third will relapse or progress necessitating further therapy. Children younger than 3 years have higher progression rates and poorer prognosis. BRAF mutations and fusions are common and affect prognosis and thus, adjuvant therapy decisions.

Figure 21.2 shows the radiotherapy planning images of two cases of recurrent posterior fossa and residual spinal pilocytic astrocytoma.

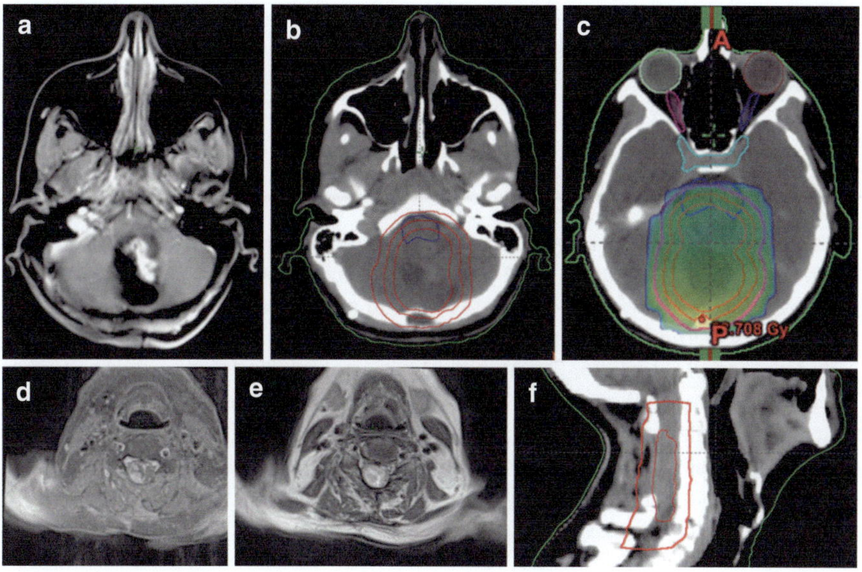


**Fig. 21.2** (**a**) Postoperative case of pilocytic astrocytoma in a 9 year old child with recurrent symptoms and an enhancing lesion in posterior fossa with invasion of brainstem, which was deemed unresectable. (**b**) She was planned for salvage radiotherapy. The gross tumor volume, clinical target volume, and planning target volume are demonstrated. (**c**) A dose of 50.4 gray (Gy) in 28 fractions was delivered by conformal radiotherapy. (**d**) Postoperative case of pilocytic astrocytoma of the spine in a young male with significant residual on T1 contrast enhanced MRI and (**e**) T2 weighted MRI. (**f**) The residual spinal tumor (light red, inner volume) was deemed unresectable, and hence, a dose of 50.4 Gy was planned to the planning target volume (outer volume, bright red)

Opticochiasmatic and Hypothalamic Gliomas: Sequelae of NF-1 should be screened for, and if in doubt, genetic testing can be performed. Optic nerve gliomas have better long-term outcomes than optic chiasmal/hypothalamic lesions. NF-1-associated lesions behave better. Vision impairment is earlier and quicker in sporadic lesions. Treatment decisions should factor the child's age, disease location and symptoms, and NF-1 status. Optic nerve lesions without extension to optic canal or chiasm may need serial imaging for follow-up and examination for progression in size or symptoms. Symptomatic or progressive lesions can be offered a trial of chemotherapy especially in very young children to stabilize the course and delay RT. Various combinations have been used with encouraging responses. Nearly 60% patients may not need RT till 5 years with this approach [20]. Surgery is offered only in case of mass effect or proptosis, or if the vision in that eye is already lost. For posterior tumors with hydrocephalus, debulking or ventriculoperitoneal shunting may be needed. Attempts should be made to obtain biopsy in all posteriorly located tumors if not associated with NF-1. Targeted therapy addressing MAPK pathway may be used as an alternative to chemotherapy, but durability of responses is unknown. MEK1/MEK2 inhibitors (trametinib and selumetinib) are preferred over BRAF inhibitors (vemurafenib and dabrafenib) and are effective in sporadic as well as NF-1 lesions in reducing (20%) or stabilizing (80%) tumor size [21]. In sporadic tumors, RT may be offered if the trial of chemotherapy fails to delay progression. In NF-1, RT should be avoided as far as possible due to risk of malignant conversion.

### 21.6.2 Subependymal Giant Cell Astrocytomas (SEGA)

These are WHO grade 1 tumors arising in periventricular region from subependymal nodules near the foramen of Monro. They can be unilateral or bilateral and have a strong association with tuberous sclerosis (an autosomal dominant neurocutaneous disorder harboring mutations of TSC or TSC2 genes, and the classic triad including mental retardation, seizures, and hamartomas involving multiple organs). They present at a median age of 11 years and are more common in males. Owing to their location, they may cause obstructive hydrocephalus and present with features of raised ICP such as headache, vomiting, blurred vision or diplopia, seizures (new or worsening), and change in personality. On imaging, the tumor classically appears as an intraventricular mass, with specks of calcification. MRI shows periventricular lesions showing T1 hypointensity, T2/FLAIR hyperintensity, with contrast enhancement in 10%. Multiple cortical tubers/subependymal nodules may be seen, Diagnosis of SEGA requires a serial increment in size of these nodules or obstructive symptoms; histopathology cannot differentiate SEGA from subependymal nodules. SEGA have a slow growth rate and may occasionally have invasion of parenchyma or perilesional edema; occasionally lesions may be seen in atypical locations such as hypothalamus or pineal. When symptoms are absent, imaging may be repeated every 1–3 years.

Histologically these tumors contain large gemistocytic, spindles, and ganglion-cell like astrocytes with immunoreactivity for both glial and neuronal markers. Dysregulation of mTOR signaling underlies the basic mechanism for their development, and therapy directed towards this pathway is used in the management of these patients.

Early surgical excision is considered for symptomatic (intractable seizures) or growing SEGA to avoid complications due to raised ICP. If GTR is achieved, it is curative. An incomplete resection may not prevent further tumor growth. Surgery in larger tumors carries the risk of motor weakness, stroke, memory loss, or dependence on ventriculoperitoneal shunt; if these are anticipated, medical management using mTOR inhibitors (rapamycin, everolimus) for reducing or stabilizing the tumor may be used; the effect, however, wanes on discontinuation of the drug. These drugs may interact with AEDs causing low platelets, immune suppression, and impairment of wound healing; hence, monitoring and judicious use are necessary. RT is usually not recommended. Some investigators have used gamma knife (peripheral dose 11–13 Gy) for progressive tumors unfit for surgery or medical therapy [22].

A Surveillance, Epidemiology, and End Results (SEER) database analysis showed that age <18 years and surgery had better survival while gender, tumor location/size, surgical extent, or delivery of RT did not have an impact on survival [23].

## 21.7 Pediatric Type Diffuse LGG

These lesions share many characteristics with adult diffuse gliomas. Tumors with diffuse infiltration and lacking the classical features mitotic activity, microvascular proliferation, and necrosis come under this category. As per WHO 2021 classification, these are categorized into four main types as described in Table 21.1.

These tumors can occur throughout the CNS, but the most common location is in the cerebral hemispheres followed by diencephalon, brainstem, and cerebellum; spinal cord is the least common location. Overall, these tumors have very good survival rate, but the location of tumor is one of the important predictors of survival. Deep-seated midline tumors are usually not amenable to GTR and adjuvant therapy is needed.

Over the last decade, a multitude of molecular markers have been identified, which also have therapeutic as well as prognostic significance. The most reported molecular events in pediatric diffuse LGG include:

1. IDH 1/2 mutations.
2. TP53 mutations.
3. BRAF mutations.
4. CDKN2A/p16 deletion.
5. H3F3A mutation.
6. MYB/MYBL1.
7. FGFR1 mutation.

### 21.7.1 Diffuse astrocytoma, MYB or MYBL1-altered

This tumor type frequently involves cerebral hemispheres. On imaging, these are seen as lobulated and infiltrative masses showing T1 iso- to hypointensity, heterogeneous T2/FLAIR hyperintensity, no contrast enhancement, and no diffusion restriction on DWI/ADC sequences.

### 21.7.2 Angiocentric gliomas

Angiocentric gliomas are rare tumors involving children and young adults and their typical presentation is with intractable seizures. On imaging, they are well-delineated supratentorial tumors that tend to expand the affected gyri and most of them are in cortical or subcortical location. On MRI, these lesions show T1 hypointensity with hyperintensity at periphery and T2/FLAIR hyperintensity with extension along vessels towards ventricles and show no contrast enhancement. On microscopic examination, the tumors shows spindle shaped bipolar cells with a perivascular orientation. One of their prominent features is subpial growth along the surface of the cortex. Surgery is curative.

### 21.7.3 Polymorphous Low-Grade Neuroepithelial Tumors of the Young (PLNTY)

This tumor mainly affects children and young adults and most commonly occurs in the temporal lobe. On MRI, this tumor shows T1 iso- to hypointensity, heterogeneous T2/FLAIR hyperintensity with salt and pepper sign (due to calcification), slight or no contrast enhancement, and blooming on T2/SWI sequences. Association with cortical dysplasia is common. On histology, they show infiltrative growth, oligodendroglioma (ODG)-like components, frequent calcification, and CD34 positivity. Unlike ODG, these tumors are IDH wild and lack 1p/19q codeletions but may have BRAFV600E mutation or FGFR2/FGFR3 translocation. Ki-67 is low (<5%).

Molecular alterations with MAPK pathway activation may be present. Surgery is curative. GTR leads to good seizure relief. Even with STR, tumors may remain stable over long periods. Role of adjuvant therapy is unclear due to recent nomenclature as well as inherent indolent behavior.

### 21.7.4 Diffuse Low-Grade Glioma, MAPK Pathway-Altered

These rare tumors comprise <2% of pLGG. They present with seizures (median age 14 years) [24]. On MRI, they are well-defined tumors, with T1 hypointensity, heterogeneous T2 hyperintensity, and no contrast enhancement or diffusion restriction.

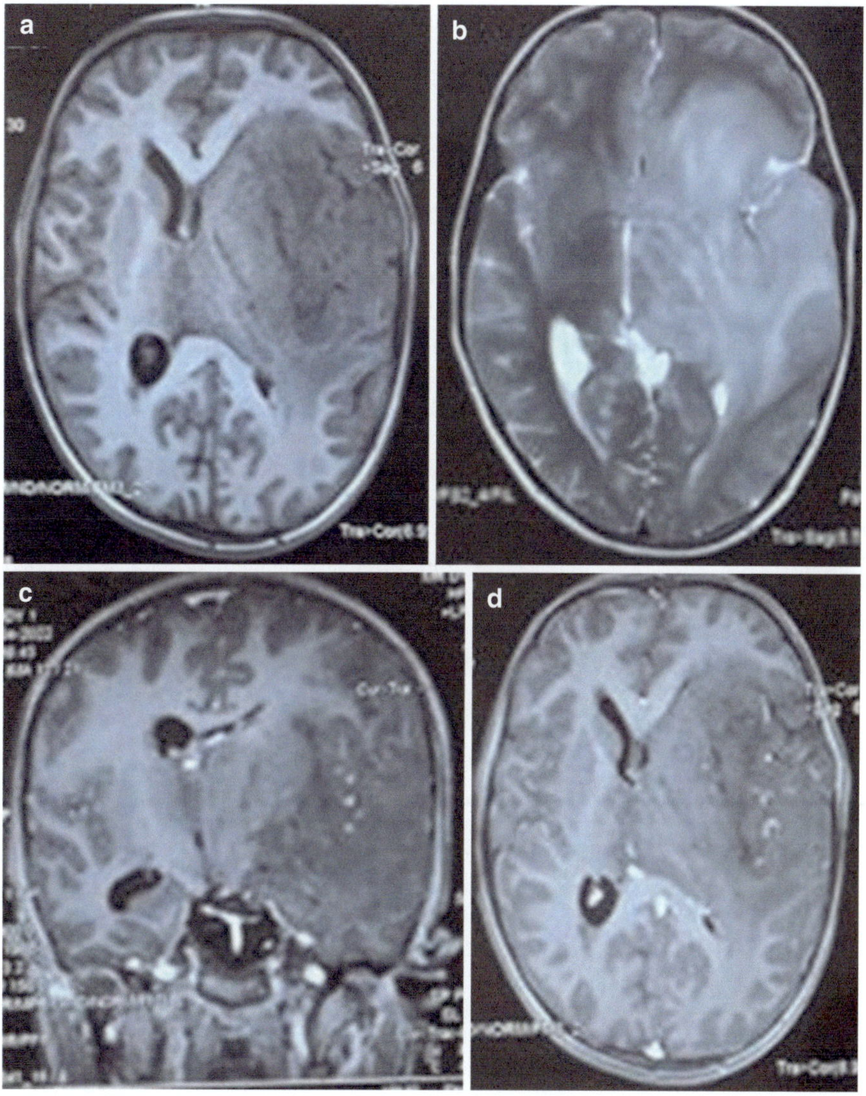

**Fig. 21.3** (**a**) Left fronto-temporo-parietal diffuse low-grade glioma that is hypointense on T1W MRI, (**b**) hyperintense on T2W MRI, (**c**, **d**) but without contrast enhancement

Pathology shows tumors with bland glial proliferations with minimal atypia, an infiltrating growth pattern and astrocytic, ODG, or mixed phenotypic features. On IHC, these are GFAP positive, OLIG2/IDH1/CD34 negative, with retained ATRX. KI-67 is low. Several genetic alterations are seen including FGFR1 duplications, fusion, and BRAFV600E mutation. Surgery is curative and relieves epilepsy as well (Fig. 21.3).

## 21.8 Glioneuronal and Neuronal Tumors

It encompasses tumors with distinct morphological features. Most frequently seen tumors in this category are discussed below.

### 21.8.1 Dysembryoplastic Neuroepithelial Tumors (DNET)

These are WHO grade 1 tumors, seen predominantly in children. Most common location is cortical in temporal lobe and their common presentation is seizures, which are sometimes refractory to anti-epileptic drugs Tumors are associated with fibrous cortical dysplasia and hemimegalencephaly in 50% cases. CT shows a hyperdense calcified lesion, and MRI shows a well-demarcated, multilobulated T1 hypointense and T2 hyperintense lesion, with enhancement in 30% cases. There is no edema or mass effect, but MRI shows choline peaks and no diffusion restriction. Histopathology shows glial nodules, glioneuronal elements, and cortical dysplasia. Although ODG-like areas may be evident, IDH mutation and 1p/19q codeletion are absent. FGFR alterations may be present. Surgical management entails extended lesionectomy (excision of abnormal dysplastic cortex along the lesion) but may not be feasible in larger tumors. Tumors are slow growing and adjuvant therapy has no role. Epilepsy may recur even in the absence of tumor regrowth after surgery [25].

### 21.8.2 Ganglioglioma (WHO Grade I)

They are rare tumors (<1% CNS tumors) presenting at a median age of 12 years and more often in males, with seizures, and have a temporal lobe location.

Histopathology shows mixed astrocytic and neuronal elements, with many showing BRAF alterations. MRI shows T1 iso- to hypointensity and T2 hyperintensity in a solid-cystic or solid mass, with variable enhancement, extensive calcification, cortical dysplasia, but no edema or mass effect. Complete resection is curative. They have a favorable prognosis. SEER database shows a 95% 5-year OS in non-brainstem lesions. Need for adjuvant RT is rare for inoperable tumors, especially in brainstem, either at presentation or at recurrence.

### 21.8.3 Desmoplastic Infantile Astrocytoma and Ganglioglioma

These are tumors of infancy, most detected earlier than 18 months of age, with increasing head circumference, seizures, and focal neurologic changes. MRI demonstrates a multilobar tumor in supratentorial location, with heterogeneity on T2 sequences (hyperintense cystic elements and hypointense but enhancing solid elements). Characteristic features include involvement of superficial cerebral cortex and leptomeninges, dural attachment, and a desmoplastic reaction. MRS reveals a high choline/NAA ratio, enhanced perfusion, and low ADC values in diffusion experiments. Mixed ganglionic and astrocytic cells are visible in histology. A high number of mitoses may be a sign of the presence of primitive cells and may resemble malignant astrocytomas. BRAF mutations may occasionally be present. Curative resection is feasible in one-third patients. Even after partial resection, observation is the norm. Chemotherapy might be necessary after multiple recurrences that are not salvageable with surgery. The long-term outlook is favorable. Midline (hypothalamic) tumors may be more aggressive.

## References


1. Ostrom QT, Price M, Ryan K, Edelson J, Neff C, Cioffi G, Waite KA, Kruchko C, Barnholtz-Sloan JS. CBTRUS statistical report: pediatric brain tumor foundation childhood and adolescent primary brain and other central nervous system tumors diagnosed in the United States in 2014-2018. Neuro Oncol. 2022;24(Suppl 3):iii1–iii38.
2. Louis DN, Perry A, Wesseling P, Brat DJ, Cree IA, Figarella-Branger D, Hawkins C, Ng HK, Pfister SM, Reifenberger G, Soffietti R, von Deimling A, Ellison DW. The 2021 WHO classification of tumors of the central nervous system: a summary. Neuro Oncol. 2021;23(8):1231–51.
3. Wisoff JH, Sanford RA, Heier LA, Sposto R, Burger PC, Yates AJ, et al. Primary neurosurgery for pediatric low-grade gliomas: a prospective multi-institutional study from the Children's Oncology Group. Neurosurgery. 2011;68(6):1548–55.
4. Bale TA, Rosenblum MK. The 2021 WHO classification of tumors of the central nervous system: an update on pediatric low-grade gliomas and glioneuronal tumors. Brain Pathol. 2022;32(4):e13060.
5. Chalil A, Ramaswamy V. Low grade gliomas in children. J Child Neurol. 2016;31(4):517–22.
6. Shaw EG, Wisoff JH. Prospective clinical trials of intracranial low-grade glioma in adults and children. Neuro Oncol. 2003;5(3):153–60.
7. Eaton BR, Yock TI. Radiation for pediatric low-grade gliomas: who will benefit and how late is soon enough? Neuro Oncol. 2020;22(8):1068–9.
8. Acharya S, Liu JF, Tatevossian RG, Chiang J, Qaddoumi I, Gajjar A, Walker D, Harreld JH, Merchant TE, Ellison DW. Risk stratification in pediatric low-grade glioma and glioneuronal tumor treated with radiation therapy: an integrated clinicopathologic and molecular analysis. Neuro Oncol. 2020;22(8):1203–13.
9. Packer RJ, Ater J, Allen J, Phillips P, Geyer R, Nicholson HS, Jakacki R, Kurczynski E, Needle M, Finlay J, Reaman G, Boyett JM. Carboplatin and vincristine chemotherapy for children with newly diagnosed progressive low-grade gliomas. J Neurosurg. 1997;86(5):747–54.
10. Ater JL, Zhou T, Holmes E, Mazewski CM, Booth TN, Freyer DR, Lazarus KH, Packer RJ, Prados M, Sposto R, Vezina G, Wisoff JH, Pollack IF. Randomized study of two chemotherapy regimens for treatment of low-grade glioma in young children: a report from the Children's Oncology Group. J Clin Oncol. 2012;30(21):2641–7.
11. Al-Jilaihawi S, Lowis S. A molecular update and review of current trials in paediatric low grade gliomas. Pediatr Neurosurg. 2023;58:290. https://doi.org/10.1159/000533703.
12. Burkhard C, Patre PLD, Schüler D, Schüler G, Yaşargil MG, Yonekawa Y, et al. A population-based study of the incidence and survival rates in patients with pilocytic astrocytoma. J Neurosurg. 2003;98(6):1170–4.
13. Czyzyk E, Jozwiak S, Roszkowski M, Schwartz RA. Optic pathway gliomas in children with and without neurofibromatosis 1. J Child Neurol. 2003;18(7):471–8.
14. Mazloom A, Hodges JC, Teh BS, Chintagumpala M, Paulino AC. Outcome of patients with pilocytic astrocytoma and leptomeningeal dissemination. Int J Radiat Oncol Biol Phys. 2012;84(2):350–4.
15. Yahanda AT, Patel B, Sutherland G, et al. A multi-institutional analysis of factors influencing surgical outcomes for patients with newly diagnosed grade I gliomas. World Neurosurg. 2020;135:e754–64.

16. Bornhorst M, Frappaz D, Packer RJ. Pilocytic astrocytomas. Handb Clin Neurol. 2016;134:329–44.
17. Collins VP, Jones DT, Giannini C. Pilocytic astrocytoma: pathology, molecular mechanisms and markers. Acta Neuropathol. 2015;129(6):775–88.
18. Xi G, Li YD, Grahovac G, et al. Targeting CD133 improves chemotherapeutic efficacy of recurrent pediatric pilocytic astrocytoma following prolonged chemotherapy. Mol Cancer. 2017;16(1):21.
19. Merchant TE, Kun LE, Wu S, Xiong X, Sanford RA, Boop FA. Phase II trial of conformal radiation therapy for pediatric low-grade glioma. J Clin Oncol. 2009;27(22):3598–604.
20. Laithier V, Grill J, Le Deley MC, Ruchoux MM, Couanet D, Doz F, Pichon F, Rubie H, Frappaz D, Vannier JP, Babin-Boilletot A, Sariban E, Chastagner P, Zerah M, Raquin MA, Hartmann O, Kalifa C, French Society of Pediatric Oncology. Progression-free survival in children with optic pathway tumors: dependence on age and the quality of the response to chemotherapy—results of the first French prospective study for the French Society of Pediatric Oncology. J Clin Oncol. 2003;21(24):4572–8.
21. Giotta Lucifero A, Elbabaa SK, Baldoncini M, Bruno N, Savasta S, Marseglia GL, Luzzi S. Novel "T-dimension" therapies for pediatric optic pathway glioma: a timely, targeted, and tailored treatment trend. Pediatr Neurosurg. 2022;57(3):161–74.
22. Park KJ, Kano H, Kondziolka D, et al. Gamma Knife surgery for subependymal giant cell astrocytomas. J Neurosurg. 2011;114(3):808–13.
23. Nguyen HS, Doan NB, Gelsomino M, et al. Subependymal giant cell astrocytoma: a surveillance, epidemiology, and end results program-based analysis from 2004 to 2013. World Neurosurg. 2018;118:e263–8.
24. Fabbri VP, Caporalini C, Asioli S, Buccoliero A. Paediatric-type diffuse low-grade gliomas: a clinically and biologically distinct group of tumours with a favourable outcome. Pathologica. 2022;114(6):410–21.
25. O'Brien DF, Farrell M, Delanty N, Traunecker H, Perrin R, Smyth MD, Park TS, Children's Cancer and Leukaemia Group. The Children's Cancer and Leukaemia Group guidelines for the diagnosis and management of dysembryoplastic neuroepithelial tumours. Br J Neurosurg. 2007;21(6):539–49.

# Intracranial Germ Cell Tumors

# 22

K. P. Haresh, V. R. Anjali, Astha Srivastava, Subhash Gupta, and Shikha Goyal

## 22.1 Introduction

Germ cell tumors (GCTs) are malignant neoplasm originating from the primordial germ cell at different stages of development. They may arise in gonads (testis and ovary) or extragonadal sites (intracranial, mediastinal, sacrococcygeal area). The extragonadal location of GCTs is explained by the presence of ectopic germline cells during the migration of primordial germ cells. The location of extragonadal GCTs is usually in the midline of the body. Intracranial GCTs (icGCTs) account for 3–5% of pediatric primary central nervous system tumors in Europe and North America and 11–15% in East Asia [1]. icGCTs show male preponderance, except in suprasellar germinomas, which are seen more frequently in females.

## 22.2 Clinical Presentation

The most common location of icGCTs is the pineal region (50–60%) followed by the suprasellar region (30–40%), basal ganglia, ventricles, thalamus, and cerebrum [2]. It can occur as a bifocal disease (5–10%), where the tumor is present in both the pineal and suprasellar regions. Signs and symptoms vary depending on the location of the tumor and tumor size.

Tumors in the pineal region can obstruct the cerebrospinal circulation, resulting in obstructive hydrocephalus, features of raised intracranial tension, headache, nausea, and vomiting requiring shunt placement. Other symptoms include vertical

K. P. Haresh (✉) · V. R. Anjali · A. Srivastava · S. Gupta
Department of Radiotherapy and Oncology, AIIMS, New Delhi, India

S. Goyal
Department of Radiotherapy and Oncology, Postgraduate Institute of Medical Education and Research, Chandigarh, India





R. Madan et al. (eds.), *Evidence Based Practice in Pediatric Radiation Oncology*, https://doi.org/10.1007/978-981-96-4872-6_22

gaze palsy, nystagmus, and pupillary hyporeflexia (Parinaud syndrome) by the involvement of dorsal midbrain structures.

Suprasellar region tumors due to compression can present with hypothalamic-pituitary dysfunction leading to diabetes insipidus, pubertal retardation, isolated growth hormone deficiency, precocious puberty, and hypopituitarism. Due to compression of optic chiasma, they can present with bitemporal hemianopia or other visual abnormalities and visual field defects.

## 22.3 Imaging

Magnetic resonance imaging of the brain with spine screening is used to assess the location and extent of the disease. Pre- and post-contrast T1- and T2-weighted images of the brain with spine screening are necessary for evaluation of extent. iGCTs appear isointense or slightly hypo-intense lesions on T1-weighted images and appear hyper-intense on T2-weighted images. Germinomas usually enhance homogeneously, whereas teratomas are more heterogeneous, with cystic components.

## 22.4 Tumor Markers

Both serum and cerebrospinal fluid (CSF) tumor markers for alpha fetoprotein (AFP) and human chorionic gonadotrophin (HCG) are performed. For secreting non-germinomatous germ cell tumors (NGGCT), International Society of Paediatric Oncology (SIOP) criteria of serum/cerebrospinal fluid (CSF) AFP levels >25 ng/mL and/or HCG >50 IU/L in Europe, and Children's Oncology Group (COG) criteria for AFP >10 ng/mL and HCG >100 IU/L values in United States are taken along with typical radiological findings for treating patients without biopsy.

## 22.5 Biopsy and CSF Cytology

A biopsy is not mandatory for tumors with raised tumor marker (secretory type) and typical radiological findings. Whereas biopsy is essential in non-secretory tumors, with slight/non-characteristic tumor marker elevation and discrepancy in radiology, CSF cytology is essential for all patients before starting treatment.

## 22.6 Pathology and Immunohistochemistry

Intracranial GCTs are classified in germinomas and non-germinomatous germ cell tumor (NGGCT). NGGCT is divided into embryonal carcinoma, yolk sac tumor, choriocarcinoma, and teratomas. Germinomas show large monomorphous round cells with clear cytoplasm immunoreactive for PLAP, CD 117, OCT4, NANOG, and negative for SOX2. Isolated syncytiotrophoblast cells may be seen in germinomas because of which small raise in HCG (<50 mlU/mL) is seen in some germinomas which should not be mistaken for choriocarcinoma. Embryonal carcinoma has poorly differentiated cells with marked nuclear atypia, necrosis, and high mitotic activity. They are positive for OCT4, NANOG, and SOX 2. Yolk sac tumors are heterogeneous with atypical cells in variable architecture. They can have a reticular pattern or endodermal sinus pattern characterized by Schiller-Duval bodies. They are positive for AFP and glypican3. Choriocarcinomas have an admixture of cytotrophoblast and syncytiotrophoblast and are positive for HCG. Teratomas can be mature (contains mature adult type of tissue from the three embryonic layers), immature (contains fetal/embryonic tissue from the embryonic layers), or teratomas with malignant transformation (with various epithelial and mesenchymal non-germ cell tumor cells). Mixed germ cell tumors have at least two different subtypes of germ cell elements.

## 22.7 Risk Stratification

In Europe and North America, icGCT is divided into two groups (germinomas and NGGCT), while in Japan, they use a three risk group classification (good, intermediate, and poor).

## 22.8 Staging

Like other pediatric brain tumors, they are staged into localized or metastatic. The disease is considered to be metastatic if CSF cytology is positive for tumor cells or any spinal drop metastasis is present. No formal staging system is available. About 20% of patients have metastases at presentation.

## 22.9 Treatment

### 22.9.1 Role of Surgery

The role of surgery is limited in icGCTs. Surgery may include biopsy for lesions that do not have any raised tumor markers and lack characteristic radiology or may be considered for symptomatic obstructive hydrocephalus. Endoscopic third ventriculostomy (ETV) is preferred; if not feasible, then externalized ventricular drainage is preferred over ventriculoperitoneal shunt. Surgery is the preferred option for diagnosed mature and immature teratoma without malignant transformation. In patients with growing teratoma syndrome, surgical excision provides excellent treatment. It may be considered as a second look procedure after completion of chemotherapy to remove residual NGGCT or teratoma.

### 22.9.2 Germinoma

Germinomas are highly radiotherapy and chemotherapy-responsive tumors. In the 1960s, patients were treated with CSI using an empirical dose of 36–40 gray (Gy) with a boost to the primary up to 50–60 Gy, like other brain tumors. The cure rates were more than 90% at 10 years but at the cost of the long-term treatment-related toxicities. Given excellent outcomes and the treated group being children and adolescents, efforts were started on dose and volume reduction to minimize the morbidity.

Shibamoto et al. evaluated 84 patients treated between 1963 and 1992 and showed that the dose can be reduced to 40–45 Gy, without compromising the outcome. The 10-year relapse free survival (RFS) was 88%, 92%, and 83% for a median dose of 42, 50, and 60 Gy, respectively, for the primary tumor [3].

Reduced dose CSI was successfully used in MAKEI 83/86 study (CSI 36 Gy followed by boost of 14 Gy) and MAKEI 89 study (CSI 30 Gy followed by boost 15 Gy), with 5-year overall survival (OS) of 100% and 92 ± 4.6%, respectively [4].

Subsequent to the success of dose reduced CSI, attempts were made to reduce the treatment volume to whole brain irradiation (WBRT) or whole ventricle irradiation (WVRT) and the outcomes are still maintained while reducing toxicity, especially in localized germinoma [5]. On further studies, it has been shown that CSI may be limited to metastatic germinoma.

The pattern of relapse following WBRT or WVRT with boost and CSI was evaluated by Rogers et al. The recurrence rate was 7.6% and 3.8%, respectively, with no increased risk of spinal metastases (2.9% vs. 1.2%) [6]. Similarly, Haas Kogan et al. in 2003 recommended WVRT with tumor bed boost, with excellent 5 year OS and progression free survival (PFS) of 88% and 93%, respectively [7].

SIOP CNS GCT 96 prospective trial evaluated CSI alone and further dose reduction with chemotherapy followed by RT. Reducing dose RT alone to 24 Gy CSI followed by 16 Gy boost to primary showed excellent 5-year event free survival (EFS) and PFS of 94% and 97%, respectively. The same study also evaluated chemotherapy with carboplatin/etoposide alternating with etoposide/ifosfamide followed by focal radiotherapy. They showed that chemotherapy followed by reduced field RT including the ventricles is also an option [8].

Together with data from SIOP CNS GCT 96, SFOP, and relapse patterns from other studies [9, 10] the standard radiotherapy target volume-WVRT became the standard. With the use of upfront chemotherapy, the role of response-adapted RT was evaluated, in SIOP GCT CNS II and ACNS1123. The current standard of care for localized germinoma is as follows:

- Neoadjuvant chemotherapy (two carboplatin/etoposide alternating with two cycles of ifosfamide/etoposide) followed by whole ventricular RT and +/– focal boost.
  - If complete response (CR) after chemotherapy, then WVRT 24 Gy in 15 fractions alone.

  - If partial response (PR) after chemotherapy, WVRT 24 Gy in 15 fractions followed by focal boost 16 Gy in10 fractions.
- If radiotherapy alone is considered, then WVRT 24 Gy in 15 fractions and boost to the tumor to a total dose of 45 Gy.

Figure 22.1 shows a case of corpus callosal germinoma with response to chemotherapy and the radiotherapy plan.

#### 22.9.2.1 Metastatic Germinoma

Bifocal tumors are treated as localized disease if CSF and MRI are negative for any other disease.

For metastatic germinoma, treatment philosophy varies across continents. In USA, treatment includes systemic chemotherapy (2 cycles carboplatin/etoposide followed by 2 cycles cisplatin/cyclophosphamide if less than complete response) followed by CSI 24 Gy in 15 fractions and boost to primary and metastatic sites 16 Gy (ACNS 0232). The EFS was 98% at 5 years. In Europe, for metastatic germinoma, the standard of care includes CSI 24 Gy with a boost to primary and metastatic site 16 Gy without chemotherapy (SIOP CNS GCT II). Further studies on response-adapted radiotherapy dose modification are still evolving.

### 22.9.3 Non Germinomatous Germ Cell Tumors

NGGCTs need an aggressive treatment than germinomas. The optimum management is still evolving. The treatment approach is multimodal and includes radiotherapy, chemotherapy, and tumor excision if indicated. Upfront surgical excision and attaining gross total resection (GTR) are uniquely recommended for the management of pure CNS mature teratoma, immature teratomas, and the growing teratoma syndrome [11].

Neoadjuvant chemotherapy and radiotherapy facilitate achieving gross total resection (GTR) by reducing the tumor volume, vascularity, and malignant components [12]. COG and SIOP study groups advocate "second-look" surgery for patients with less than complete response (CR) to neoadjuvant chemotherapy, intending to decrease recurrence rates while avoiding the chances of upfront radical surgical excision [13]. MAKEI 89 trial reported no significant association between upfront GTR and survival. In infants and very young children, chemotherapy only regimens are used exclusively to avoid long-term neuropsychological and neurocognitive sequelae.

Since the 1980s, platinum-based chemotherapy has shown to be effective in NGGCT. The most effective chemotherapy agents include cisplatin, carboplatin, etoposide, and cyclophosphamide. There are no randomized trials that compare carboplatin and cisplatin inclusive of patients with CNS-NGGCT. However, carboplatin is often preferred over cisplatin in induction chemotherapy regimens to avoid ototoxicity, nephrotoxicity, and neurotoxicity.

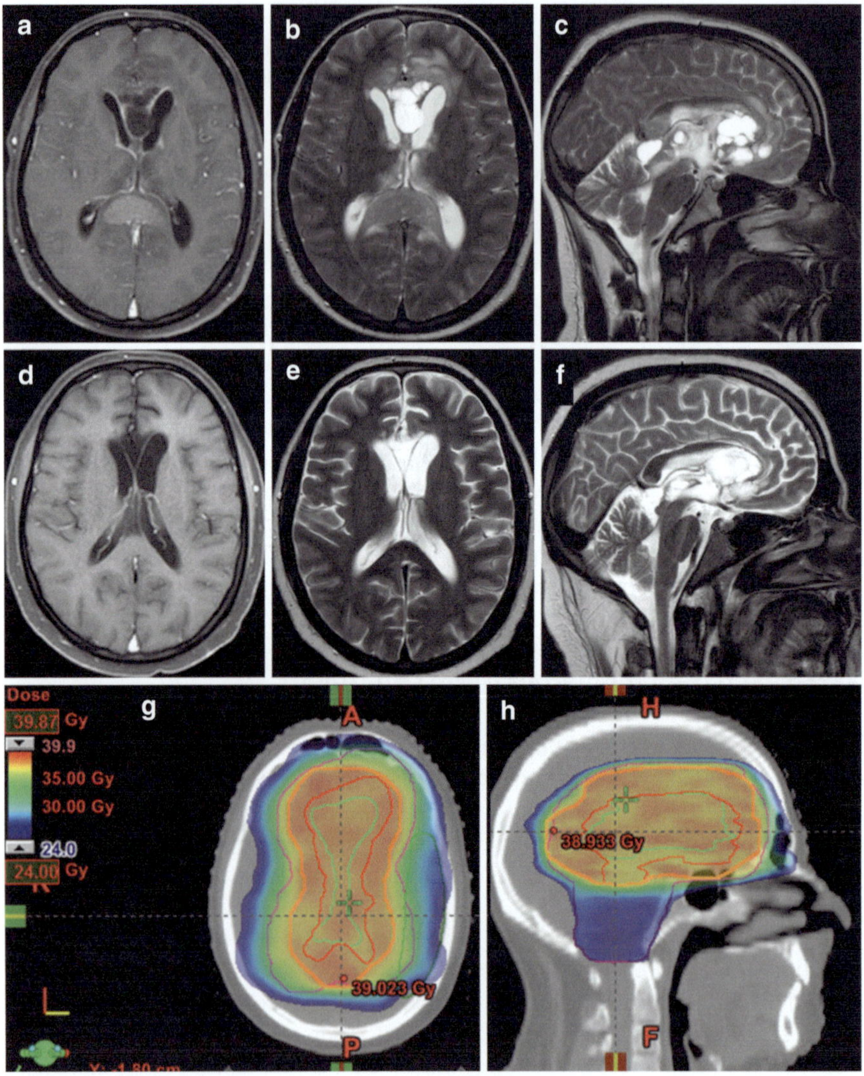


**Fig. 22.1** A 35-year-old young male presented with history of headache and MRI showed a solid-cystic heterogeneously enhancing lesion involving frontal lobe and corpus callosum. (**a**) Axial T1 contrast, (**b**) axial T2-weighted, and (**c**) sagittal T2-weighted images showing the extent of disease at baseline. After four cycles of chemotherapy, there was considerable reduction with small residual component seen on (**d**) axial T1 contrast, (**e**) axial T2-weighted, and (**f**) sagittal T2-weighted images. The patient was planned for radical radiotherapy. RT planning CT scan in (**g**) axial and (**h**) sagittal orientations shows the target volume (baseline tumor in red, residual tumor in light green). A dose of 24 gray (Gy) in 12 fractions was delivered to whole ventricles (magenta outline) followed by a boost of 12 Gy in 6 fractions to PTV 36 (orange outline, encompassing residual tumor)

Radiotherapy alone has reported 20–40% OS, while chemotherapy followed by radiotherapy leads to 60–70% survival. In the ACNS0122 trial, 102 patients received 6 cycles of carboplatin/etoposide alternating with ifosfamide/etoposide and second-look surgery followed by CSI 36 Gy and tumor boost till 54 Gy [14]. The 5-year EFS and OS rates were 84% and 93%, respectively, for this approach.

Retrospective studies have shown that CSI has a positive and independent protective value in avoiding distant relapse [15, 16]. There are no guidelines on the optimal irradiation dosage and field that are mandatory, conjointly with chemotherapy, specifically for patients with localized tumors. In North America, chemotherapy followed by CSI 30 Gy in 20 fractions and boost 24 Gy in 15 fractions is the standard of care, while the European approach is to deliver focal-RT 54 Gy in 30 fractions after chemotherapy for localized NSGCT. For disseminated or metastatic icGCT, chemotherapy followed by CSI 30 Gy in 20 fractions and a boost to the primary and metastatic sites of 24 Gy in 15 fractions is delivered.

## 22.10 Relapse

Patients with relapsed NGGCT have a poor prognosis compared with relapsed CNS germinoma. Approximately 30% of NGGCTs recur following primary treatment and local recurrence is the most common. Patients with refractory or recurrent germinomas are offered high-dose chemotherapy with autologous hematopoietic stem-cell rescue [17]. Patients who managed to receive high-dose chemotherapy and stem cell transplant had a 4- to 5-year survival rate in the range of 30–42%. Patients attaining minimal residual disease (MRD) have better results than those who had less than CR before receiving high-dose chemotherapy and stem cell rescue. Reirradiation and high-dose chemotherapy is still an option for relapsed germinomas. But the role of radiotherapy in relapsed CNS-NGGCT is debatable. While re-irradiating, the time interval from prior irradiation, treatment field, dose prescribed in prior treatment, size, site of the relapsed tumor, and the adjacency of organs at risk to bypass long-term neurocognitive and neuroendocrine side effects should be considered.

## 22.11 Long-Term Toxicity

The location of intracranial GCT itself is responsible for early development of endocrine and neurologic complaints. Since most of these are curable, delayed treatment effects hold relevance.

Although data on effects of radiotherapy in GCTs is sparse, it is known that cranial radiotherapy in these tumors can cause neurocognitive deficits, increases risk of future strokes and second malignancies [18]. With reduction in irradiation volumes with multimodal therapy, the incidence of neurocognitive effects may reduce in future. Use of cisplatin chemotherapy may lead to hearing deficits (especially when combined with cranial irradiation), renal impairment, peripheral neuropathy, infertility, and hypogonadism. Endocrine deficiencies (central hypothyroidism, diabetes insipidus, growth hormone deficiency, hypogonadism) resulting from disease process and accentuated by therapy occur in half the patients and may need long-term correction. Incidence of second cancers at 25 years seems high at 4–6%.

## 22.12 Indian Data on Intracranial GCTs

Incidence in Indian tertiary hospital series (0.43%) seems to match the Western data (0.3–0.6%) [19]. A large series from AIIMS New Delhi reported a median age of 12 years with male preponderance and pineal location being the most common. Germinomas were twice as common compared to nongerminomatous tumors. Another series from NIMHANS Bangalore reported a similar incidence, higher median age (16.5 years) and a higher proportion of nongerminomatous tumors (44%) [20]. In this series, females had poorer survival. A smaller series from PGIMER Chandigarh showed the data from radiation oncology department, where in addition to radiotherapy [21], ~80% had received chemotherapy. Germinoma histology and pineal location were prognostic for overall survival.

## References

1. Zapotocky M, Ramaswamy V, Lassaletta A, Bouffet E. Adolescents and young adults with brain tumors in the context of molecular advances in neuro-oncology. Pediatr Blood Cancer. 2018;65(2):e26861.
2. Echevarría ME, Fangusaro J, Goldman S. Pediatric central nervous system germ cell tumors: a review. Oncologist. 2008;13(6):690–9.
3. Shibamoto Y, Takahashi M, Abe M. Reduction of the radiation dose for intracranial germinoma: a prospective study. Br J Cancer. 1994;70:984–9.
4. Bamberg M, Kortmann RD, Calaminus G, et al. Radiation therapy for intracranial germinoma: results of the German cooperative prospective trials MAKEI 83/86/89. J Clin Oncol. 1999;17:2585–92.
5. Aoyama H, Shirato H, Kakuto Y, et al. Pathologically-proven intracranial germinoma treated with radiation therapy. Radiother Oncol. 1998;47:201–5.
6. Rogers SJ, Mosleh-Shirazi MA, Saran FH. Radiotherapy of localised intracranial germinoma: time to sever historical ties? Lancet Oncol. 2005;6:509–19.
7. Haas-Kogan DA, Missett BT, Wara WM, Donaldson SS, Lamborn KR, Prados MD, Fisher PG, Huhn SL, Fisch BM, Berger MS, Le QT. Radiation therapy for intracranial germ cell tumors. Int J Radiat Oncol Biol Phys. 2003;56(2):511–8. https://doi.org/10.1016/s0360-3016(02)04611-4. Erratum in: Int J Radiat Oncol Biol Phys. 2003 Sep 1;57(1):306. PMID: 12738328.
8. Calaminus G, Kortmann R, Worch J, Nicholson JC, Alapetite C, Garrè ML, Patte C, Ricardi U, Saran F, Frappaz D. SIOP CNS GCT 96: final report of outcome of a prospective, multinational nonrandomized trial for children and adults with intracranial germinoma, comparing craniospinal irradiation alone with chemotherapy followed by focal primary site irradiation for patients with localized disease. Neuro Oncol. 2013;15(6):788–96. https://doi.org/10.1093/neuonc/not019. Epub 2013 Mar 3. PMID: 23460321; PMCID: PMC3661100.
9. Aoyama H, Shirato H, Ikeda J, Fujieda K, Miyasaka K, Sawamura Y. Induction chemotherapy followed by low-dose involved-field radiotherapy for intracranial germ cell tumors. J Clin Oncol. 2002;20(3):857–65.

10. Baranzelli MC, Patte C, Bouffet E, Couanet D, Habrand JL, Portas M, et al. Nonmetastatic intracranial germinoma: the experience of the French Society of Pediatric Oncology. Cancer. 1997;80(9):1792–7.
11. Noudel R, Vinchon M, Dhellemmes P, Litré CF, Rousseaux P. Intracranial teratomas in children: the role and timing of surgical removal. J Neurosurg Pediatr. 2008;2:331–8.
12. Kanamori M, Kumabe T, Saito R, et al. Optimal treatment strategy for intracranial germ cell tumors: a single institution analysis. J Neurosurg Pediatr. 2009;4:506–14.
13. Calaminus G, Frappaz D, Kortmann RD, et al. Outcome of patients with intracranial non-germinomatous germ cell tumors—lessons from the SIOP-CNS-GCT-96 trial. Neuro Oncol. 2017;19:1661–72.
14. Goldman S, Bouffet E, Fisher PG, et al. Phase II trial assessing the ability of neoadjuvant chemotherapy with or without second-look surgery to eliminate measurable disease for nongerminomatous germ cell tumors: a Children's Oncology Group Study. J Clin Oncol. 2015;33(22):2464–71.
15. Breen WG, Blanchard MJ, Rao AN, Daniels DJ, Buckner JC, Laack NNI. Optimal radiotherapy target volumes in intracranial nongerminomatous germ cell tumors: long-term institutional experience with chemotherapy, surgery, and dose- and field-adapted radiotherapy. Pediatr Blood Cancer. 2017;64:e26637.
16. Kim JW, Kim WC, Cho JH, et al. A multimodal approach including craniospinal irradiation improves the treatment outcome of high-risk intracranial nongerminomatous germ cell tumors. Int J Radiat Oncol Biol Phys. 2012;84:625–31.
17. Malone K, Croke J, Malone C, Malone S. Successful salvage using combined radiation and ABMT for patients with recurrent CNS NGGCT following failed initial transplant. BMJ Case Rep. 2012;2012:bcr2012006298.
18. Acharya S, DeWees T, Shinohara ET, Perkins SM. Long-term outcomes and late effects for childhood and young adulthood intracranial germinomas. Neuro Oncol. 2015;17(5):741–6.
19. Kakkar A, Biswas A, Kalyani N, et al. Intracranial germ cell tumors: a multi-institutional experience from three tertiary care centers in India [published correction appears in Childs Nerv Syst. 2016 Nov;32(11):2181]. Childs Nerv Syst. 2016;32(11):2173–80.
20. Borde TD, Arimappamagan A, Srinivas D, et al. Intracranial germ cell tumors: spectrum of disease in an Indian cohort and management strategies. J Neurosci Rural Pract. 2018;9(3):291–7.
21. Kumar N, Madan R, Dracham CB, et al. Multimodality treatment for central nervous system germ cell tumors: disease spectrum and management strategies—a tertiary care center experience from India. Clin Neurol Neurosurg. 2021;202:106481.

# Brainstem Glioma

# 23

Namrata Das, G. Y. Srinivasa, Chirag Ahuja, and Apinderpreet Singh

## 23.1 Introduction

The brainstem is the conduit connecting the cerebrum to cerebellum. It harbours multiple vital centres and origins of cranial nerve nuclei. Gliomas can arise from any of its three components, namely, the midbrain, pons and medulla oblongata, making it a tricky site for surgical manipulation. Broadly brainstem gliomas fall in two categories: low-grade focal brainstem glioma (FBSG) and diffuse intrinsic pontine glioma (DIPG). FBSGs comprising 20% cases have pathological features and a favourable clinical course resembling low-grade gliomas in other regions of the brain. Surgical management with tissue diagnosis is mainstay except for tectal gliomas, with chemotherapy and radiotherapy reserved for inoperable, symptomatic or progressive cases. DIPGs, which make up 80% of all cases resemble high grade gliomas on imaging, have a rapid clinical course and radiotherapy is the only modality of treatment that has proven to have a survival benefit. Unlike other sites, diagnosis is often radiological and the onus is upon the multidisciplinary team to correctly diagnose and risk-stratify patients with history, clinical cues and optimal magnetic resonance imaging (MRI) [1–3].

N. Das
Department of Radiotherapy and Oncology, AIIMS, New Delhi, India

G. Y. Srinivasa (✉)
Department of Radiotherapy and Oncology, PGIMER, Chandigarh, India

C. Ahuja
Department of Radiodiagnosis, PGIMER, Chandigarh, India

A. Singh
Department of Neurosurgery, PGIMER, Chandigarh, India



R. Madan et al. (eds.), *Evidence Based Practice in Pediatric Radiation Oncology*, https://doi.org/10.1007/978-981-96-4872-6_23

## 23.2 Epidemiology

Brainstem gliomas predominantly affect children making up 10–20% of all paediatric central nervous system tumours. It is commoner in the first decade of life and slightly higher in females. An Indian series of more than a hundred patients showed two peaks in age distribution occurring at 6–10 years and 36–45 years with pons being the commonest site [4–6].

## 23.3 Classification: Pathology

Various classifications have been used to describe brainstem gliomas. A traditional descriptive grouping based on imaging and locations group brainstem gliomas (BSG) into four types: focal, dorsal exophytic, cervicomedullary and diffuse intrinsic. These have implications in management. Pathologically, these gliomas are either high grade (WHO Grade 3, 4) or low grade (WHO 1,2). Merging location and pathology, two broad types of brainstem gliomas are important to differentiate: (1) diffusely infiltrative gliomas, high grade, unfavourable prognosis and (2) focal, exophytic, cervicomedullary lesions, low grade, favourable prognosis [5, 7–10].

## 23.4 Management

### 23.4.1 Diagnosis

#### 23.4.1.1 Clinical Features

Symptoms can be subtle, especially in children, like failure to thrive due to frequent vomiting, poor school performance due to diplopia to classic midbrain syndromes like Parinaud's syndrome. Cranial nerve deficits manifest in the form of diplopia, compensatory head tilt, altered facial expressions, dysphonia, etc. A thorough neurological examination helps localise cranial nerve deficits, elicit cerebellar signs and often reveal pyramidal weakness. An acute presentation is associated with DIPGs and portends a poor prognosis. Low-grade gliomas often have subtle symptoms which might be present for months to years.

#### 23.4.1.2 Imaging in Brainstem Gliomas

Most paediatric brainstem gliomas (70%) are centred in the pons unlike in adults, where most (60%) are medullary in location. MRI and Computed Tomography (CT) form the primary cross-sectional modalities for their evaluation.

##### CT

The tumour appears hypo- to isodense in character, causing brainstem expansion. These lesions usually don't enhance following contrast administration. Adjoining mass effect may lead to compression of the fourth ventricle leading to hydrocephalus. Haemorrhage within the lesion is relatively rare and seen in higher-grade aggressive tumours.

### MRI

Due to its excellent soft tissue details, MRI is the preferred modality for tumour diagnosis, characterisation and follow-up. Brainstem gliomas are hypointense on T1 weighted imaging and hyperintense on T2/fluid attenuated inversion recovery (FLAIR), showing no or relatively faint patchy enhancement with gadolinium [11]. Adult gliomas may sometimes show moderate enhancement. Necrotic foci are seen as focally increased T2 signal areas. No significant restriction is noted on diffusion-weighted imaging (DWI). Gradient-echo-based or susceptibility-weighted imaging (SWI) may show intratumoral susceptibility inducing foci signifying microhaemorrhages. Due to relatively higher cell turnover, MR spectroscopy demonstrates raised choline peak with reversal of Cho/NAA and Cho/Cr ratios. Higher ratios indicate a higher grade of tumour. Perfusion-weighted imaging like dynamic susceptibility contrast imaging (DSCI), dynamic contrast enhancement (DCE) and arterial spin labelling (ASL) aids in the depiction of tumour blood supply and perfusion pattern (Fig. 23.1) [12]. Most of these lesions show low to intermediate perfusion values (relative cerebral blood volume, rCBV). Occasionally, areas of intralesional hyperperfusion are seen indicative of aggressive transformation. Perfusion imaging may guide the site of biopsy if diagnosis is in doubt. The tumour is often expansile, with

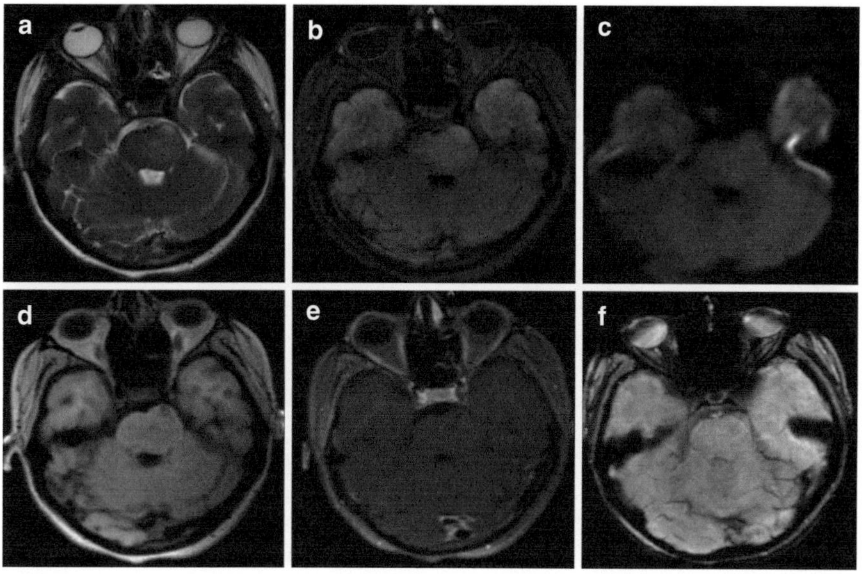


**Fig. 23.1** Pontine glioma-Axial T2 (**a**) and FLAIR (**b**) weighted MR images showing an expansileT2/FLAIR hyperintense lesion in the left pontine region showing no diffusion restriction (**c**). The tumour is iso-hypointense on T1-weighted image (**d**) and shows faint contrast enhancement (**e**). Few tiny susceptibility inducing foci suggesting microhaemorrhages are seen on SWI (**f**)

indistinct margins. Anterior expansion is more common and may sometimes lead to engulfment of the basilar artery (considered a specific sign for glioma). The relationship of the lesion with various brainstem tracts may be highlighted by diffusion tensor imaging (DTI), which helps to differentiate displacement from infiltration. Leptomeningeal or non-contiguous parenchymal dissemination, uncommon in DIPGs, may be seen in H3 K27 M-mutant midline gliomas. Radiogenomics-based tumour identification and characterisation helps to significantly improve accuracy of diagnosis of gliomas and attempts at histopathological diagnosis based on deep learning based image algortihms [13].

Brainstem gliomas may have to be differentiated from brainstem encephalitis, demyelination and osmotic demyelination at times. Expansile nature, relatively heterogeneous appearance, indistinct margins with metabolite abnormalities (increased choline on MR perfusion) and areas of hyperperfusion in an appropriate clinical setting are more specific for gliomas [14].

***Post-radiation Follow-Up Imaging*** Radiation induces injury to the tumour cells, which may result in increased lesion enhancement with areas of necrosis and resultant expansion leading to mass effect on the adjoining tissues. This effect needs to be differentiated from tumour growth, which may be difficult with conventional MRI. Multiparametric MRI may help in distinction of tumour progression from pseudoprogression and radiation-induced effects. Increased choline values on MR spectroscopy with raised perfusion indices are indicative of tumour growth, in contrast to lower rCBV and choline values seen in radiation-induced changes [15].

#### 23.4.1.3 Biopsy and Role of Surgery

The need of histological diagnosis is an indication for surgery in BSG in certain situations. Though advanced imaging modalities have helped in classifying the disease, a histological diagnosis is helpful in equivocal cases.

(a) *DIPG* is diagnosed on radiological appearance only and considered non-operable with poor overall prognosis, but as per WHO 2016 classification, the H3K27M mutation confirmation is essential for its diagnosis which can be only sampled in obtained tumour tissue. Hence, the role of histopathology cannot be ruled out completely if such a lesion is suspected.
(b) *Diagnostic dilemma*: In certain focal and diffuse lesions, the diagnostic dilemma might exist between neoplastic, demyelinating, inflammatory and/or infective lesions, necessitating a tissue diagnosis, particularly in the adult population. In neoplastic lesions too, the presence of lymphomas, germ cell tumours, radiation necrosis, hemangioblastomas, metastases, etc., has been identified apart from low- and high-grade astrocytomas. The histological diagnosis in such diverse situations becomes mandatory for deciding the future course of management.

While planning the surgery for BSG, the surgeon must consider different anatomical factors for safe corridors to access the tumour. In modern day practice, the surgical planning is facilitated by various adjuncts like pre-operative Diffusion

Tensor Imaging (DTI) demonstrating the tracks, intraoperative neuronavigation guidance, intraoperative MRI and neurophysiological monitoring, which help surgeons decide the appropriate approach, cause minimal deficits and achieve maximal safe resection. Certain factors like pre-operative basilar artery encasement, facial nerve involvement, vertical extension of tumour along brainstem and involvement of pontine crossing fibres are associated with poor overall survival (OS) and surgical morbidity [1]. To obtain the diagnosis or to plan excision, surgical intervention can be broadly categorised into three approaches:

1. Open surgery: This type of approach can be considered predominantly for lesions like dorsally exophytic tumours, vascular malformations with bleed/mass effect, predominantly cystic lesions and/or lesions approaching the surface. Various safe entry zones to the brainstem have been described for such lesions.
2. Stereotactic guided biopsy: For diffuse lesions and for lesions where the surgical excision would be too morbid, the stereotactic guided biopsy can be considered as a safer option [16].
3. Endoscopic guided biopsy: For lesions like ventrally placed pontine and medullary lesions, endonasal endoscopic biopsy under neuronavigation and neurophysiological guidance can be considered a good, safe and minimally invasive technique. Endoscopic trans-ventricular biopsy can help in select cases with intraventricular extension and obstructive hydrocephalus [17].

### 23.4.2 Treatment

#### 23.4.2.1 Diffuse Intrinsic Pontine Glioma (DIPG)

Radiation therapy (RT) is the only modality that has shown a survival benefit. The benefit, however, is temporary and recurrences occur within 3–6 months. A Cochrane review studying the role of radiotherapy in DIPG found no difference in outcomes or toxicity with conventional fractionation versus hyper- or hypofractionation. However, the authors did emphasise the need of better designed, multi-institutional trials to better characterise the role of RT. Systemic agents active against high-grade gliomas have been tried. However, till date, no agent has shown a proven benefit and one should be wary of the additional toxicities. Early addition of corticosteroids is often necessary.

## 23.5 Radiation Therapy

### 23.5.1 Indication

All patients regardless of age should be treated with RT.

### 23.5.2 RT Planning

- CT-based conformal planning should to be performed for all patients. For RT planning, a contrast-enhanced CT scan is taken with the patient immobilised with a thermoplastic shell. In paediatric patients requiring sedation or general anaesthesia for treatment, treatment should be done in experienced centres in view of proximity of the disease to vital centres.
- Tumour volume delineation: Diagnostic MRI images are to be fused with planning CT images for accurate tumour delineation. Gross tumour volume (GTV) is delineated on T1 contrast-enhanced and T2/FLAIR sequences. The clinical target volume (CTV) is obtained by adding a 1–2 cm margin. A 0.3–0.5 cm margin (based on institutional norms) is given to the CTV to obtain the final planning target volume (PTV) (Fig. 23.2).
- Technique: Traditionally, bilateral parallel opposed fields were used for treatment and gave uniform coverage at the expense of higher temporal lobe and bilateral cochlear doses. Using 3D conformal radiotherapy (3D-CRT) and intensity modulated radiotherapy (IMRT) using image guidance, doses to organs at risk can be reduced, which will have an impact on quality of life in the small number of long-term survivors.
- Dose, fractionation: 54–60 gray (Gy) total dose with conventional fractionation (1.8–2 Gy/fraction) is the usual dose prescribed in keeping with other high-grade gliomas.

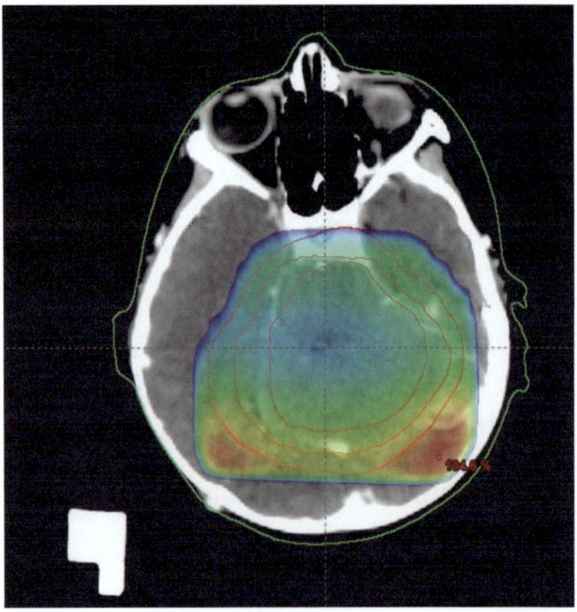

**Fig. 23.2** Concentric contours showing gross tumour volume (GTV), clinical target volume (CTV) and planning target volume (PTV) with dose colour wash showing 95–107% of prescribed dose in a 3D-CRT plan

- Organ at risk (OAR) constraints: Optic chiasma, pituitary gland, bilateral cochlea, spinal cord, bilateral optic nerves, eyeballs and lens are the OARs that need to be spared during RT planning.

### 23.5.3 Results, Prognosis, Survival

Radiotherapy improves OS in DIPG. In 1991, Langmoen et al. showed a doubling of survival in irradiated versus non-irradiated patients (280 days versus 140 days) [2].

Median survival of DIPG is <1 year while in surgically treated patients, prognosis would depend on histology. Long-term survival beyond 5 years is <5%. Older patients >10 years with long evolution history and absence of cranial nerve deficits may have better outcomes.

### 23.5.4 Follow-Up, Radiotherapy Sequelae

Since the disease carries a poor long-term survival, survivors with delayed sequelae are not common. However, the cranial nerve palsies or other neural deficits usually persist for the duration of life. High temporal lobe exposure to radiotherapy may produce cognitive impairment although the magnitude has not been systematically evaluated.

### 23.5.5 Future Research

- Altered fractionation: Both hyperfractionated and hypofractionated radiotherapy have been tested against conventional fractionation in prospective randomised control trials. However, none have shown superiority in terms of survival or toxicity profile as per a Cochrane systematic review though adequately powered studies are limited [18]. Mandell et al. randomised 130 participants to conventional RT (54 Gy in 6 weeks, 1.8 Gy per fractions) and hyperfractionated RT (70.2 Gy in 6 weeks, twice a day treatment of 1.17 Gy per fraction). The OS, response rates and toxicities were comparable between both arms [19]. Zaghloul et al. tested the same with hypofractionated RT randomising patients to conventional (54 Gy in 6 weeks) and hypofractionated RT (39 Gy in 13 fractions and 3 Gy per fraction). The trial showed equivalence of both with a numerically higher OS in the conventional group (9.5 months versus 7.8 months) [20].
- Systemic treatment: Multiple systemic agents have been tried with RT. Temozolomide in the concurrent and adjuvant setting with conventional and hypofractionated radiotherapy has not shown a survival benefit [21, 22]. ONC201 has shown promising control in anecdotal data on diffuse midline gliomas and is being evaluated in phase 2 studies.

## 23.5.6 Brainstem Gliomas Except DIPG

### 23.5.6.1 Surgery

The surgery for brainstem gliomas has a limited role considering the eloquence and the associated postoperative morbidity. Historically, the intrinsic brainstem gliomas have been considered as a relative contraindication to surgery and had remained a nightmare for the treating physician. However, with recent advancements in the imaging modalities, neuronavigation and other technology, the role of surgery in treating/obtaining histological diagnosis has come into play for some selected cases [23, 24]. The goals of surgery in BSG can be categorised as:

1. Treating hydrocephalus: Though hydrocephalus is a relatively late feature of intrinsic brainstem gliomas, in certain locations like tectal plate gliomas and dorsally exophytic tumours, the patients usually present with hydrocephalus and raised Intracranial pressure. Cerebrospinal fluid (CSF) diversion initially with either endoscopic third ventriculostomy (ETV) or a ventriculo-peritoneal shunt in such situations becomes important. The ETV has the advantage of obtaining a tumour tissue for histopathology as well if it is accessible.
2. To obtain maximal tumour debulking and relieve the mass effect: In certain situations like dorsally exophytic lesions (with or without focal intrinsic component), the tumours fill the fourth ventricle and often cause obstructive hydrocephalus, invariably requiring a CSF diversion procedure. Since the exophytic component is variable and is accessible, the surgical debulking of such lesions is feasible with neurophysiological monitoring.

With better understanding of the disease and the advancing technology, the surgical results have improved overtime, but BSG surgery remains a formidable challenge even now. Larger studies and further evaluation are required to improve outcomes further.

In the St. Jude's hospital experience exceeding two decades, 52 patients with focal brainstem gliomas were analysed. The majority were located in the midbrain (42%), followed by pons (29%) and medulla (29%). A biopsy was obtained in all cases and surgical extirpation was possible in half of them. With a median follow-up of 10 years, the 10 years event free survival (EFS) and OS was 52% and 90%, respectively. RT was given in 11 patients who progressed after surgery [3].

An Indian surgical series operated on 40 patients of focal intrinsic (intraxial) brainstem gliomas with longstanding duration of symptoms (more than 6 months) and good neurological status. Microsurgical techniques, intraoperative evoked potentials and brain mapping were used when appropriate. MRI imaging showed no residual tumour in 23 patients and minimum residual disease in another 5. Survival characteristics could not be commented upon due to limited follow up data [6].

## 23.6 Conclusion

Brainstem gliomas are a rare and heterogeneous group of paediatric tumours with thc majority having a rapid course and poor prognosis. DIPG is a site where active translational research is required to understand and target the biology of the disease because present standards of care do not provide long time cure.

## References

1. Green AL, Kieran MW. Pediatric brainstem gliomas: new understanding leads to potential new treatments for two very different tumors. Curr Oncol Rep. 2015;17(3):436.
2. Langmoen IA, Lundar T, Storm-Mathisen I, Lie SO, Hovind KH. Management of pediatric pontine gliomas. Childs Nerv Syst. 1991;7(1):13–5.
3. Klimo P Jr, Pai Panandiker AS, Thompson CJ, et al. Management and outcome of focal low-grade brainstem tumors in pediatric patients: the St. Jude experience. J Neurosurg Pediatr. 2013;11(3):274–81.
4. Patil N, Kelly ME, Yeboa DN, et al. Epidemiology of brainstem high-grade gliomas in children and adolescents in the United States, 2000-2017. Neuro Oncol. 2021;23(6):990–8.
5. Freeman CR, Farmer JP. Pediatric brain stem gliomas: a review. Int J Radiat Oncol Biol Phys. 1998;40(2):265–71.
6. Kansal S, Jindal A, Mahapatra AK. Brain stem glioma—a study of 111 patients. Indian J Cancer. 1999;36(2–4):99–108.
7. Hargrave D, Bartels U, Bouffet E. Diffuse brainstem glioma in children: critical review of clinical trials. Lancet Oncol. 2006;7(3):241–8.
8. Fisher PG, Breiter SN, Carson BS, et al. A clinicopathologic reappraisal of brain stem tumor classification. Identification of pilocystic astrocytoma and fibrillary astrocytoma as distinct entities. Cancer. 2000;89(7):1569–76.
9. Epstein FJ, Farmer JP. Brain-stem glioma growth patterns. J Neurosurg. 1993;78(3):408–12.
10. Robertson PL, Allen JC, Abbott IR, Miller DC, Fidel J, Epstein FJ. Cervicomedullary tumors in children: a distinct subset of brainstem gliomas. Neurology. 1994;44(10):1798–803.
11. Tisnado J, Young R, Peck KK, Haque S. Conventional and advanced imaging of diffuse intrinsic pontine glioma. J Child Neurol. 2016;31(12):1386–93.
12. Abrigo JM, Fountain DM, Provenzale JM, et al. Magnetic resonance perfusion for differentiating low-grade from high-grade gliomas at first presentation. Cochrane Database Syst Rev. 2018;1:CD011551.
13. Calmon R, Dangouloff-Ros V, Varlet P, et al. Radiogenomics of diffuse intrinsic pontine gliomas (DIPGs): correlation of histological and biological characteristics with multimodal MRI features. Eur Radiol. 2021;31(12):8913–24.
14. Duran-Peña A, Ducray F, Ramirez C, et al. Adult brainstem glioma differential diagnoses: an MRI-based approach in a series of 68 patients. J Neurol. 2022;269(8):4349–62.
15. Kessler AT, Bhatt AA. Brain tumour post-treatment imaging and treatment-related complications. Insights Imaging. 2018;9(6):1057–75.
16. Jung IH, Chang KW, Park SH, et al. Stereotactic biopsy for adult brainstem lesions: a surgical approach and its diagnostic value according to the 2016 World Health Organization classification. Cancer Med. 2021;10(21):7514–24.
17. Topczewski TE, Di Somma A, Culebras D, et al. Endoscopic endonasal surgery to treat intrinsic brainstem lesions: correlation between anatomy and surgery. Rhinology. 2021;59(2):191–204.
18. Hu X, Fang Y, Hui X, Jv Y, You C. Radiotherapy for diffuse brainstem glioma in children and young adults. Cochrane Database Syst Rev. 2016;(6):CD010439.
19. Mandell LR, Kadota R, Freeman C, Douglass EC, Fontanesi J, Cohen ME, Kovnar E, Burger P, Sanford RA, Kepner J, Friedman H, Kun LE. There is no role for hyperfractionated radiother-

apy in the management of children with newly diagnosed diffuse intrinsic brainstem tumors: results of a Pediatric Oncology Group phase III trial comparing conventional vs. hyperfractionated radiotherapy. Int J Radiat Oncol Biol Phys. 1999;43(5):959–64.

20. Zaghloul MS, Eldebawy E, Ahmed S, et al. Hypofractionated conformal radiotherapy for pediatric diffuse intrinsic pontine glioma (DIPG): a randomized controlled trial. Radiother Oncol. 2014;111(1):35–40.
21. Jalali R, Raut N, Arora B, et al. Prospective evaluation of radiotherapy with concurrent and adjuvant temozolomide in children with newly diagnosed diffuse intrinsic pontine glioma. Int J Radiat Oncol Biol Phys. 2010;77(1):113–8.
22. Izzuddeen Y, Gupta S, Haresh KP, Sharma D, Giridhar P, Rath GK. Hypofractionated radiotherapy with temozolomide in diffuse intrinsic pontine gliomas: a randomized controlled trial. J Neurooncol. 2020;146(1):91–5.
23. Faulkner H, Arnaout O, Hoshide R, et al. The surgical resection of brainstem glioma: outcomes and prognostic factors. World Neurosurg. 2021;146:e639–50.
24. Holzapfel J, Kandels D, Schmidt R, et al. Favorable prognosis in pediatric brainstem low-grade glioma: report from the German SIOP-LGG 2004 cohort. Int J Cancer. 2020;146(12):3385–96.

# Gamma Knife Radiosurgery for Intracranial Pathologies of the Pediatric Population

24

Harsh Deora, Manjul Tripathi, and Siddharth Kumar

## 24.1 Introduction

Stereotactic radiosurgery (SRS) has evolved to be a pivotal tool in neurosurgery, particularly valuable in treating tumors located in deep and intricate regions of the brain, such as the skull base and areas with critical neurovascular structures. Initially, the use of SRS was met with considerable skepticism due to concerns over long-term radiation side effects and its tolerability, especially in children. However, as technology and understanding of radiation effects have progressed, SRS has gained acceptance as a safer, precise, and effective treatment option for brain and skull base tumors [1].

In pediatric neurosurgery, where a multimodal approach is often required to manage brain tumors, complete surgical resection frequently poses challenges. In many cases, attempting a complete resection carries a significant risk of severe side effects due to the delicate nature of the developing brain and its complex surroundings. Additionally, chemotherapy has shown limited efficacy in treating many pediatric brain tumors, necessitating alternative therapeutic options. Conventional surgical and radiation treatments may adversely affect a child's neurological and physical development, leading to a heightened demand for approaches that minimize these risks [2–5].

H. Deora
Department of Neurosurgery, National Institute of Mental Health and Neurosciences, Bangalore, India

M. Tripathi (✉)
Deparment of Neurosurgery, Gamma Knife Radiosurgery, Neurosurgery Office, Postgraduate Institute of Medical Education and Research, Chandigarh, India

S. Kumar
Department of Neurosurgery, Postgraduate Institute of Medical Education and Research, Chandigarh, India



R. Madan et al. (eds.), *Evidence Based Practice in Pediatric Radiation Oncology*, https://doi.org/10.1007/978-981-96-4872-6_24

With its precise delivery of radiation to targeted areas, SRS has become an increasingly viable alternative in pediatric cases despite its initial prevalence in adult treatment. The development of technologies such as the Gamma Knife has contributed significantly to SRS's suitability for pediatric patients. The Gamma Knife's high degree of conformality allows for targeted radiation that minimizes exposure to surrounding healthy tissue, a critical benefit in pediatric patients where preserving normal brain development is essential [6, 7].

Stereotactic radiation can be administered in a single session (as in standard SRS) or through a hypo-fractionated approach (hfSRS). The latter involves delivering up to five fractions of radiation over 5 days, with a 24-h interval between sessions. This hypo-fractionated approach allows for a more controlled and potentially safer method of treatment in some pediatric cases, balancing the precision of SRS with a fractionated dosage to manage tumors effectively while reducing the risk of damaging healthy tissue [8, 9].

The growing acceptance of SRS in pediatric neurosurgery highlights its role as an effective, targeted treatment that complements traditional methods without the high risk of developmental impact. As SRS continues to evolve, its application in children will likely expand, offering promising alternatives for managing challenging brain and skull base tumors with a focus on preserving quality of life and long-term health.

## 24.2 Radiobiology of Gamma Knife Radiosurgery (GKRS)

Gamma Knife Radiosurgery (GKRS) stands apart from traditional radiotherapy primarily because it does not adhere to the conventional radiobiological principles known as the "5Rs": repair, redistribution, repopulation, reoxygenation, and radiosensitivity. These principles typically govern the effects of lower-dose, fractionated radiation treatments but are less applicable to the high-dose, single-session nature of GKRS, where doses often exceed 10 Gy. The primary effect of GKRS at these high doses is linked to the heightened sensitivity of endothelial cells, which are prone to radiation-induced apoptosis and vascular injury, contributing significantly to the therapeutic outcomes [10].

Standard radiobiological models, like the linear-quadratic (LQ) model used in traditional radiotherapy, do not effectively predict the biological effects of single high-dose radiosurgery sessions like those in GKRS. The LQ model, designed to estimate cell survival across multiple low-dose fractions, does not accurately reflect cell response to the concentrated radiation dose used in stereotactic radiosurgery (SRS). Recognizing this gap, Park and colleagues developed the Universal Survival Curve (USC). This model merges the linear-quadratic approach for the "shoulder" of the dose-response curve—where cell survival rates drop off more gradually—with the multi-target model, which better represents cell response to the high-dose range utilized in GKRS and other SRS applications. Through this hybrid approach, the USC can more accurately depict the response of the tumor and other target tissues to the single, high-dose GKRS treatment [11].

The USC framework also allows for calculating the biological effective dose (BED) and the single fraction equivalent dose (SFED). These measures are essential in translating the biological impact of GKRS into comparable terms with traditional fractionated treatments. BED reflects the accumulated effect of a given radiation dose on tissue, considering factors like total dose and fractionation. At the same time, SFED provides a dose metric representing a single fraction with an equivalent biological effect to a given fractionated schedule. This is particularly useful in clinical settings. SFED enables practitioners to compare the efficacy of various radiotherapy regimens and optimize treatment for conditions like arteriovenous malformations, benign tumors, and selected malignant tumors where GKRS is commonly applied [12].

## 24.3 Arteriovenous Malformations (AVMs)

In pediatric patients, arteriovenous malformations (AVMs) are the leading cause of intracranial hemorrhage (ICH), accounting for 50% of hemorrhagic strokes in children. Pediatric hemorrhage carries a mortality rate of 22%, alongside a long-term risk of morbidity and mortality [9]. AVMs located in deep or functionally critical (eloquent) brain areas pose a significant challenge for surgical intervention due to a high morbidity rate of 70–90%. As a result, Gamma Knife Radiosurgery (GKRS) is often recommended for such cases.

The International Gamma Knife Research Foundation (IGKRF) conducted a pooled analysis showing a 63% rate of AVM obliteration with GKRS at an average follow-up period of 92 months in patients under 18 years [9]. This approach presented a low risk of permanent radiation damage, estimated at 3%. A dose-response effect was observed in the IGKRF series, indicating that a marginal radiosurgery dose of at least 22 Gy significantly enhances the likelihood of a favorable outcome. The AVM obliteration rate was notably higher at this dose, with a reported success of 78% versus 47% for lower doses and obliteration rates of 81.6% versus 51.4%. Additionally, unpublished findings from this group indicate a 3% incidence of rebleeding at a median follow-up of 5.6 years. Studies by Nicole et al. and Dinca et al. [10], analyzing outcomes in UK cohorts, reported 88% and 70% obliteration rates, respectively, with permanent complication rates of 11% and a 1.1% risk of radiation necrosis.

Furthermore, evidence suggests that pediatric AVMs respond more favorably to radiation compared to those in adults. Smaller AVMs, with a volume under 10 cc, also demonstrate higher obliteration rates while minimizing the risk of radiation-induced necrosis.

**Cavernous Malformations** Cavernous malformations in functionally sensitive brain regions, such as the thalamus and brainstem, are potential candidates for Gamma Knife Radiosurgery (GKRS). Although surgical intervention is traditionally preferred for cavernous malformations due to its immediate reduction of rebleeding risk and improvement in seizure control, surgery in deep-seated, eloquent brain areas carries a substantial risk of morbidity and mortality, which can be permanent in approximately 15–35% of cases. GKRS offers a valuable alternative for reducing the risk of re-bleeding 2 years post-treatment when it targets the lesion precisely without affecting the surrounding hemosiderin ring or developmental venous anomaly (DVA) [11]. Additionally, GKRS has been shown to enhance control over epilepsy associated with cavernous malformations.

## 24.4 Craniopharyngiomas

Craniopharyngiomas are benign but challenging intracranial tumors due to their slow-growing yet locally invasive nature, which often results in substantial morbidity [12]. Achieving a complete resection is complex, and even when possible, studies show that recurrence rates can reach 20–27% [13]. Because of their proximity to critical structures such as the pituitary gland and optic nerves, aggressive surgery carries a significant risk of hormonal disturbances, visual impairment, and cognitive decline. Consequently, a combined approach involving cyst aspiration, Ommaya reservoir placement, limited excision, and radiotherapy has yielded better functional outcomes in cognition, vision, and endocrine health [14].

Kobayashi and colleagues [15] conducted a significant study, reporting 98 cases of craniopharyngiomas treated with Gamma Knife radiosurgery (GKRS), delivering a median marginal dose of 11.5 Gy. Patients had a minimum follow-up of 6 months and a median follow-up of 63 months. In this cohort, 38 patients were 15 years old or younger, and the reported progression-free survival (PFS) rates at 5 and 10 years were 60.8% and 53.8%, respectively. Only 6% of patients experienced deterioration in visual or endocrine function, highlighting the relative safety and efficacy of GKRS in treating this condition. Other studies with a minimum of 4 years of follow-up report tumor control rates ranging from 67% to 100% [16–18]. Solid lesions tend to respond better to radiosurgery than cystic ones, and dosage considerations are often based on the tolerance levels of nearby optic structures.

Radiation therapy for skull base tumors, including craniopharyngiomas, carries a risk of radiation-induced optic neuropathy. An analysis of 1578 skull base tumors identified doses to the optic apparatus exceeding 12 Gy in one session, 20 Gy in three sessions, and 25 Gy in five sessions as predictive factors for optic neuropathy [15]. Radiosurgery-induced hypothalamic dysfunction occurs at rates of approximately 2–8% [16–20], whereas traditional radiotherapy frequently results in hormone deficiencies: growth hormone deficiency is the most common, affecting 45–100% of cases, followed by gonadotropin deficiency (30%), TSH deficiency (6–25%), and ACTH deficiency (22%) [20]. These findings underscore the role of GKRS as a preferable treatment option in many cases of craniopharyngioma.

## 24.5 Pediatric Gliomas

In the treatment of pediatric gliomas, particularly pilocytic astrocytomas, and recurrent gliomas, GKRS has shown promising results. In a series by Grabb et al., 25 pediatric patients with a mean age of 8.5 years were treated with a mean peripheral dose of 15.2 Gy, with a follow-up of 22 months. Survival rates were 100% for this cohort's pilocytic and grade II gliomas [21]. Similarly, Boethius et al. reported that 19 patients, averaging 10.6 years of age, were diagnosed with pilocytic astrocytomas. Treated with a mean dose of 11.3 Gy over an average follow-up of 5.9 years, the study reported a 100% survival rate but noted a 26% incidence of adverse radiation effects (ARE). One patient required additional surgery due to radionecrosis, and another required decompression for a symptomatic cyst [22]. Weintraub et al. evaluated 24 cases with a mean age of 11 years and mixed histology types. The patients received a mean dose of 15 Gy and were followed for an average of 5.9 years. This study showed a 96% survival rate, although 12.5% required further surgery, with more extensive tumor volume found to be predictive of progression [23].

## 24.6 Choroid Plexus Tumors

For choroid plexus tumors, GKRS is generally applied in cases of incomplete resection. Although its use in pediatric cases is limited to scattered case reports, doses generally range from 14 to 19 Gy [24]. Surgical resection remains the primary treatment option; however, GKRS is a viable alternative when total resection is impossible.

## 24.7 Vestibular Schwannomas

In pediatric patients, vestibular schwannomas (VS) differ significantly from those in adults, as they are often associated with neurofibromatosis type 2 (NF2) rather than being sporadic. Outcomes for pediatric VS in NF2 patients are generally less favorable than those seen in adults with sporadic VS. Additionally, NF2 patients who receive radiation therapy may have an increased risk of malignant transformation of the tumor following radiation exposure.

## 24.8 Ependymoma

The primary treatment strategy for intracranial ependymoma is to achieve maximal safe resection followed by radiotherapy. For recurrent ependymomas (rEPN), Gamma Knife Radiosurgery (GKRS) has demonstrated benefits in improving patient outcomes. Stauder et al. [25] studied 26 patients, including 12 individuals aged 18 or younger, who received a median radiation dose of 18 Gy through

GKRS. Three years following treatment, the patients experienced a local control rate of 72%, while the median overall survival (OS) reached 5.5 years. Similarly, Kano et al. [26] evaluated GKRS for recurrent ependymomas, administered a median marginal dose of 15 Gy, and documented a 3-year progression-free survival (PFS) rate of 42%. However, they observed a high rate of remote relapse, with an 80.3% occurrence at 3 years, underscoring a significant challenge in achieving durable control of the disease in this context.

## 24.9 Medulloblastoma

Radiosurgery in medulloblastoma is typically reserved for recurrent disease cases or as an initial boost for residual tumors. Patrice et al. [27] examined 11 patients treated for recurrent medulloblastoma and three patients treated for residual disease, utilizing a median peripheral dose of 12 Gy. With a median follow-up period of 27 months, all patients who underwent treatment for residual disease were alive and showed no evidence of disease recurrence. In contrast, over half of those treated for recurrence succumbed to progressive disease. This trend is reflected in other studies [28, 29] that have assessed radiosurgery efficacy in medulloblastoma. These studies generally demonstrate favorable local control rates; however, disease recurrence typically occurs outside the volume treated with stereotactic radiosurgery (SRS), highlighting the critical role of optimizing systemic therapy for comprehensive disease management. Toxicity reports have varied across studies, with the most extended follow-up in a particular series [29] involving three patients monitored for 30, 39, and 48 months, during which no toxicity was reported.

## 24.10 Malignant Diseases

Currently, metastasis is the most common indication for global Gamma Knife Radiosurgery (GKRS). However, the application of radiosurgery for metastatic diseases within the pediatric population requires further prospective evaluation to determine its full efficacy and safety profile. The lack of extensive, dedicated studies in this demographic underscores a need for focused research to establish guidelines specific to pediatric patients with metastatic malignancies (Fig. 24.1).

## 24.11 Inflammatory Pathologies

Stereotactic radiosurgery (SRS) has also been explored in treating specific inflammatory pathologies, such as Langerhans cell histiocytosis and Rosai-Dorfman disease [30]. Although promising, additional studies are necessary to assess the potential benefits of combining concurrent chemotherapy with radiosurgery and to compare this combination against conventional treatment options. Prospective trials are crucial to understanding the best approach for managing these inflammatory

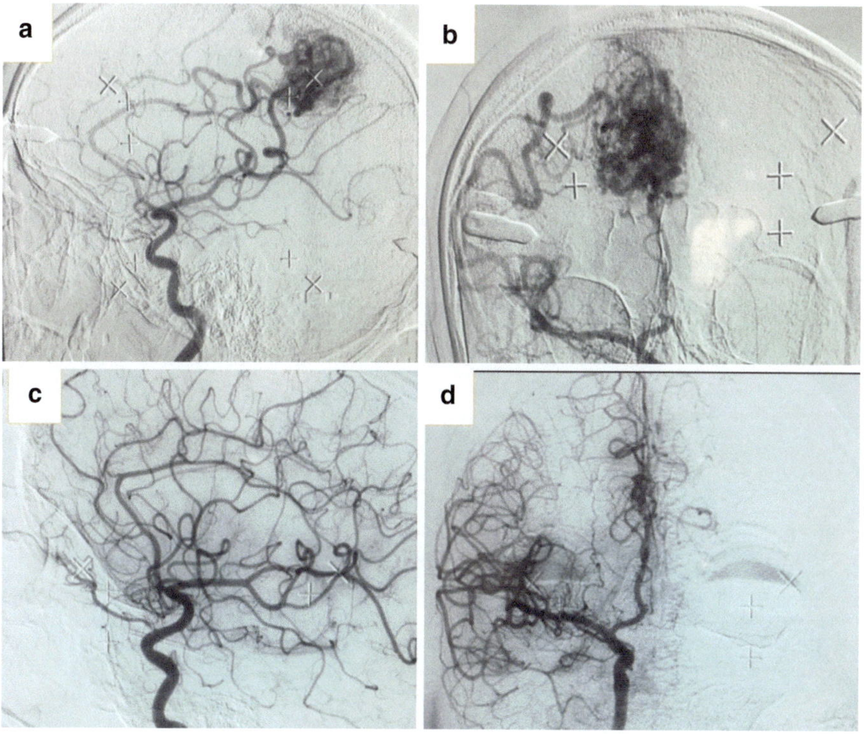


**Fig. 24.1** (**a**, **b**) Pre GKRS lateral and AP view of DSA of a pediatric AVM; and (**c**, **d**), follow-up DSA after 2 years showing complete obliteration after primary GKRS (*AVM* arteriovenous malformation, *DSA* digital subtraction angiography, *GKRS* gamma knife radiosurgery)

diseases with SRS, potentially establishing it as a valuable adjunct or alternative to existing therapies.

## 24.12 Functional Indications: Hypothalamic Hamartoma (HH)

Hypothalamic hamartoma (HH) often manifests in patients with symptoms like seizures and precocious puberty, with an average age of presentation at 2.8 years. Treatment options are diverse, encompassing both surgical and non-surgical approaches. Available interventions include surgical resection, stereotactic radiosurgery (SRS), radiofrequency thermocoagulation, laser interstitial thermal therapy, and stereotactic brachytherapy. Among these, SRS is commonly considered a first-line treatment for Regis type 1–3 lesions, primarily due to its favorable safety and lower risk of complications than other approaches.

The efficacy of SRS in controlling seizures has been supported by studies, notably from Abla et al. and the Marseille group. These studies demonstrate improved seizure control outcomes in approximately 60–70% of HH patients treated with

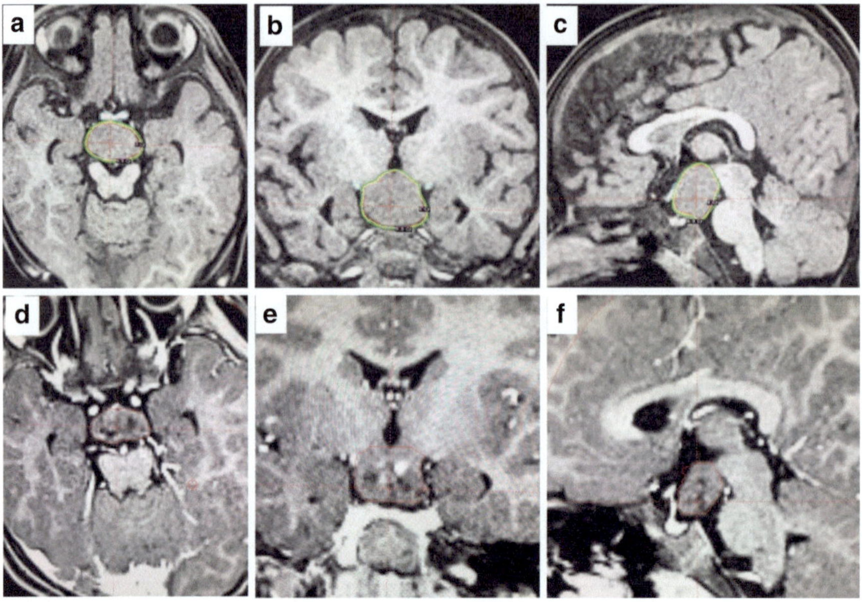


**Fig. 24.2** (**a–c**) Axial, coronal, and sagittal MRI showing hypothalamic hamartoma at the time of radiosurgery; and (**d–f**) corresponding post radiosurgery images after 2 years showing patchy necrosis inside the hamartoma

SRS. Additionally, hormonal outcomes appear more favorable with SRS when compared to conventional surgical methods, suggesting it may offer a superior quality of life for patients who experience hormonally driven symptoms like precocious puberty [31–33].

In a recent study, three pediatric patients were treated with a primary hypo-fractionated Gamma Knife Radiosurgery (GKRS) protocol, delivering therapy over 2–3 consecutive days. The treatment regimen included marginal doses ranging from 8.1 to 9.2 Gy at a 50% isodose to target the entire volume of the hamartoma across 2–3 fractions. Results indicated a substantial volumetric reduction in HH, ranging from 32% to 48%, alongside the development of patchy necrosis within the hamartoma tissue (Fig. 24.2).

This recent study highlights the effectiveness of hypo-fractionated GKRS, offering promising therapeutic outcomes, particularly for children with HH who require precision and reduced adverse effects in their treatment.

## 24.13 Emerging Indications

**Corpus Callosotomy** Currently, radiosurgical callosotomy serves a mainly palliative role, particularly as an alternative to traditional microsurgical callosotomy for patients with drug-resistant epilepsy. This approach is especially beneficial in

Lennox-Gastaut syndrome cases and patients experiencing frequent drop attacks. Radiosurgery for callosotomy is focused on a small target area, precisely the anterior two-thirds of the corpus callosum, which helps to mitigate seizure activity effectively [3, 34].

**Radiosurgical Third Ventriculostomy** Radiosurgical third ventriculostomy presents a significant advancement over conventional techniques due to its non-invasive nature and eliminating the need for general anesthesia. This approach was notably utilized by Gutierrez-Aceves and colleagues [35] in treating a patient with midbrain glioma and mild obstructive hydrocephalus. In this case, the radiosurgical lesioning was precisely applied to the third ventricle floor, targeting the area between the mammillary body and the infundibular recess. A prescription isodose of 120 Gy at 100% was administered, demonstrating this method's potential for effectively managing specific obstructive conditions within the ventricular system.

**Ophthalmic Indications** Gamma Knife radiosurgery (GKRS) is also emerging as a viable treatment option for pediatric glaucoma. In this indication, GKRS targets the ciliary bodies, helping lower intraocular pressure to within normal limits, alleviating pain, and allowing the patient to retain functional vision. This non-invasive method may provide a durable solution for pediatric patients with refractory glaucoma where conventional interventions are either insufficient or unfeasible.

**Movement Disorders** Radiosurgical thalamotomy offers a practical option for managing specific movement disorders, including Holmes tremor and post-traumatic tremor [36]. This technique can modulate motor pathways and reduce tremor severity by targeting the thalamus. However, radiosurgical pallidotomy has seen reduced usage due to the variable response rates observed in the iron-rich globus pallidus interna, as well as the complexity posed by the dense network of lenticulostriate arteries in this area, which can lead to unpredictable outcomes [37].

## 24.14 Anesthetic Considerations for Pediatric Patients

Pediatric patients undergoing radiosurgery often require immobilization and frame fixation anesthesia. The frame-based stereotactic approach demands a stable, four-point pin fixation to ensure rigid immobilization and a secure, fixed position on the gamma couch for the entire treatment duration. The delivery time for GKRS radiation is typically longer than that of other radiosurgery systems, such as the LINAC-based CyberKnife system [38]. While most pediatric patients can be managed with light sedation, typically using chloral hydrate, preparations for general anesthesia and ventilation are essential in cases where more profound sedation is required. In the author's experience, children over ten generally cooperate reasonably and tolerate the procedure, similar to adults [39].

## 24.15 Radiation Toxicity in Pediatric SRS

Pediatric patients exhibit differential tolerance and sensitivity to radiation, raising concerns about radiation-induced toxicity, mainly when radiosurgery (SRS) is utilized for benign conditions in this age group. One significant risk associated with SRS in children is the potential development of radiation-induced second malignancies (RISM). The extended life expectancy in pediatric patients means they have a longer timeframe during which radiation-induced cancers could develop, making RISM a concern despite the low incidence. Factors influencing the likelihood of developing RISM include the patient's age, sex, the volume of tissue exposed to low-dose radiation, and genomic stability. In a study estimating global SRS treatment for benign conditions, the incidence of SRS-induced tumors was 0.04% at a 15-year follow-up [40]. Additionally, a comprehensive international analysis of 5000 patients undergoing SRS for benign conditions revealed a 0.0006% risk of malignant transformation and a 0.0002% risk of radiation-induced malignancy [3]. Therefore, the overall risk of RISM remains exceedingly low compared to SRS's therapeutic advantages.

## 24.16 Safety of SRS

Data on SRS's safety in pediatric patients is limited, especially concerning critical structures such as the optic chiasm and brainstem. These areas are particularly vulnerable to radiation exposure. In one study, Baumann and colleagues [41] reported no lasting visual complications in 2 pediatric patients who received over 8 Gy to the optic chiasm. Similarly, only 1 out of 16 patients who received a maximum dose of 16 Gy to the brainstem experienced temporary brainstem edema. These findings indicate that, although sensitive, critical structures can tolerate specific radiation doses without severe long-term effects. However, younger patients may still face neurocognitive risks following irradiation, underscoring the need for prospective research focused on determining appropriate radiation dosages for pediatric populations across various clinical indications [42].

## 24.17 Endocrine Dysfunction as a Side Effect of SRS

Endocrine disruption is a relatively common side effect of SRS in pediatric patients, especially in pituitary adenoma cases. One study examining SRS for pituitary adenomas reported that hypopituitarism, a condition where the pituitary gland fails to produce adequate hormones, was the most frequent adverse event, with an estimated incidence of 21.0% (95% CI: 15–27%). Conversely, visual dysfunction or other cranial nerve injuries were less common in 0–7% of cases [43]. Given the potential impact on growth and development in children, endocrine dysfunction following SRS necessitates vigilant, long-term follow-up in pediatric cases to monitor and manage any emerging hormonal deficiencies effectively.

## 24.18 Conclusion

Stereotactic radiosurgery (SRS) has demonstrated significant potential in treating pediatric patients, providing a level of accuracy and precision highly suitable for this sensitive group. With the unique ability to target lesions with minimal impact on surrounding healthy tissues, SRS represents a valuable therapeutic option that aligns well with the critical need for tissue-sparing interventions in children.

Despite its evolving nature, SRS has become essential in pediatric oncology, particularly in treating small and well-defined brain lesions. The high conformality of SRS reduces radiation exposure to adjacent typical structures, an especially critical factor given the heightened sensitivity of developing tissues in younger patients. SRS offers both immediate and potentially long-term advantages by minimizing complications associated with radiation in children, such as cognitive and developmental effects, which can be more pronounced than in adults. To solidify the role of SRS in pediatric treatment paradigms, it is essential to conduct long-term, multicenter, randomized controlled trials. These studies are critical to rigorously assess outcomes, adverse effects, and survival benefits compared to other treatment modalities in diverse pediatric populations. Such trials would enable the establishment of standardized protocols, potentially increasing the accessibility of SRS as an option for children with brain tumors and other intracranial conditions.

A promising direction for future research lies in expanding the applications of SRS to include functional disorders and managing oligometastatic disease in conjunction with systemic therapies. Combining SRS with biologics and immunotherapy presents an innovative approach that may enhance treatment efficacy in metastatic cases, particularly where traditional chemotherapy or whole-brain radiotherapy poses excessive risks to pediatric patients. This integrative approach can potentially tailor treatments more effectively to children's unique pathophysiological and immune characteristics.

## References

1. Park HJ, Griffin RJ, Hui S, et al. Radiation-induced vascular damage in tumors: implications of vascular damage in ablative hypofractionated radiotherapy (SBRT and SRS). Radiat Res. 2012;177:311–27.
2. Lo SS, Fakiris AJ, Abdulrahman R, et al. Role of stereotactic radiosurgery and fractionated stereotactic radiotherapy in pediatric brain tumors. Expert Rev Neurother. 2008;8(1):121–32.
3. Park C, Papiez L, Zhang S, et al. Universal survival curve and single fraction equivalent dose: useful tools in understanding potency of ablative radiotherapy. Int J Radiat Oncol Biol Phys. 2008;70:847–52.
4. Hladky JP, Lejeune JP, Blond S, Pruvo JP, Dhellemmes P. Cerebral arteriovenous malformations in children: report on 62 cases. Childs Nerv Syst. 1994;10(5):328–33.
5. Broderick J, Talbot GT, Prenger E, Leach A, Brott T. Stroke in children within a major metropolitan area: the surprising importance of intracerebral hemorrhage. J Child Neurol. 1993;8(3):250–5.
6. Kano H, Kondziolka D, Flickinger JC, et al. Stereotactic radiosurgery for arteriovenous malformations, part 2: management of pediatric patients. J Neurosurg Pediatr. 2012;9(1):1–10.

7. Ding D, Starke RM, Kano H, et al. International multicenter cohort study of pediatric brain arteriovenous malformations. Part 1: predictors of hemorrhagic presentation. J Neurosurg Pediatr. 2017;19(2):127–35.
8. Bajwa SJ, Bajwa SK, Bindra GS. The anesthetic, critical care and surgical challenges in the management of craniopharyngioma. Indian J Endocrinol Metab. 2011;15(2):123–6. https://doi.org/10.4103/2230-8210.81944.
9. Yen CP, Sheehan JP, Schwyzer L, Schlesinger D. Hemorrhage risk of cerebral arteriovenous malformations before and during the latency period after GAMMA knife radiosurgery. Stroke. 2011;42(6):1691–6.
10. Nicolato A, Lupidi F, Sandri MF, et al. Gamma knife radiosurgery for cerebral arteriovenous malformations in children/adolescents and adults. Part II: differences in obliteration rates, treatment-obliteration intervals, and prognostic factors. Int J Radiat Oncol Biol Phys. 2006;64(3):914–21.
11. Abla AA, Lekovic GP, Garrett M, et al. Cavernous malformations of the brainstem presenting in childhood: surgical experience in 40 patients. Neurosurgery. 2010;67(6):1589–99. https://doi.org/10.1227/NEU.0b013e3181f8d1b2.
12. Lévêque M, Carron R, Bartolomei F, Régis J. Radiosurgical treatment for epilepsy associated with cavernomas. Prog Neurol Surg. 2013;27:157–65. https://doi.org/10.1159/000341785.
13. Aquilina K, Merchant TE, Rodriguez-Galindo C, Ellison DW, Sanford RA, Boop FA. Malignant transformation of irradiated craniopharyngioma in children: report of 2 cases. J Neurosurg Pediatr. 2010;5(2):155–61.
14. Jeon C, Kim S, Shin HJ, et al. The therapeutic efficacy of fractionated radiotherapy and gamma-knife radiosurgery for craniopharyngiomas. J Clin Neurosci. 2011;18(12):1621–5.
15. Kobayashi T. Long-term results of gamma knife radiosurgery for 100 consecutive cases of craniopharyngioma and a treatment strategy. Prog Neurol Surg. 2009;22:63–76.
16. Lee CC, Yang HC, Chen CJ, et al. Gamma knife surgery for craniopharyngioma: report on a 20-year experience. J Neurosurg. 2014;121(Suppl):167–78.
17. Niranjan A, Kano H, Mathieu D, Kondziolka D, Flickinger JC, Lunsford LD. Radiosurgery for craniopharyngioma. Int J Radiat Oncol Biol Phys. 2010;78(1):64–71.
18. Xu Z, Yen CP, Schlesinger D, Sheehan J. Outcomes of gamma knife surgery for craniopharyngiomas. J Neurooncol. 2011;104(1):305–13.
19. Milano MT, Grimm J, Soltys SG, et al. Single- and multi-fraction stereotactic radiosurgery dose tolerances of the optic pathways. Int J Radiat Oncol Biol Phys. 2021;110(1):87–99. https://doi.org/10.1016/j.ijrobp.2018.01.053. S0360–3016(18)30125-1.
20. Appelman-Dijkstra NM, Kokshoorn NE, Dekkers OM, et al. Pituitary dysfunction in adult patients after cranial radiotherapy: systematic review and meta-analysis. J Clin Endocrinol Metab. 2011;96:2330–40.
21. Grabb PA, Lunsford LD, Albright AL, Kondziolka D, Flickinger JC. Stereotactic radiosurgery for glial neoplasms of childhood. Neurosurgery. 1996;38:696–702.
22. Boëthius J, Ulfarsson E, Rähn T, Lippittz B. Gamma knife radiosurgery for pilocytic astrocytomas. J Neurosurg. 2002;97(5 Suppl):677–80.
23. Weintraub D, Yen CP, Xu Z, Savage J, Williams B, Sheehan J. Gamma knife surgery of pediatric gliomas. J Neurosurg Pediatr. 2012;10:471–7.
24. Faramand A, Kano H, Niranjan A, et al. Stereotactic radiosurgery for choroid plexus tumors: a report of the international radiosurgery research foundation. Neurosurgery. 2020;88:791. https://doi.org/10.1093/neuros/nyaa538. PMID: 33372216.
25. Stauder MC, Ni Laack N, Ahmed KA, Link MJ, Schomberg PJ, Pollock BE. Stereotactic radiosurgery for patients with recurrent intracranial ependymomas. J Neurooncol. 2012;108(3):507–12.
26. Kano H, Yang HC, Kondziolka D, et al. Stereotactic radiosurgery for pediatric recurrent intracranial ependymomas. J Neurosurg Pediatr. 2010;6(5):417–23.
27. Patrice SJ, Tarbell NJ, Goumnerova LC, Shrieve DC, Black PM, Loeffler JS. Results of radiosurgery in the management of recurrent and residual medulloblastoma. Pediatr Neurosurg. 1995;22(4):197–203.

28. King D, Connolly D, Zaki H, Lee V, Yeomanson D. Successful treatment of metastatic relapse of medulloblastoma in childhood with single session stereotactic radiosurgery: a report of 3 cases. J Pediatr Hematol Oncol. 2014;36(4):301–4.
29. Woo C, Stea B, Lulu B, Hamilton A, Cassady JR. The use of stereotactic radiosurgical boost in the treatment of medulloblastomas. Int J Radiat Oncol Biol Phys. 1997;37(4):761–4.
30. Faramand A, Niranjan A, Flickinger J, et al. Salvage gamma knife stereotactic radiosurgery for recurrent intracranial Langerhans cell histiocytosis: a 36-year saga. World Neurosurg. 2020;144:205–8.
31. Abla AA, Shetter AG, Chang SW, et al. Gamma knife surgery for hypothalamic hamartomas and epilepsy: patient selection and outcomes. J Neurosurg. 2010;113(Suppl):207–14.
32. Regis J, Scavarda D, Tamura M, et al. Epilepsy related to hypothalamic hamartomas: surgical management with special reference to gamma knife surgery. Childs Nerv Syst. 2006;22:881–95.
33. Tripathi M, Maskara P, Sankhyan N, et al. Safety and efficacy of primary hypofractionated gamma knife radiosurgery for giant hypothalamic hamartoma. Indian J Pediatr. 2021;88:1086. https://doi.org/10.1007/s12098-020-03637-w.
34. Tripathi M, Maskara P, Rangan VS, Mohindra S, De Salles AAF, Kumar N. Radiosurgical corpus callosotomy: a review of literature. World Neurosurg. 2021;145:323–33. https://doi.org/10.1016/j.wneu.2020.08.205. Epub 2020 Sep 3. PMID: 32891831.
35. Gutierrez-Aceves GA, Rodriguez-Camacho A, Celis-Lopez MA, Moreno-Jimenez S, Herrera-Gonzalez JA. Frameless radiosurgical third ventriculostomy: technical report. Surg Neurol Int. 2020;11:398. Published 2020 Nov 18. https://doi.org/10.25259/SNI_247_2020.
36. Tripathi M, Mehta S, Singla R, et al. Vim stereotactic radiosurgical thalamotomy for drug-resistant idiopathic Holmes tremor: a case report. Acta Neurochir. 2021;163(7):1867–71.
37. Tripathi M, Sharan S, Mehta S, et al. Gamma knife radiosurgical pallidotomy for dystonia: not a fallen angel. Neurol India. 2019;67(6):1515–8.
38. Tripathi M, Deora H, Sadashiva N, Batish A, Mohindra S. Disinfecting gamma gantry during the coronavirus pandemic: another area 51. Stereotact Funct Neurosurg. 2020;98(5):358–60.
39. Tripathi M, Rekhapalli R, Batish A, et al. Safety and efficacy of primary multisession dose fractionated gamma knife radiosurgery for jugular paragangliomas. World Neurosurg. 2019;131:e136–48.
40. Postow MA, Callahan MK, Barker CA, et al. Immunologic correlates of the abscopal effect in a patient with melanoma. N Engl J Med. 2012;366:925–31.
41. Baumann GS, Wara WM, Larson DA, et al. Gamma knife radiosurgery in children. Pediatr Neurosurg. 1996;24:193–201.
42. Paddick I, Cameron A, Dimitriadis A. Extracranial dose and the risk of radiation-induced malignancy after intracranial stereotactic radiosurgery: is it time to establish a therapeutic reference level? Acta Neurochir. 2020;163:971. https://doi.org/10.1007/s00701-020-04664-4.
43. Kotecha R, Sahgal A, Rubens M, et al. Stereotactic radiosurgery for non-functioning pituitary adenomas: meta-analysis and international stereotactic radiosurgery society practice opinion. Neuro Oncol. 2020;22:318–32.

# Management of Renal Neoplasms 25

Pooja Sethi, Pritam Singha Roy, Treshita Dey, and Renu Madan

**Introduction** Pediatric renal tumors account for 3–11% of childhood cancers [1]. These can be broadly classified into two main types: Wilms tumor and non-Wilms renal tumors. Wilms tumor (WT) is the most common pediatric renal tumor, accounting for approximately 90% of cases. Overall, it has a good prognosis, and the majority of children with WT can be successfully treated with a combination of surgery, chemotherapy, with or without radiation therapy (RT). Non-Wilms renal tumors are relatively less common and include clear cell sarcoma of the kidney (CCSK), rhabdoid tumor of the kidney (RTK), and renal cell carcinoma (RCC). These tumors are often more aggressive than WT and require more intensive treatment. An Indian report on non-Wilms pediatric renal tumor showed a 19% incidence among all diagnosed renal cancer, most common being CCSK (39.4%), RCC (19.3%), RTK (12.8%), and Ewings sarcoma (15.6%) [2]. Treatment options and outcomes for pediatric renal tumors have significantly improved over the years, leading to improved outcome and better quality of life. In this chapter, we will discuss the management of renal neoplasm in children with main emphasis on Wilms tumor.

P. Sethi (✉)
Department of Radiotherapy, JIPMER, Puducherry, India

P. Singha Roy
Pediatric Hematology-Oncology, Medica Superspecialty Hospital, Kolkata, India

T. Dey · R. Madan
Department of Radiotherapy and Oncology, Postgraduate Institute of Medical Education and Research, Chandigarh, India



R. Madan et al. (eds.), *Evidence Based Practice in Pediatric Radiation Oncology*, https://doi.org/10.1007/978-981-96-4872-6_25

## 25.1 Diagnostic Workup in a Child with Suspected Renal Mass

Most of the children with WT present with abdominal mass or swelling. Other symptoms may include abdominal pain, hematuria, fever, and hypertension [3]. Although lung is the most common site of metastasis, very rarely patients present with respiratory difficulty.

The evaluation of a child with suspected renal mass starts with a detailed clinical examination, including a focused search for hypertension, dysmorphic feature, pupillary abnormality, genital ambiguity, or varicocele. Physical examination often reveals a smooth, firm, and non-tender mass situated on one side of abdomen which rarely crosses midline. Once the diagnosis of WT is suspected, subsequent examination should be performed gently since vigorous examination may lead to capsule rupture and tumor spillage, which requires more intensive therapy.

The initial investigations encompass an abdominal ultrasound with a color Doppler study of the renal vessels, complete blood count, serum chemistry, and coagulation profile. The blood work confirms adequate renal function, supports subsequent chemotherapy, and excludes the rare occurrence of acquired von Willebrand's disease [4]. The subsequent steps in the evaluation include abdominal cross-sectional imaging, confirmation of the diagnosis, and staging. Details of the imaging and histopathology are discussed elsewhere. A 2D echocardiography is indicated preceding the first dose of anthracycline. The assessment of differential renal function with a dimercapto succinic acid (DMSA) scan and selective renal angiography is essential if nephron-sparing surgery (NSS) is considered.

## 25.2 Evaluation for a Predisposing Syndrome

Merely 10–15% of sporadic WT develop on a background of a germline predisposition. Hence, routine evaluation for genetic predisposition is unwarranted. However, bilateral or multicentric disease, nephroblastomatosis, or any clinical stigmata of a predisposing syndrome, such as anisocoria, genital ambiguity, nephrotic syndrome, hemihypertrophy, or macroglossia, should invoke a syndromic evaluation [5].

## 25.3 Staging

A high-resolution, non-contrast computed tomography of the chest is the investigation of choice to screen for pulmonary metastasis. Metastatic nodules are well-circumscribed, round, non-calcified, and peripherally located. A nodule with a transverse diameter of ≥3 mm is considered metastatic. The staging evaluation for CCSK or RTK should additionally include bone scintigraphy and brain imaging, given their propensity for bone and brain metastasis. Staging of the Wilms tumor is shown in Table 25.1 [6].

**Table 25.1** Staging of Wilms tumor

| Stage | COG (before chemotherapy) | SIOP (after chemotherapy) |
|---|---|---|
| 1 | • Tumor limited to kidney, completely resected, resection margins clear<br>• Vessels of renal sinus not involved beyond 2 mm<br>• No tumor rupture before or during surgery | • Tumor limited to kidney or surrounded by fibrous pseudocapsule<br>• Capsule or pseudocapsule may be involved (but doesn't reach till the outer surface) but tumor completely resected with clear margins<br>• Tumor may be protruding into pelvic system but not infiltrating the walls<br>• Vessels of renal sinus not involved<br>• Intrarenal vessels may be involved |
| 2 | • Tumor extending beyond kidney but completely resected with clear margins<br>• Tumor thrombus may be present outside renal vessels, but thrombus should be completely removed with the tumor | • Tumor extending beyond kidney or penetrates capsule/pseudocapsule but completely resected with clear margins<br>• Infiltrates renal sinus or vessels/lymphatics outside kidney but completely resected<br>• Infiltrates adjacent structures or IVC but completely resected |
| 3 | • Incomplete excision (microscopic or gross residual)<br>• Abdomino-pelvic lymph nodes positive<br>• Diffuse peritoneal contamination or peritoneal implants<br>• Tumor biopsy or local spillage | • Incomplete excision (microscopic or gross residual)<br>• Abdomino-pelvic lymph nodes positive<br>• Tumor rupture before or during surgery<br>• Penetrates peritoneum<br>• Surgical (wedge) biopsy prior to chemotherapy<br>• Tumor thrombi at resection margin or tumor removed piecemeal by surgeon |
| 4 | Hematogenous metastasis or metastasis to lymph nodes outside abdominopelvic region | Hematogenous metastasis or metastasis to lymph nodes outside abdominopelvic region |
| 5 | Bilateral renal involvement at diagnosis | Bilateral renal involvement at diagnosis |

## 25.4 Prognostic Factors

The two primary "western" academic bodies concerning pediatric renal tumors, namely, the Société Internationale d'Oncologie Pédiatrique (SIOP), and the Children's Oncology Group (COG), influence the prognostic features and management strategy of childhood renal tumors across the Atlantic Ocean. Children's Oncology Group (NWTSG/COG) risk stratification is based on the age, stage, histology, tumor weight, presence of unfavorable histologies (focal or diffuse anaplasia, clear cell sarcoma of the kidney, rhabdoid kidney tumor), response to neoadjuvant chemotherapy (NACT), and molecular studies (combined loss of heterozygosity [LOH] at 1p &16q) [7, 8].

Société Internationale d'Oncologie Pédiatrique (SIOP) risk stratification is based upon age, the initial response to NACT, stage, and histology (low, intermediate, and high risk) [9]. Older age translates to an inferior survival given a higher prevalence of anaplastic histology and unfavorable biomarkers rather than having an independent prognostic value [10].

## 25.5 Management of WT

Treatment of WT remains a paradigm for multimodal management except in selected patients where surgery alone is adequate. The COG and SIOP approaches differ in several facets of management, albeit both eventuate in comparable outcomes. The strategic differences between the two schools will be emphasized in the subsequent sections wherever necessary.

## 25.6 Role of Systemic Therapy

The European countries adhere to the approach prescribed by SIOP, which endorses the administration of NACT followed by nephrectomy for children >6 months old. On the contrary, the North America-based COG advocates for upfront nephrectomy unless the procedure is considered unacceptably morbid. The intensity of adjuvant therapy is adjusted for age, stage, histology, and tumor biomarkers [11].

## 25.7 Synopsis of the SIOP Approach (UMBRELLA SIOP-RTSG 2016 Protocol)

### 25.7.1 Neo-Adjuvant Chemotherapy

Patients with the localized disease receive two-drug (dactinomycin and vincristine) NACT over 4 weeks. Three-drug (doxorubicin, dactinomycin, and vincristine) NACT is administered over 6 weeks for metastatic disease.

### 25.7.2 Adjuvant Chemotherapy

- **Localized disease:** The histological risk-stratification and local stage dictate the adjuvant chemotherapy (Table 25.2). The extent of NACT-induced tumor necrosis and the composition of the viable residual tumor are taken into consideration for the risk stratification. Very low-risk tumors, such as stage I, low-risk histology disease, carry excellent outcomes even without adjuvant therapy. On the other end of the spectrum, advanced local stage or high-risk histology warrants prolonged adjuvant chemotherapy spanning 7–9 months. The use of anthracycline is restricted to high-risk histology WTs or large volume (post-NACT tumor volume ≥500 mL), stage II/III, non-epithelial, non-stromal predominant WTs.
- **Metastatic disease:** The intensity of adjuvant chemotherapy is decided based on the response of the metastatic disease to NACT, the feasibility of metastatec-

**Table 25.2** Plan of adjuvant chemotherapy for Wilms tumor (SIOP)

<table>
<tr><th colspan="2" rowspan="2">Stage</th><th colspan="3">Histology</th></tr>
<tr><th>Low risk</th><th>Intermediate risk</th><th>High risk</th></tr>
<tr><td colspan="2">I</td><td>Adjuvant chemotherapy unwarranted</td><td>AV × 4 weeks</td><td>AVD[a] × 27 weeks</td></tr>
<tr><td colspan="2">II</td><td colspan="2" rowspan="2">AV[b] × 27 weeks</td><td rowspan="6">Four-drug regimen (alternating cycles of cyclophosphamide-doxorubicin[c] and carboplatin-etoposide, over 34 weeks)</td></tr>
<tr><td colspan="2">III</td></tr>
<tr><td rowspan="4">IV</td><td>Metastatic CR or VGPR at week 10 or complete metastatectomy</td><td colspan="2">AVD[d] × 27 weeks</td></tr>
<tr><td rowspan="3">Single or multiple inoperable residual metastases (biopsy from a representative lung nodule decides the chemotherapy regimen)</td><td colspan="2">Low-risk histology, necrotic: AVD[d]</td></tr>
<tr><td colspan="2">Low-risk histology, viable or intermediate-risk histology, necrotic: AVD[e]</td></tr>
<tr><td colspan="2">Intermediate-risk histology, viable: four-drug regimen</td></tr>
</table>

AV, actinomycin D, vincristine; AVD, actinomycin D, vincristine, doxorubicin; COG, Children's Oncology Group; CR, complete response; SIOP, Société Internationale d'Oncologie Pédiatrique; VGPR, very good partial response

Cumulative doses of doxorubicin: [a]250 mg/m$^2$, [c]300 mg/m$^2$, [d]150, and [e]250 mg/m$^2$

[b] Inclusion of doxorubicin is indicated for large volume (post-NACT tumor volume ≥500 mL), stage II/III, non-epithelial, non-stromal predominant tumors

tomy, and the tumor histology. Low-risk histology of the primary tumor or achievement of metastatic remission following NACT (±metastatectomy) translates to a superior disease-free survival, allowing de-intensification of adjuvant therapy. A metastatic remission is defined as a complete radiological resolution or histologically documented necrosis of the nodule(s) post-NACT or complete surgical removal of the viable residual nodule(s). Residual unresectable viable metastatic nodule(s) or high-risk histology portend inferior survival requiring augmentation of adjuvant treatment.

## 25.8 Synopsis of the COG Approach

The COG advocates for universal upfront nephrectomy, except when the anticipated burden of surgical morbidity seems repugnant. However, in specific situations, COG recommend for NACT instead of primary nephrectomy, such as (a) tumor infiltration into the contiguous organs, (b) an extension of tumor thrombus beyond the retrohepatic IVC, (c) surgeon's anticipation of intraoperative tumor spillage, or (d) pulmonary compromise due to extensive metastases. NACT is also prescribed in patients with bilateral WT to facilitate NSS.

The adjuvant chemotherapy is decided on the age, stage of disease, histology, and tumor biomarkers (Table 25.3). The presence of adverse biomarkers in

**Table 25.3** Plan of adjuvant chemotherapy for Wilms tumor (COG)

| Stage | Histology | | | |
|---|---|---|---|---|
| | Favorable | | Focal anaplasia | Diffuse anaplasia |
| I | AV[a] × 19 week | | AVD × 25 weeks | AVD × 25 weeks |
| | AVD[b] × 25 weeks in the presence of LOH 1p/16q | | | |
| II | AV × 19 weeks | | AVD × 25 weeks | VDCyCE[c] × 31 weeks |
| | AVD × 25 weeks in the presence of LOH 1p/16q | | | |
| III | AVD × 25 weeks | | AVD × 25 weeks | VDCyCE × 31 weeks |
| | VDACyE[d] × 31 weeks in the presence of LOH 1p/16q | | | |
| IV | Metastatic CR at week 6 | AVD × 25 weeks | VDCyCE × 31 weeks | VDCyCEI[e] × 36 weeks |
| | No metastatic CR at week 6 | VDACyE × 31 weeks | | |
| | In the presence of LOH 1p/16q; irrespective of metastatic response at week 6 | VDACyE × 31 weeks | | |

AV, actinomycin D, vincristine; AVD, actinomycin D, vincristine, doxorubicin; COG, Children's Oncology Group; CR, complete response; LOH, loss of heterozygosity; VDACyE, vincristine, doxorubicin, actinomycin D, cyclophosphamide, etoposide; VDCyCE, vincristine, doxorubicin, cyclophosphamide, carboplatin, etoposide; VDCyCEI, vincristine, doxorubicin, cyclophosphamide, carboplatin, etoposide, irinotecan

[a]AV, [b]AVD, [c]VDACyE, [d]VDCyCE, [e]VDCyCEI regimen are also referred as EE4A, DD4A, regimen M, regimen UH-1, and regimen UH-2, respectively

favorable histology disease warrants augmentation of therapy [7, 8]. A highly selected group of young children (<2 years) with stage I, small (weight <550 g), favorable histology tumor are spared from adjuvant chemotherapy without compromising on the excellent survival [12].

### 25.8.1 Comparison of SIOP Vis-à-Vis COG Approach

- Advantages of the SIOP approach
  - Reduced risk of intraoperative tumor rupture due to NACT-induced tumor shrinkage
  - Opportunity to assess the chemo-responsiveness of disease
- Advantages of the COG approach
  - Possible avoidance of chemotherapy in selected patients with very low-risk disease
  - Avoidance of empirical treatment with ineffective chemotherapy for non-Wilms renal malignancy, such as CCSK or MRT
  - Opportunity of a precise assessment of tumor biology, given the availability of chemotherapy-naïve tumor tissue [4, 11]

## 25.9 Role of Surgery

A curative approach for pediatric renal tumors must always include surgery, and total tumor excision is unquestionably the cornerstone of care and prognosis. Surgery helps in providing complete tumor removal, staging, and evaluation of tumor characteristics. Various major international groups have created and supported evidence-based recommendations for surgical excision of WT. SIOP 93-01/ German Society of Paediatric Haematology and Oncology recommend that unilateral WT to be treated by complete tumor nephrectomy. The tumor should be removed en bloc to avoid tumoral spillage into peritoneal cavity.

WT patients may be at risk for renal impairment due to nephrotoxic chemotherapeutic drugs and RT. Hence, recent literature has recommended the use of NSS as a possible alternative to the conventional radical nephrectomy approach for a selected group of patients [13]. SIOP WT-2001 protocol recommends NSS for peripherally located non-infiltrating tumors, which can be surgically removed with clean margins [14]. However, the long-term advantages of maintaining renal parenchyma must be weighed against the potential negative effects of NSS on immediate outcomes, particularly in terms of overall and event-free survival. It is also crucial to take lymph node sampling during surgery. The current accepted practice is to sample the ipsilateral nodes.

Similar to WT, unilateral nephrectomy forms an essential component in the combined modality treatment for CCSK and RTK [15].

## 25.10 Role of Radiotherapy

Friedlander of Cincinnati introduced radiation therapy in the 1950s for Wilms tumor as an adjunct to surgery. The preoperative RT approach in SIOP Protocols was based on reducing the risk of intraoperative spillage and facilitating tumor resection by downsizing the tumor. SIOP-5 established the role of pre-operative chemotherapy as efficacious as pre-operative RT; henceforth, preoperative chemotherapy became the standard of care in SIOP trials instead of pre-op RT [16]. The current role of RT in WT is mainly limited to high-risk categories, i.e., some stage 2 patients, stage 3 patients, and those with unfavorable histologies.

Due to differences in staging and risk categorization of NWTSG and SIOP models, indications and doses for radiotherapy as per NWTSG and SIOP are listed separately, as shown below in Tables 25.4 and 25.5 [7–9].

### 25.10.1 General Considerations for Radiotherapy

Timing for initiation of RT is by day 10 post-surgery, no later than day 14, considering day of surgery as day 0. Delay of >10 days is associated with significantly higher abdominal relapse rate, especially in patients with unfavorable histology as per results of NWTSG 1, 3 and 4 [17, 18].

**Table 25.4** Radiotherapy for localized disease in Wilms tumor

| NWTSG/COG | Dose and site | SIOP | Dose and site |
|---|---|---|---|
| Upfront nephrectomy with planned lymph node sampling/dissection except in selected conditions[a]<br>Followed by postop RT and chemotherapy | | For patients with age >6 months, Preoperative chemotherapy (vincristine and actinomycin D) × 4 weeks<br>Followed by surgery and histologic risk assessment[b] followed by postop RT and chemotherapy | |
| Timing of radiotherapy: start by Day 10 and no later than 14 days, if surgery day is 0, concurrently with chemotherapy | | Timing of radiotherapy: flank/abdominal RT 2 weeks from surgery | |
| Stage III[c], FH | 10.8 Gy @ 1.8 Gy/# to flank; 10.8 Gy boost if gross residual disease post-surgery **(AREN0532)** | Stage III-Intermediate risk **(SIOP 2001)** | 14.4 Gy @ 1.8 Gy/#flank; 10.8 Gy boost for lymph node involvement or gross residual disease after surgery (total dose-25.2 Gy) |
| Stage I–III, FA<br>Stage I–II, DA<br>Stage I–III CCSK<br>Stage I–III RTK, Infants less than 12 months | 10.8 Gy @ 1.8 Gy/# to flank; 10.8 Gy boost if gross residual disease post-surgery | Stage II–III[d], High risk<br>Except Stage II blastemal-predominant type histology **(SIOP 2001)** | 25.2 Gy @ 1.8 Gy/# flank; 10.8 Gy boost for gross residual disease after surgery |
| Stage III, DA<br>Stage I–III RTK | 19.8 Gy @ 1.8 Gy/# to Flank | | |

*LOH* loss of heterozygosity of 1p and 16q, *FH* favorable histology, *FA* focal anaplasia, *DA* diffuse anaplasia

[a] Pre-operative chemotherapy can be considered in special conditions such as solitary kidney/horseshoe kidney, tumor thrombus in the inferior vena cava above the level of the hepatic veins, and when the child presents with respiratory distress due to extensive pulmonary metastases or in infants with Denys-Drash or Frasier syndrome (to delay the need for dialysis) followed by surgery at week 6 or 12 based on response to treatment [7–9]

[b] Low risk (mesoblastic nephroma, completely necrotic nephroblastoma, or cystic partially differentiated nephroblastoma), intermediate risk (regressive, epithelial, stromal, mixed, or focal anaplastic nephroblastoma), and high risk (blastemal or diffuse anaplastic nephroblastoma, CCSK, RTK)

[c] Whole abdomen RT (WAR): If stage III by virtue of preoperative tumor rupture, cytology proven ascites, peritoneal mets found at surgery, intraoperative tumor spill outside tumor bed 10.5 Gy @ 1.5 Gy/# to whole abdomen with 10.5 Gy supplemental boost to gross residual disease if any or if diffuse unresectable peritoneal implants-21 Gy @ 1.5 Gy/# to whole abdomen

[d] Whole abdomen RT: If stage III by virtue of diffuse peritoneal mets or diffuse gross perioperative—21 Gy to whole abdomen with consideration of boost to limited area. In children under 1 year of age, total dose should be reduced to 10–12 Gy

- Supine position, reproducible immobilization, need for anesthesia in very young children.
- Simulation, CT scans: 3–5 mm slice thickness.
- Co-registration of radiotherapy planning CT scan with preoperative or prechemotherapy diagnostic images.

**Table 25.5** Radiotherapy for metastatic sites in Wilms tumor

| NWTSG | Dose and target volume | SIOP-2001 | Dose and target volume |
|---|---|---|---|
| Upfront nephrectomy with planned lymph node sampling/dissection or pre-operative chemotherapy with DD4A Regimen (Vincristine, Actinomycin D and Doxorubicin) × 6 weeks | | Preoperative chemotherapy (vincristine, actinomycin D and doxorubicin) × 6 weeks | |
| Timing for flank/abdomen RT—by week 2 if upfront nephrectomy and by week 7 in pre-chemo group<br>Timing for lung mets—by week 7 in both groups with upfront surgery or pre-chemo group after assessment at week 6 | | Timing for RT: flank/abdominal RT 2 weeks from surgery or at week 9, if planned along with pulmonary RT<br>– The order of the chemotherapy blocks can be altered if necessary to allow doxorubicin not to be given within 14 days of RT, depending on when it can be arranged<br>– Pneumocystis carinii pneumoniae prophylaxis with cotrimoxazole in case of pulmonary RT | |
| Local site RT in Stage IV and V - according to local stage will receive radiotherapy in both groups | | | |
| Isolated lung mets with LOH 1p/16q or lung mets with no LOH and persistent at week 6 of induction chemotherapy **(AREN 0533)** | 12 Gy @ 1.5 Gy/# to whole lung,<br>10.5 Gy@ 1.5 Gy/# if age <12 month,<br>Followed by 4 cycles of cyclophosphamide/ etoposide (Regimen M) | Lung mets: If persistent mets at week 9 of induction chemotherapy and cannot be completely excised in low and intermediate histological risk category or in patients with high-risk histology category irrespective of metastatic response at week 9 | 15 Gy @ 1.5 Gy/# (with correction of tissue heterogeneity) to whole lung (WLI) including the apices and costo-diaphragmatic recesses ±10–15 Gy boost for residual disease post-surgery |
| Brain metastasis **(AREN 0532)** | 21.6 Gy @ 1.8 Gy/# to whole brain + 10.8 Gy, IMRT/stereotactic boost if age <16 years,<br>30.6 Gy to whole brain if age >=16years | Brain mets: regardless of response to chemotherapy | 25.5 Gy to whole brain (WBI) ± Boost 4.5 Gy @ 1.5 Gy/# |

(continued)

**Table 25.5** (continued)

| NWTSG | Dose and target volume | SIOP-2001 | Dose and target volume |
|---|---|---|---|
| Bone metastasis **(AREN 0532)** | 25.2Gy @ 1.8 Gy/# to the lesion + 1 cm margin if age <16 years, 30.6 Gy if age >=16years | Bone mets: regardless of response to chemotherapy | 30 Gy @ 3 Gy/# -Focal RT with 3 cm margin |
| Liver metastasis **(AREN 0532)** | Focal mets-19.8 Gy @ 1.8 Gy/# to mets with 2 cm margin ± 5.4–10.8 Gy boost, Diffuse mets-19.8 Gy @ 1.8 Gy/# to whole liver | Liver mets which do not respond completely to chemotherapy and which cannot be completely resected with negative margins | 20 Gy to site of R1 Metastasis @ 1.5 Gy/# with a margin of 2 cm |
| Lymph-node metastasis **(AREN 0532)** | Resected-10.8 Gy, Unresected-19.8 Gy | | |
| Recurrent **(AREN 0532)** | Flank/WAR: primary and supplementary doses same as mentioned in Table 25.4 for localized site | Recurrent | 15 Gy (except initial stage 1 and presently in CR after chemotherapy and surgery for recurrence) ± boost for postop residual disease |

*WLI* whole lung irradiation, *WBI* whole brain irradiation, WAR whole abdomen radiotherapy, CR complete response

- Discussion with the operating surgeon or refer to operative notes for any tumor spillage or peritoneal implantation.
- Unresected gross lymph nodes should be treated.
- Fraction size of 1.8 Gy/# is preferred unless large field like whole abdomen radiotherapy (in case of toxicity or children aged less than 2 years, dose per fraction should be lowered to 1.5 Gy or even to 1.25 Gy).
- In case multiple areas need to be treated (i.e., local plus metastatic sites), simultaneous treatment should be preferred to avoid any gap or overlap of fields.
- The full width of the vertebral bodies should be encompassed in the treatment volume with homogenous dose distribution to prevent the risk of scoliosis (where indicated, like in flank radiation or paraaortic lymph node irradiation).
- To prevent late toxicities, appropriate use of shielding blocks is recommended at sites such as Testicular, bilateral femoral heads, bilateral acetabulum, heart, contralateral kidney, shoulder joints, and hip joints [19].
- Myelotoxicity should be monitored weekly.

## 25.11 Target Volume for Radiotherapy

### 25.11.1 2D Radiotherapy

**Flank Irradiation** Ideally intravenous pyelogram should be done to assess the site of the contralateral renal pelvis.

Field borders:

- Superior: If tumor extending to upper pole—Up to dome of diaphragm, if the tumor at the lower pole—1 cm above the superior pole of the kidney.
- Inferior: 1 cm below the lowermost extent of the tumor
- Medial: Include the full width of the vertebral bodies
- Lateral: Include the abdominal wall

Field borders of whole abdomen irradiation:

- Superior: Dome of the diaphragm, using customized blocking—shield portions of the heart (beyond a 1 cm margin from the diaphragm)
- Inferior: Bottom of obturator foramen
- Flash laterally (Shield - Contralateral kidney, bilateral acetabulum and femoral heads)

**Paraaortic Lymph Node RT** The entire length of the paraaortic lymph node chain should be included in the treatment volume in case of pathological involvement of lymph nodes. The upper border should be kept at the crus of the diaphragm, the lower border at the bottom of L5 vertebra, and laterally include the full width of vertebra.

### 25.11.2 Conformal RT

#### 25.11.2.1 AREN0532 Guidelines

Flank Irradiation

- Gross tumor volume (GTV): Gross residual disease and or tumor bed
- Clinical target volume (CTV): 1 cm for primary radiotherapy treatment and 0.5 cm for supplemental radiation (boost radiation)
- Planning target volume (PTV): Internal Margin for breathing movements: 0.5 cm; setup margin: 0.5–1 cm (institutionally defined)
- Planning organ at risk volume (PRV) for critical organ at risk—at least 0.5 cm

#### 25.11.2.2 SIOP-2001

Flank Irradiation:

- GTV includes the post-chemotherapy and pre-operative macroscopic tumor.
- CTV- GTV + 10 mm (1 cm margin is beyond clips) (editing at anatomical barriers of resistance), goal to achieve homogeneous irradiation across the full width of the vertebral bodies.
- PTV individualized as per institute policy should be at least 1 cm considering breathing movements

Boost for residual macroscopic disease CTV: This includes the post-operative macroscopic residual disease with a margin of 1 cm.

Whole abdominal RT CTV: This includes the coverage of entire abdomen from the dome of the diaphragm to the pelvic floor (lower border of obturator foramen).

## 25.12 Management of Bilateral WT

Treating bilateral WT is targeted to achieve the best possible chemoreduction to facilitate NSS. The response to NACT is monitored with serial ultrasound imaging at 4–6 weeks intervals. In case of poor response or progression, the NACT is intensified, typically with the incorporation of anthracycline. Surgery is postponed until the tumor regression continues, albeit not beyond 12 weeks [9].

## 25.13 Side Effects of Radiotherapy: Acute and Long Term

Acute: Loose stools, nausea, fatigue, diarrhea

Long term: Bowel adhesions, infertility (more in females treated with whole abdomen with both ovaries and uterus in the field, more common in boys on cyclophosphamide), mamma hypoplasia, scoliosis, slipped capital femoral epiphysis, hypertension (secondary to fibrosis of contralateral renal artery), cardiomyopathy, congestive heart failure, renal failure, radiation pneumonitis (due to pulmonary RT), second malignancy (leukemia and breast cancer) [7–9, 19, 20].

## 25.14 Ongoing and Future Research to Reduce/Eliminate RT in Renal Tumors

- Umbrella Protocol by The Renal Tumour Study Group of the International Society of Paediatric Oncology (SIOP-RTSG) is assessing the prognostic significance of genomic changes within the tumor and blastemal component volume that persists preoperative chemotherapy. Whole lung radiation dose is reduced from 15 to 12 Gy in intermediate-risk histology category patients as per the results of COG trials demonstrating high relapse-free and overall survival in favorable histology [20].

- Possibility of eliminating flank radiation in Stage 1 Diffuse anaplasia Wilms tumor or stage 1 CCSK with the use of intensive three-drug chemotherapy should be tested prospectively, considering early salvage options in case of relapse [21].

## 25.15 Toxicities of Chemotherapy

Chemotherapy-induced nausea, vomiting, vincristine-related neuropathy, and neutropenic sepsis are the commonly encountered toxicities. Hematological toxicities are frequent in children with high-risk or metastatic disease. The hepatic veno-occlusive disease is an infrequent, however, dreadful complication of dactinomycin [22]. Late effects, especially prevalent among patients with high-risk or metastatic disease, include anthracycline-related cardiomyopathy, alkylator-induced infertility, and second malignancy.

## 25.16 Supportive Care

Control of hypertension, nutritional rehabilitation, and amelioration of chemotherapy toxicities are instrumental in achieving a favorable outcome. Prophylaxis with granulocyte-colony stimulating factor is indicated in patients experiencing grade 4 neutropenia or protracted count recovery leading to treatment delay. Prophylaxis for *Pneumocystis jirovecii* pneumonia is indicated in patients with high-risk diseases.

## 25.17 Non-Wilms Renal Malignancies of Childhood

CCSK, MRT, congenital mesoblastic nephroma (CMN), and renal cell carcinoma (RCC) collectively account for <20% of pediatric renal tumors. The typical age of presentation of CCSK is 2–5 years, overlapping with WT. CMN presents in early infancy, MRT in young children (<2 years), and RCC in adolescence [23, 24]. Marked paraneoplastic hypercalcemia in an infant with renal mass indicates a possibility of MRT or CMN [25].

The adjuvant therapy for CCSK and MRT follows the chemotherapy protocol for high-risk renal tumors. A complete surgical excision remains the mainstay of curative treatment in non-metastatic pediatric RCC and CMN. Systemic therapy for RCC is restricted for metastatic disease, multikinase inhibitor sunitinib being the agent of choice [26].

## 25.18 Challenges in the LMICs

The challenges unique in the LMICs include (a) delayed presentation to the healthcare facility, leading to a greater tumor burden, (b) higher risk of intraoperative tumor spillage and other surgical morbidities, (c) greater prevalence of metastatic disease, and (d) comorbidities, such as malnutrition or infection in a substantial proportion of patients. Limited access to centers with expertise in managing childhood cancer and state-of-art diagnostic facilities are additional challenges [4, 27].

## References


1. Libes J, Hol J, de Neto JCA, Vallance KL, van Tinteren H, Benedetti DJ, et al. Pediatric renal tumor epidemiology: global perspectives, progress, and challenges. Pediatr Blood Cancer. 2023;70(1):1–10.
2. Qureshi SS, Bhagat M, Verma K, Yadav S, Prasad M, Vora T, et al. Incidence, treatment, and outcomes of primary and recurrent non-Wilms renal tumors in children: report of 109 patients treated at a single institution. J Pediatr Urol. 2020;16(4):475.e1–9.
3. Fernandez C, Geller JI, Ehrlich PF, et al. Renal tumors. In: Pizzo P, Poplack D, editors. Principles and practice of pediatric oncology. 6th ed. St. Louis: Lippincott Williams & Wilkins; 2011. p. 861.
4. Spreafico F, Fernandez CV, Brok J, et al. Wilms tumour. Nat Rev Dis Primers. 2021;7(1):1–21.
5. Turner JT, Brzezinski J, Dome JS. Wilms tumor predisposition [updated 2022 Mar 24]. In: Adam MP, Ardinger HH, Pagon RA, et al., editors. GeneReviews®. Seattle, WA: University of Washington, Seattle; 1993-2022.
6. Metzger ML, Dome JS. Current therapy for Wilms' tumor. Oncologist. 2005;10:815.
7. Dix DB, Fernandez CV, Chi YY, et al. Augmentation of therapy for combined loss of heterozygosity 1p and 16q in favorable histology Wilms tumor: a Children's Oncology Group AREN0532 and AREN0533 study report. J Clin Oncol. 2019;37(30):2769–77.
8. Dix DB, Seibel NL, Chi YY, et al. Treatment of stage IV favorable histology Wilms tumor with lung metastases: a report From the Children's Oncology Group AREN0533 Study. J Clin Oncol. 2018;36:1564–70.
9. Groenendijk A, van Tinteren H, Jiang Y, et al. Outcome of SIOP patients with low- or intermediate-risk Wilms tumour relapsing after initial vincristine and actinomycin-D therapy only—the SIOP 93-01 and 2001 protocols. Eur J Cancer. 2022;163:88–97.
10. Gooskens SL, Segers H, Pritchard-Jones K, et al. The clinical relevance of age at presentation in nephroblastoma. In: van den Heuvel-Eibrink MM, editor. Wilms tumor. Brisbane: Codon Publications; 2016.
11. Gleason JM, Lorenzo AJ, Bowlin PR, et al. Innovations in the management of Wilms' tumor. Ther Adv Urol. 2014;6:165–76.
12. Fernandez CV, Perlman EJ, Mullen EA, et al. Clinical outcome and biological predictors of relapse after nephrectomy only for very low-risk Wilms tumor: a report from Children's Oncology Group AREN0532. Ann Surg. 2017;265:835–40.
13. Termuhlen AM, Tersak JM, Liu Q, Yasui Y, Stovall M, Weathers R, et al. Twenty-five year follow-up of childhood Wilms tumor: a report from the Childhood Cancer Survivor Study. Pediatr Blood Cancer. 2011;57(7):1210–6.
14. Wilde JCH, Aronson DC, Sznajder B, Van Tinteren H, Powis M, Okoye B, et al. Nephron sparing surgery (NSS) for unilateral wilms tumor (UWT): the SIOP 2001 experience. Pediatr Blood Cancer. 2014;61(12):2175–9.

15. Argani P, Perlman EJ, Breslow NE, et al. Clear cell sarcoma of the kidney: a review of 351 cases from the National Wilms Tumor Study Group Pathology Center. Am J Surg Pathol. 2000;24(1):4–18.
16. Bhatnagar S. Management of Wilms' tumor: NWTS vs SIOP. J Indian Assoc Pediatr Surg. 2009;14(1):6–14.
17. Kalapurakal JA, Li SM, Breslow NE, Beckwith JB, Macklis R, Thomas PRM, et al. Influence of radiation therapy delay on abdominal tumor recurrence in patients with favorable histology Wilms' tumor treated on NWTS-3 and NWTS-4: a report from the National Wilms' Tumor Study Group. Int J Radiat Oncol Biol Phys. 2003;57(2):495–9.
18. D'Angio GJ, Tefft M, Breslow N, Meyer JA. Radiation therapy of Wilms' tumor: results according to dose, field, post-operative timing and histology. Int J Radiat Oncol Biol Phys. 1978;4(9–10):769–80.
19. Blitzer GC, Bradley KA. Four ways to decrease late toxicity from pelvic radiation therapy in children and young adults. Pract Radiat Oncol. 2021;11(6):434–40.
20. van den Heuvel-Eibrink MM, Hol JA, Pritchard-Jones K, et al. Rationale for the treatment of Wilms tumour in the UMBRELLA SIOP–RTSG 2016 protocol. Nat Rev Urol. 2017;14:743–52.
21. Fajardo RD, van den Heuvel-Eibrink MM, van Tinteren H, Spreafico F, Acha T, Bergeron C, et al. Is radiotherapy required in first-line treatment of stage I diffuse anaplastic Wilms tumor? A report of SIOP-RTSG, AIEOP, JWiTS, and UKCCSG. Pediatr Blood Cancer. 2020;67(2):e28039.
22. Cesaro S, Spiller M, Sartori MT, et al. Veno-occlusive disease in pediatric patients affected by Wilms tumor. Pediatr Blood Cancer. 2011;57:258–61.
23. Craig KM, Poppas DP, Akhavan A. Pediatric renal cell carcinoma. Curr Opin Urol. 2019;29:500–4.
24. Dome JS, Gooskens SL, van den Heuvel-Eibrink MM. Non-Wilms pediatric renal tumors. In: Pritchard-Jones K, Dome JS, editors. Renal tumors of childhood: biology and therapy. Pediatric oncology. Berlin: Springer; 2014. p. 249–69.
25. Kerdudo C, Aerts I, Fattet S, et al. Hypercalcemia and childhood cancer: a 7-year experience. J Pediatr Hematol Oncol. 2005;27:23–7.
26. Ray S, Jones R, Pritchard-Jones K, et al. Pediatric and young adult renal cell carcinoma. Pediatr Blood Cancer. 2020;67:e28675.
27. Israels T, Moreira C, Scanlan T, et al. SIOP PODC: clinical guidelines for the management of children with Wilms tumour in a low income setting. Pediatr Blood Cancer. 2013;60:5–11.

# Rhabdomyosarcoma

# 26

Varshu Goel, Anurita Srivastava, Archana Agarwal, Narayan Adhikari, and Mayank Agarwal

Rhabdomyosarcoma (RMS) is a soft tissue sarcoma (STS) of skeletal muscle phenotype arising from primitive mesenchymal cell, rhabdomyoblast. It is the most common childhood and adolescent STS with slight male predominance, with only 1% of adulthood tumors being RMS [1]. The age distribution is binomial, with higher incidence among 2–4 years of age and 12–16 years. Incidence is lower in the Asian population. Most cases are sporadic; however, some association is found with familial syndromes such as neurofibromatosis type 1, Li-Fraumeni, Beckwith-Wiedemann, Costello, Noonan, and *DICER1* syndrome [2].

## 26.1 Etiology and Epidemiology

Though the exact etiology remains unknown, risk factors include in utero radiation exposure or parental use of recreational drugs during pregnancy. Children have more head and neck involvement, whereas extremity RMS is more common in adolescents. Botryoid RMS occurs in hollow viscera, usually in children. Pleomorphic RMS arises in the extremities and mainly affects adults. Common metastatic sites for RMS include lung, bone marrow, and lymph nodes.

---

V. Goel
Department of Radiotherapy, IRCH, AIIMS, New Delhi, India

A. Srivastava (✉) · A. Agarwal
Department of Radiotherapy, Maulana Azad Medical College, New Delhi, India

N. Adhikari · M. Agarwal
DrNB Medical Oncology, Medanta Gurugram, India



R. Madan et al. (eds.), *Evidence Based Practice in Pediatric Radiation Oncology*,
https://doi.org/10.1007/978-981-96-4872-6_26

## 26.2 Histopathology

Histological types of RMS include embryonal (approximately 60%), alveolar (approximately 20%), pleomorphic (approximately 10%), spindle/sclerosing (approximately 10%), and sarcoma not otherwise specified (NOS), with the first four variants described in the 2020 update of the World Health Organization (WHO) classification of soft tissue and bone tumors [3]. The botryoid and spindle cell types have a superior prognosis, the embryonal type shows an intermediate prognosis, and the alveolar and undifferentiated types have a poor prognosis. The pathological identification of RMS is often difficult due to its similarity to the other small, blue, round cell tumors of bone and soft tissue such as lymphoma, osteosarcoma, chondrosarcoma, and the Ewing's family of tumors. Various immunohistochemical, molecular genetics and ultra-structural techniques may be needed to confirm the diagnosis of RMS. Immunohistochemistry (IHC) is a useful tool to establish the diagnosis as RMS tumors are usually positive for myogenin, desmin, sarcomeric actin, and myoglobin, while they are negative for NKX2.2, CD99, CD45, CK, S100, and NSE. Alveolar EMS shows a FOXO1 rearrangement, t(2;13) (q35;q14) for PAX3-FOXO1 fusion or t(1;13) (p36;q14) for PAX7-FOXO1 fusion and N-myc amplification [4]. Embryonal rhabdomyosarcoma may show loss of heterozygosity (LOH) at the 11p15 locus, the site of the IGF-II gene, in about 80% of cases [5].

## 26.3 Clinical Manifestations

The presenting signs and symptoms of RMS are site specific and depend on patient's age, distant metastases, and other factors. For example, orbital tumors may present as proptosis or ophthalmoplegia; parameningeal tumors may present with nasal obstruction, cranial nerve palsy, or headache; genitourinary tumors may present as hematuria, urinary obstruction, constipation; extremity tumors may present as a painful mass, with or without associated erythema of the overlying skin.

## 26.4 Evaluation

Post histological confirmation of diagnosis, it is essential to assess the extent of disease both locally and distantly. Metastatic workup is tailored as per the clinical and histologic findings. Firstly, CT or MRI scan of the primary site of tumor is performed. CT scan of the thorax for locally advanced disease and/or involved nodes and CT whole abdomen for below diaphragm primaries is indicated. Bone scan and bilateral bone marrow aspirate and biopsy is required in case of positive findings on CT chest, nodal involvement, or locally advanced disease with unfavorable histology. Lumbar puncture for CSF cytology is performed in case of intracranial extension of para-meningeal or orbital disease.

## 26.5 Risk Stratification

Treatment in RMS is based on prognostic stratification using combined information from (a) the pre-treatment TNM (tumor, nodes, metastasis) staging assessment and (b) the post-resection pathological staging or the clinical group (CG) system along with factors like age, histology, and presence or absence of FOXO1 fusion gene (Table 26.1). As per the TNM system, *favorable sites* are orbit, nonparameningeal head and neck, biliary tract, and genitourinary (non-bladder/prostate), while all others such as extremities, retroperitoneum, bladder–prostate, trunk, cranial parameningeal sites, and retroperitoneum are designated as *unfavorable*. FOXO1 fusion is the most important prognostic factor in both localized and metastatic disease.

### 26.5.1 Prognosis

RMS prognosis depends on multiple clinical, biologic, and pathologic factors as listed. Adults generally have poorer 5-year overall survival compared with children (27% versus 61%) [10, 11]. Parameningeal and extremity tumors tend to have a worse prognosis than other sites.

## 26.6 Treatment

**Evidence** The Intergroup Rhabdomyosarcoma studies I–V have contributed to the formulation of the treatment strategies among various risk categories over the last two decades with the aim to maximize tumor control and minimize the treatment-related toxicities [7, 12–14].

**General Principles of Treatment** Traditionally, treatment of RMS is based on risk stratification based on pretreatment stage (TNM) and the Clinical Group classification. The survival of RMS patients has improved significantly in the last decade due to multimodality management (Table 26.2).

Role of surgery is to achieve complete resection while preserving function and cosmesis. Surgery should be attempted only if complete removal of gross disease can be achieved, else it is no better than biopsy alone [9]. Complete resection entails removal of tumour with an uninvolved rim of tissue all around (at least 0.5 cm margin). If R0 resection is not achievable, then use of neoadjuvant chemotherapy followed by local therapy by either surgery or radiotherapy is recommended. Use of second-look surgery in children after chemotherapy for the purpose of documenting response to chemotherapy carries no survival advantage and is to be used selectively; however, when it documents response histologically, it can help reduce radiotherapy dose in CG III disease. Any radiologically enlarged or palpable node needs to be surgically excised and assessed histologically.

**Table 26.1** Staging and risk group stratification

| **TNM staging** [6] | | | | |
|---|---|---|---|---|
| **Stage** | **Site** | **Size (a or b)** | **Lymph node involvement** | **Distant spread** |
| 1 | Favorable | Any | Any | No |
| 2 | Unfavorable | a ≤5 cm | $N_0$ or $N_x$ | No |
| 3 | Unfavorable | a ≤5 cm | Yes | No |
| | | b >5 cm | Any | No |
| 4 | Any | Any | Any | Yes |
| **Clinical groups by the intergroup rhabdomyosarcoma study group (IRSG)** [7] | | | | |
| | **I** | **II** | **III** | **IV** |
| | Localized (T1) and completely resected | Locally extensive tumor (T2) | Localized or locally extensive tumor | Any size primary, any nodal status, with distant metastases irrespective of surgical approach |
| (a) | Confined to site of origin | Localized, microscopic residual disease | Gross residual after biopsy only | |
| (b) | Infiltrating beyond site of origin | Locally extensive (nodal spread), completely resected | Gross residual after ≥50% debulking | |
| (c) | | Locally extensive (nodal spread), microscopic residual | | |
| **New risk group classification with FOXO1 fusion status** [8, 9] | | | | |
| **Risk group** | **Stage** | **Group** | **Age** | **Fusion** |
| Low | 1 | I–II | Any | FOXO1− |
| | 1 | III (orbit) | | |
| | 2 | I–II | | |
| Intermediate | 1 | III (non-orbit) | Any | FOXO1− |
| | 3 | I–II | | FOXO1− |
| | 2–3 | III | | FOXO1− |
| | 1–3 | I–III | | FOXO1+ |
| | 4 | IV | <10 years | FOXO1− |
| High | 4 | IV | >10 years | FOXO1− |
| | | | Any | FOXO1+ |

Role of Chemotherapy: Use of chemotherapy for cytoreduction and eradication of both micro- and macroscopic disease has improved outcomes. Main chemotherapy regimens in the treatment of RMS include the VAC/VAI (vincristine, actinomycin-D, and cyclophosphamide/ifosfamide) regimens, the former being preferred in North America, while the latter in Europe. Depending on disease stratification, the doses and duration of the regimens are modified. For low risk patients, two-drug (VA) regimen for 15 cycles over 45 weeks or combination of VAC/VA × 8 cycles

**Table 26.2** Site-wise treatment [15–17]

| Favorable or unfavorable | Site | Histology | Lymph node involvement | Surgery | Radiotherapy | Comments |
|---|---|---|---|---|---|---|
| Favorable | Orbit | Embryonal (80–90%) | Rare | Biopsy only<br>Routine LN sampling not required | 45 Gy | |
| | Non-parameningeal (head and neck) | Embryonal (majority) and alveolar for cheek and scalp | 10–20% | Surgical resection for superficial tumors of the scalp, parotid, and for some oral cavity and oropharynx | RT alone for invasive or deep-seated tumors | No prophylactic nodal irradiation |
| Unfavorable | Parameningeal | Embryonal (70%) | 15–20% | Infiltrative and rarely surgically resectable | 50.4 Gy<br>Begin at week 4 | 30% with intracranial extension |
| | Bladder prostate | Embryonal | 20–30% to hypogastric and external iliac nodes >para-aortic nodes | Not preferred unless located at dome of bladder | Induction chemotherapy followed by RT for organ preservation | PET/CT for staging and cystoscopic biopsy may allow for diagnosis |
| | Paratesticular | Embryonal | 25% | Radical inguinal orchiectomy and ipsilateral (trans-abdominal) nerve-sparing retroperitoneal lymph node dissection (RPLND) for patients ≥10 years old. Under 10 years, RPLND only if radiographically node positive | Postoperative radiation 41.4 Gy to para-aortic chain and 50.4 Gy to gross nodes | Avoid transscrotal approach |
| | Extremity and trunk | Alveolar (60–70%) | 30–40%<br>Sentinel node biopsy if $cN_0$ | Wide resection with negative margins is mainstay either upfront or DPE | Same[a] | |
| **General recommendations for all sites** | **Surgical resection** with 5 mm margin when feasible or delayed primary excision (DPE) | | | | | |
| | **Radiotherapy** for local control to all except completely resected embryonal tumors without any involved lymph nodes | | | | | |
| | Induction **chemotherapy** can be utilized to reduce the disease burden to facilitate surgical resection and reduce RT volumes | | | | | |

[a] Same implies as per general recommendations for all sites

over 24 weeks or three-drug (VAC) regimen for 14 cycles over 40 weeks are recommended. For intermediate and high risk categories, 3 drug (VAC) × 14 cycles over 40 weeks is recommended. Patients with high-risk (metastatic) disease are treated primarily with chemotherapy. Still, hypofractionated SBRT and debulking surgery can play a role in local control of the primary and metastatic disease depending on location, symptoms, and response to systemic therapy.

Role of Radiotherapy (RT): RT has been established as an instrumental tool in decreasing disease recurrence rates. Use of conformal techniques is essential to minimize irradiation of normal tissues. The location of primary, extent of residual post-surgery, histology, response to chemotherapy, and the risk group stratification are considered in deciding the dose and timing of radiotherapy.

It is, thus, recommended in all cases except low-risk, completely resected embryonal tumors without nodal involvement and FOXO1 fusion negative and should not be omitted, even in younger children less than 2 years of age [18].

Timing of RT varies as per presentation, risk group, and systemic chemotherapy. In tumours with intracranial extension, sudden vision loss or cord compression should receive urgent RT [19], whereas low-risk patients start RT at week 13 [20], intermediate-risk patients at week 4 [21], and high-risk patients at week 20 [19]. RT doses up to 36 Gy are delivered to completely resected tumors with alveolar subtype, 41.4 Gy to resected nodal regions, and 50.4 Gy to gross disease and can be escalated to 59.4 Gy for patients with diffuse anaplasia or bulky disease (>5 cm) with less than complete response (<CR) on chemotherapy.

As per the RT techniques available, the important steps include simulation, anesthesia assistance (pediatric), delineation of target volumes and organs-at-risk (OARs), plan evaluation, plan implementation, daily localization, and management of toxicities during and after RT.

**Simulation** It is the first and most crucial step, especially for pediatric patients, both from the perspective of treatment planning and anesthesia care. The various pre-exposure therapies for acclimatization of children include departmental tours, audiovisuals of the radiation process, mask modifications/decorations, among others [22]. During planning computed tomography (CT) simulation and radiation treatment, comforting modalities are used, such as stuffed animals, music or audiobooks [23], two-way communication with caregiver, child-friendly décor and aromatherapy, end-of-treatment rewards or tokens, and dedicated playrooms with drawing material [24].

**Target Volumes** A suitable radiotherapy plan warrants careful attention to dose and target volumes. Three-dimensional (3D) and intensity-modulated RT (IMRT) planning techniques ensure adequate target coverage with reduced doses to the OARs.

- **GTV**: The gross tumor volume (GTV) is defined as the disease at the initial presentation. It is necessary to encompass the pre-chemotherapy or the pre-operative disease with adequate margins, including biopsy tracts. GTV2 is contoured as the post-chemotherapy disease in case of cone down or boost.

- **CTV**: The clinical target volume (CTV) is the margin of 0.5–1 cm to GTV with anatomically constrained borders. When lymph nodes are involved (clinically or pathologically), the entire lymph node chain is included in the CTV.
- **PTV**: The planning target volume (PTV) varies from 0.3 to 0.5 cm as per the institutional protocols and is added to the CTV to incorporate organ motion and setup errors. A cone down or a simultaneously integrated boost (SIB) can be used to target the post-chemotherapy gross tumor volume.

Though site-wise contouring guidelines can be followed for organ delineation, certain specific recommendations for RMS tumors are as follows:

- **Parameningeal Tumors**: A field reduction after 36 Gy to gross disease can be applied for tumors with significant tumor response after induction chemotherapy. Still, the initial volume should include the entire pre-chemotherapy tumor volume, areas of concern for microscopic invasion, and a clinical target volume (CTV) margin (typically 0.5–1 cm). Prophylactic nodal radiation is typically not used in PM RMS.
- **Orbit**: Meningeal invasion can be seen when intracranial extension occurs via the superior orbital fissure. Thus, the muscle of origin should be tracked back to the insertion, as failures can occur in the posterior orbit. A 0.5–1 cm CTV is recommended tailored to the pre-treatment extent of the tumor and the post-treatment changes with regard to re-expansion of the globe after surgery or chemotherapy response. The entire orbit need not be covered if the pre-treatment tumor is localized. A dose reduction after 36 Gy can be used to help spare sensitive structures such as the lens, retina, and lacrimal gland if surgical resection or response to systemic therapy is present. Proton therapy scores over photon therapy here by avoiding exit dose.
- **Paratesticular**: After RPLND, patients with positive lymph nodes undergo post-operative radiation of 41.4 Gy to the para-aortic chain with a boost up to 50.4 Gy to the gross nodal disease. For testicular preservation, the remaining testicle can be transposed laterally into the thigh before radiation therapy and then re-implanted into the scrotum after the completion of the treatment.
- **Extremity**: Larger CTV margins are used, with the current COG protocols recommending a 1.5 cm expansion. Care should be taken to remove CTV expansion from the bone and joint spaces. Circumferential irradiation of the limb should be avoided when possible, and a strip of soft tissue along the extremity should be spared to reduce the risk of lymphedema. Regional lymph nodes are treated only when involved.
- **Trunk**: Tumors that displaced a significant amount of lung should have the GTV contoured as the pre-operative (pre-chemotherapy) tumor volume, excluding the intrathoracic tumor. All areas of pleural involvement need to be included in the GTV regardless of whether the RT is delivered pre- or post-operatively.

- **Retroperitoneum**: Bowel and other organs displaced by the tumor that has returned to the normal anatomical position following surgery or chemotherapy should not be included in the delineation of the radiation pre-treatment tumor volume, though they can be included in the CTV if concern for microscopic invasion exists. All areas of peritoneal or mesenteric involvement should be included in the GTV regardless of whether the radiation is delivered pre- or post-operatively. If whole abdominopelvic radiotherapy is required for malignant ascites or diffuse peritoneal involvement, 24 Gy at 1.5 Gy per fraction is recommended with appropriate blocking of the kidneys and liver.
- **Metastatic disease**: RT can be given to the primary site and metastatic lesions as standard fractionation or hypofractionated SBRT. For patients with lung metastases, whole lung radiation can be considered (15 Gy in 10 fractions), and for those with diffuse abdominal metastases, whole abdominal RT can be considered.

**Proton Therapy** Current Children's Oncology Group (COG) and International Rhabdomyosarcoma Study Group (IRSG) protocols recommend the use of proton therapy due to the high sensitivity of children to the late effects of radiation and the tendency of pediatric RMS to arise in close proximity to critical structures. Because the relative biologic effectiveness (RBE) of protons is nearly equivalent to that of high-energy X-rays (RBE = 1.1), the interest in protons is based primarily on the physical properties that provide favorable dosimetric distributions. The abrupt dose fall-off is seen at the distal end of the proton beam, which allows for a reduction of dose to adjacent normal tissue and an increase in the total dose that can be safely delivered to the target volume. Further, the "integral dose" or total energy deposited in a patient from radiation therapy is decreased with protons, often by two to three times [25]. This reduced exposure is of great importance when considering the secondary malignancy risk in children.

**Treatment-Related Toxicities** Acute radiation toxicities are related to the dose to the critical organs in the path of the radiation and can be managed in most cases by a careful frequent assessment during and after irradiation. Late stochastic and deterministic radiation sequelae such as dental/bone and soft tissue growth abnormalities, cataracts, gonadal dysfunction, and secondary malignancies need to be explained beforehand to the patient and caregivers.

## 26.7 Metastatic Disease

Roughly 15% of pediatric RMS patients present with metastatic disease (stage IV). The majority of metastatic lesions appear in the lungs, bone, bone marrow, and distant lymph nodes. The metastatic disease tends to appear more frequently in older patients, male sex, alveolar histology, and with bulky primary tumors (>5 cm). Survival is poor for disseminated RMS, and a pooled analysis of US and European patients treated in cooperative group studies found a 3-year OS and EFS of 37% and 27% [26]. Attempts to intensify chemotherapy through increasing cyclophosphamide doses, incorporation of novel drugs and targeted therapies, and high-dose chemotherapy with stem cell rescue have all been tried to improve outcomes for these patients.

## 26.8 Follow-Up

Close follow-up with MRI/CT imaging every 3 months in the first year of treatment completion, every 4 months in the second and third year, every 6 months in the fourth and fifth year, and annually thereafter is preferred, along with imaging of any suspected metastatic site.

## 26.9 Recurrence

Approximately 30% of patients recur despite aggressive therapy. The overall survival (OS) after relapse can range from 15% to 80%, depending on the extent and site of recurrence [27]. Other factors such as time to relapse of <18 months, prior RT, large tumor size, and alveolar histology can decrease the chances of salvage. A multidisciplinary treatment approach is utilized with second-line chemotherapy followed by local therapy with surgery and radiation as per the site and extent of the recurrence as well as prior therapy and the response to second-line chemotherapy.

## 26.10 Conclusion

Though tremendous progress has occurred in treating RMS through multimodality therapy with the studies from cooperative groups over the last few decades, there is still a possibility for improvement in outcomes with advances in radiation oncology, molecular profiling, and targeted therapy.

## References

1. Amer KM, Thomson JE, Congiusta D, Dobitsch A, Chaudhry A, Li M, et al. Epidemiology, incidence, and survival of rhabdomyosarcoma subtypes: SEER and ICES database analysis. J Orthop Res. 2019;37(10):2226–30.
2. Li H, Sisoudiya SD, Martin-Giacalone BA, Khayat MM, Dugan-Perez S, Marquez-Do DA, et al. Germline cancer predisposition variants in pediatric rhabdomyosarcoma: a report from the Children's Oncology Group. J Natl Cancer Inst. 2021;113(7):875–83.
3. Anderson WJ, Doyle LA. Updates from the 2020 World Health Organization classification of soft tissue and bone tumours. Histopathology. 2021;78(5):644–57.
4. Parham DM, Qualman SJ, Teot L, Barr FG, Morotti R, Sorensen PHB, et al. Correlation between histology and PAX/FKHR fusion status in alveolar rhabdomyosarcoma: a report from the Children's Oncology Group. Am J Surg Pathol. 2007;31(6):895–901.

5. Davicioni E, Anderson MJ, Finckenstein FG, Lynch JC, Qualman SJ, Shimada H, et al. Molecular classification of rhabdomyosarcoma—genotypic and phenotypic determinants of diagnosis. Am J Pathol. 2009;174(2):550–64.
6. Lawrence W, Anderson JR, Gehan EA, Maurer H. Pretreatment TNM staging of childhood rhabdomyosarcoma: a report of the Intergroup Rhabdomyosarcoma Study Group. Children's Cancer Study Group. Pediatric Oncology Group. Cancer. 1997;80(6):1165–70.
7. Crist WM, Anderson JR, Meza JL, Fryer C, Raney RB, Ruymann FB, et al. Intergroup rhabdomyosarcoma study-IV: results for patients with nonmetastatic disease. J Clin Oncol. 2001;19(12):3091–102.
8. Hibbitts E, Chi Y, Hawkins DS, Barr FG, Bradley JA, Dasgupta R, et al. Refinement of risk stratification for childhood rhabdomyosarcoma using FOXO1 fusion status in addition to established clinical outcome predictors: a report from the Children's Oncology Group. Cancer Med. 2019;8(14):6437–48.
9. Rhee DS, Rodeberg DA, Baertschiger RM, et al. Update on pediatric rhabdomyosarcoma: a report from the APSA Cancer Committee. J Pediatr Surg. 2020;55:1987. https://doi.org/10.1016/j.jpedsurg.2020.06.015.
10. Esnaola NF, Rubin BP, Baldini EH, Vasudevan N, Demetri GD, Fletcher CD, et al. Response to chemotherapy and predictors of survival in adult rhabdomyosarcoma. Ann Surg. 2001;234(2):215–23.
11. Gerber NK, Wexler LH, Singer S, Alektiar KM, Keohan ML, Shi W, et al. Adult rhabdomyosarcoma survival improved with treatment on multimodality protocols. Int J Radiat Oncol Biol Phys. 2013;86(1):58–63.
12. Maurer HM, Beltangady M, Gehan EA, Crist W, Hammond D, Hays DM, et al. The intergroup rhabdomyosarcoma study-I. A final report. Cancer. 1988;61(2):209–20.
13. Casey DL, Chi YY, Donaldson SS, Hawkins DS, Tian J, Arndt CA, et al. Increased local failure for patients with intermediate-risk rhabdomyosarcoma on ARST0531: a report from the Children's Oncology Group. Cancer. 2019;125(18):3242–8.
14. Raney RB, Walterhouse DO, Meza JL, Andrassy RJ, Breneman JC, Crist WM, et al. Results of the Intergroup Rhabdomyosarcoma Study Group D9602 protocol, using vincristine and dactinomycin with or without cyclophosphamide and radiation therapy, for newly diagnosed patients with low-risk embryonal rhabdomyosarcoma: a report from the Soft Tissue Sarcoma Committee of the Children's Oncology Group. J Clin Oncol. 2011;29(10):1312–8.
15. Kaseb H, Kuhn J, Babiker HM. Rhabdomyosarcoma. In: StatPearls. Treasure Island, FL: StatPearls Publishing; 2022. http://www.ncbi.nlm.nih.gov/books/NBK507721/.
16. Merchant TE, Kortmann RD, editors. Pediatric radiation oncology. Cham: Springer International Publishing; 2018. http://link.springer.com/10.1007/978-3-319-43545-9.
17. Constine LS, Tarbell NJ, Halperin EC. Pediatric radiation oncology. Philadelphia, Pa: Wolters Kluwer; 2016.
18. Defachelles AS, Rey A, Oberlin O, Spooner D, Stevens MCG. Treatment of nonmetastatic cranial parameningeal rhabdomyosarcoma in children younger than 3 years old: results from international society of pediatric oncology studies MMT 89 and 95. J Clin Oncol. 2009;27(8):1310–5.
19. Weigel BJ, Lyden E, Anderson JR, Meyer WH, Parham DM, Rodeberg DA, et al. Intensive multiagent therapy, including dose-compressed cycles of ifosfamide/etoposide and vincristine/doxorubicin/cyclophosphamide, irinotecan, and radiation, in patients with high-risk rhabdomyosarcoma: a report from the Children's Oncology Group. J Clin Oncol. 2016;34(2):117–22.
20. Walterhouse DO, Pappo AS, Meza JL, Breneman JC, Hayes-Jordan AA, Parham DM, et al. Shorter-duration therapy using vincristine, dactinomycin, and lower-dose cyclophosphamide with or without radiotherapy for patients with newly diagnosed low-risk rhabdomyosarcoma: a report from the Soft Tissue Sarcoma Committee of the Children's Oncology Group. J Clin Oncol. 2014;32(31):3547–52.
21. National Cancer Institute (NCI). A randomized phase 3 study of vincristine, dactinomycin, cyclophosphamide (VAC) alternating with vincristine and irinotecan (VI) versus VAC/VI plus temsirolimus (TORI, Torisel, NSC# 683864) in patients with intermediate risk (IR)

rhabdomyosarcoma (RMS). clinicaltrials.gov; 2022 Jul [cited 2022 Jul 14]. Report No.: NCT02567435. https://clinicaltrials.gov/ct2/show/NCT02567435.
22. Holt DE, Hiniker SM, Kalapurakal JA, Breneman JC, Shiao JC, Boik N, et al. Improving the pediatric patient experience during radiation therapy—a Children's Oncology Group Study. Int J Radiat Oncol Biol Phys. 2021;109(2):505–14.
23. Klosky JL, Tyc VL, Srivastava DK, Tong X, Kronenberg M, Booker ZJ, et al. Brief report: evaluation of an interactive intervention designed to reduce pediatric distress during radiation therapy procedures. J Pediatr Psychol. 2004;29(8):621–6.
24. Engvall G, Lindh V, Mullaney T, Nyholm T, Lindh J, Ångström-Brännström C. Children's experiences and responses towards an intervention for psychological preparation for radiotherapy. Radiat Oncol. 2018;13(1):9.
25. Ladra MM, Edgington SK, Mahajan A, Grosshans D, Szymonifka J, Khan F, et al. A dosimetric comparison of proton and intensity modulated radiation therapy in pediatric rhabdomyosarcoma patients enrolled on a prospective phase II proton study. Radiother Oncol. 2014;113(1):77–83.
26. Oberlin O, Rey A, Lyden E, Bisogno G, Stevens MCG, Meyer WH, et al. Prognostic factors in metastatic rhabdomyosarcomas: results of a pooled analysis from United States and European cooperative groups. J Clin Oncol. 2008;26(14):2384–9.
27. Chen C, Dorado Garcia H, Scheer M, Henssen AG. Current and future treatment strategies for rhabdomyosarcoma. Front Oncol. 2019;9:1458.

# Pediatric Bone Tumors

# 27

Shikha Goyal, Sanal Canute Fernandes,
and Deepam Pushpam

Pediatric bone tumors are relatively rare but can significantly impact a child's health and well-being. Diagnosis and treatment require a multidisciplinary approach involving oncologists, orthopedic surgeons, radiologists, and pathologists. They may be classified according to the tissue of origin or differentiation and according to behavior, as benign or malignant, as detailed in Table 27.1.

Clinical presentation is variable and based on tumor type and location. Pain, swelling, and limited range of motion are common symptoms. Some tumors may present with pathologic fractures. Imaging includes X-rays, MRI, and/or CT scans to visualize tumor size, location, and characteristics. Age and symptoms at presentation along with imaging features (location, appearance) may help distinguish these tumors, but these details are beyond the scope of this chapter. If imaging is not characteristic or a malignancy is suspected based on clinical presentation, diagnosis is established using either a core biopsy or an open biopsy (preferably performed by an oncosurgeon who would also be involved in future surgical management, with biopsy scar in the same plane as that for planned surgery).

Benign tumors may be managed according to growth potential and symptomatology. Those with minimal symptoms or low growth potential may be managed with observation, while those with symptoms or rapid growth/disfigurement may be managed with surgical excision. Only occasionally, when symptomatic tumors are located in sites where surgery is mutilating or there are multiple recurrences after repeated surgical management, radiotherapy may be offered if the tumors is radioresponsive (e.g., giant cell tumor, aneurysmal bone cyst, Langerhans cell histiocytosis).

S. Goyal (✉)
Department of Radiotherapy and Oncology, Postgraduate Institute of Medical Education and Research, Chandigarh, India

S. C. Fernandes · D. Pushpam
Department of Medical Oncology, AIIMS, New Delhi, Delhi, India



R. Madan et al. (eds.), *Evidence Based Practice in Pediatric Radiation Oncology*,
https://doi.org/10.1007/978-981-96-4872-6_27

**Table 27.1** Classification of bone tumors

| Type of tumor | Benign | Malignant |
|---|---|---|
| Bone forming | Osteoid osteoma<br>Osteoblastoma<br>Enostosis | Osteosarcoma<br>Adamantinoma (rare) |
| Fibro-osseous | Non-ossifying fibroma<br>Fibrous dysplasia<br>Osteofibrous dysplasia | Fibrosarcoma<br>Malignant fibrous histiocytoma |
| Cartilage forming | Enchondroma<br>Chondroblastoma<br>Chondromyxoid fibroma<br>Osteochondroma | Chondrosarcoma (rare) |
| Vascular/connective tissue | Haemangioma<br>Lymphangioma<br>Myofibrosis<br>Gorham disease | Haemangiopericytoma |
| Cystic | Simple (unicameral) bone cyst<br>Aneurysmal bone cyst | |
| Small round blue cell tumor | | Ewing sarcoma family of tumors<br>Lymphoma<br>Rhabdomyosarcoma |
| Other | Langerhans cell histiocytosis | |

For malignant tumors, treatment is more aggressive and involves a combination of systemic therapy, surgery (preferably with limb/function preservation), and radiation therapy.

Irrespective of management, long-term follow-up is required to monitor for recurrence or late effects of treatment and continuous rehabilitation to regain function and mobility post-surgery as well as to reduce long-term sequelae of radiotherapy. One important aspect to consider prior to planning therapy, especially for patients undergoing chemotherapy or radiation therapy, is fertility counseling for considering fertility preservation options.

Osteosarcoma, Ewing's sarcoma, and Langerhans cell histiocytosis (LCH) will be discussed in detail in this chapter. Rhabdomyosarcoma has been discussed in another chapter.

## 27.1 Osteosarcoma

### 27.1.1 Epidemiology

Osteosarcoma is the most common primary malignant bone tumor. It is most often seen in patients aged 15–19 years and represents ~55% of all bone tumors under 20 years. The age is typically associated with the adolescent growth spurt and thus presents at a slightly earlier age in females. There is a male preponderance (M:F = 1.4). It is occasionally associated with retinoblastoma (RB1 mutation) or Li-Fraumeni syndrome (TP53 mutation) and a history of treatment with alkylating agents, radiotherapy, or prior history of Paget's disease when presenting in adulthood. Many-a-times, a history of trauma brings it to clinical attention.

### 27.1.2 Clinical Presentation

Most common presentation is a painful swelling in metaphysis of long bones: distal femur, proximal tibia, proximal humerus, or proximal femur. Occasionally flat bones such as mandible or pelvis may be involved. Pain is waxing and waning over several weeks. Some may have a pathological fracture, but not accompanied by constitutional symptoms. The swelling is usually tender and has a soft tissue component with reduced range of motion or gait disturbances. Metastatic disease may be present in 10–20% at diagnosis; skip metastases in same bone are seen in less than 5% but carry a poorer prognosis. Even when lung metastases are present, respiratory symptoms are not common.

### 27.1.3 Imaging

On X-ray, it is seen as a metaphysial lesion with destruction of long bones (often crossing growth plates), poorly defined margins, osteoid production giving rise to a mixture of radiolucent and radiodense areas, new bone formation in periosteal region, Codman triangle, and a soft-tissue mass (with ossification in radial or sunburst pattern). MRI (T1 coronal sequence) may help define the extent of neurovascular bundle, marrow, and soft tissue involvement in addition to any skip lesions, and may aid planning biopsy or resection. CT scan of the chest and bone help detect the most common site of metastases and are used for staging. Role of whole body MRI in detecting distant skeletal lesions is evolving, as is the role of FDG PET-CECT for staging.

### 27.1.4 Lab Parameters

Nearly 50% may have raised lactate dehydrogenase and alkaline phosphatase levels. Other tests are usually non-contributory.

### 27.1.5 Biopsy

It is needed even if characteristic radiologic findings are present.

### 27.1.6 Pathology

According to WHO 2020 classification, histologic subtypes include [1].

- Low-grade central osteosarcoma (1–2%, 20–30% may progress to higher grades; treatment is typically surgery alone).
- Osteosarcoma not otherwise specified (NOS)—conventional (90%), telangiectatic, small cell.
  - Conventional osteosarcomas may be labelled osteoblastic (75–80%), chondroblastic (10–15%), or fibroblastic (10%) based on cellular component, but behavior and management do not differ.
- Parosteal osteosarcoma (uncommon in children).
- Periosteal osteosarcoma.
- High-grade surface osteosarcoma.
- Secondary osteosarcoma (rare in children, bad prognosis).

### 27.1.7 Differential Diagnoses

- Malignant bone tumors: Ewing's, lymphoma, metastases from other tumors.
- Benign bone tumors: giant cell tumor, chondroblastoma, osteoblastoma.
- Non-neoplastic lesions: osteomyelitis, LCH, aneurysmal bone cysts.

### 27.1.8 Staging

The Musculoskeletal Tumor Society (MSTS) staging system classifies tumors based on grade and compartmental involvement. Low-grade tumors are stage I, high-grade tumors are stage II, Intracompartmental location is substaged as A, while extracompartmental extension is substaged as B, for both stage I and II. If regional or distant metastases are present, tumors are labelled as stage III [2].

AJCC 8 assigns different T stage system based on tumor location (appendicular/trunk/craniofacial, pelvic or spine). For appendicular/trunk/craniofacial lesions, T1, T2, and T3 denote lesions ≤8 cm, >8 cm, and skip lesions in same bone, respectively. For spinal lesions, tumors are staged T1–4 based on number of vertebral segments involved and spinal or vascular involvement. For pelvic lesions, tumors are staged T1–4 based on number of pelvic segments involved, size, extraosseous extension, and neural foramen or vascular involvement. Nodal staging is N0 or N1 based on absence or presence of regional nodes. Metastases to lung are staged M1a, while those to bones or other sites are staged M1b. Tumor grade (G1: low grade, well differentiated; G2: high grade, moderately differentiated; G3: high grade, poorly differentiated) is also important for staging. Composite stage is I to IVB. All high-grade tumors are at least stage II. T3 lesions are stage III, lung metastases comprise stage IVA, while either regional nodes or other distant metastases comprise IVB [3].

### 27.1.9 Prognosis

The single most important prognostic marker is the presence of metastases. For patients on neoadjuvant chemotherapy, response to therapy (defined as >90% necrosis on histopathology) is prognostic for better survival (5-year survival 70–80% vs. <60%) except in patients with chondroblastic osteosarcoma [4]. Tumor location is also prognostic as it may impact feasibility and extent of surgical resection—axial and pelvic tumors have worse prognosis than appendicular tumors if incompletely resected.

### 27.1.10 Treatment

Osteosarcoma was traditionally considered a surgical disease; however, the long-term survival with surgery alone was under 20%. Addition of chemotherapy has helped improve 5-year survival to 70% when using three-drug regimes, by reducing the volume of primary disease, enabling limb salvage, and elimination of micrometastases [5]. Macrometastases should also be considered for surgical resection if feasible.

If amenable for upfront surgery with function preservation, resection with wide margins can be performed, followed by adjuvant chemotherapy. Neoadjuvant chemotherapy (NACT) does not give a survival advantage over adjuvant chemotherapy but may help in limb salvage [6]. When used, NACT is given for 10 weeks preoperatively and then continued till 29 weeks in postoperative period. The standard chemotherapy regime consists of methotrexate, adriamycin, and cisplatin combination as per control arm of EURAMOS-1 trial [7]. Studies exploring change to ifosfamide-based regimes have not proven more effective. There are no recommendations to change to alternative chemotherapy regimes for adjuvant therapy in case of poor responders to NACT.

Radiotherapy has been used at doses >60 Gy in good responders to NACT in surgically inaccessible sites with good local control and metastases-free survival [8]. Proton or carbon ion therapy may help further dose escalation in these tumors and improve local control [9]. At present, these is no role of adjuvant radiotherapy in completely resected disease. Radiotherapy may be used for palliation in symptomatic sites such as bone metastases.

### 27.1.11 Follow-Up

Local surveillance of the surgical site can be performed with plain X-rays and if needed, MRI. It is recommended that patients with treated lung metastases be followed up with NCCT chest from years 1–5 and CXR for years 6–10 [10]. Suspicion of non-pulmonary metastases based on symptoms or other imaging findings can be evaluated with FDG PET-CT. Long-term toxicity, especially cardiac effects and second neoplasms, needs to be evaluated periodically lifelong.

## 27.2 Ewing's Sarcoma

### 27.2.1 Epidemiology

Ewing's sarcoma (ES) is an aggressive, malignant bone tumor characterized by EWSR1-FLI gene fusion (t (11;22)). It is the second most common bone tumor in childhood. It is encountered in the second decade with a peak incidence at 15 years, with no gender predilection [11]. Incidence is higher in Europeans compared to Asian and African populations [12]. The most commonly involved bony sites include pelvis, femur, and tibia while the chest wall is the most common soft tissue site [11]. Historically, all small round blue cell sarcomas with characteristic immunophenotypical features were included in the Ewing family of tumors. The 2020 WHO classification places these tumors as one of 4 entities included within "Undifferentiated Small Round Cell Sarcomas of Bone and Soft Tissue," comprising of Ewing's sarcoma with FET-ETS gene fusion, round cell sarcomas having EWSR1–non-ETS fusions, CIC-rearranged sarcomas, and sarcomas with BCOR genetic alterations. The second entity has higher propensity for bony involvement and the remaining two involve soft tissues more often. All three non-ES entities are more aggressive than ES [13].

Multimodality treatment approaches have led to dramatically improved outcomes in localized Ewing's sarcoma in the last three decades, with 5-year survivals reaching 70–80%. However, outcomes for metastatic disease continue to be dismal with <30% of patients with metastatic disease surviving at 5 years.

Despite a multipronged approach, 25% of localized Ewing's sarcoma patients suffer recurrences. The prognosis for relapsed disease is extremely poor, with 5-year survival rates varying between 15 and 20% [11].

The recent decades have seen remarkable advances in the survival of patients with these aggressive tumors, especially in those with localized disease. However, the outcomes for patients with disseminated and relapsed disease continue to be poor. The lack of predictive biomarkers and models to predict recurrence risk and potential chemo-refractoriness have led to a plateauing of outcomes in this subset of patients. Targeted therapies to overcome chemoresistance and better models to predict outcomes represent a large unmet need in Ewing sarcoma.

### 27.2.2 Clinical Presentation

ES arises in long bones (femur, tibia, fibula, humerus) and pelvic bones. Involvement of spine, hands and feet, and skull is less common. Intraspinal soft tissue without bone involvement may also occur. Extraosseous ES may occur in older children and females and more commonly has axial localization. Patients present with progressive pain or swelling for weeks or months. Pain may be aggravated by activity and worse at night. Swelling, if present, may be tender. Rib lesions may extend to involve the pleura. Spinal lesions may present with neural symptoms. Nearly 10–20% have constitutional symptoms. Metastases may be present in ~20% patients at diagnosis (most common in lung); probability is higher in cases of pelvic origin, presence of fever or raised LDH, older age >12 years, and short duration of symptoms.

### 27.2.3 Imaging

Plain X-ray of involved area may show a destructive lesion with ill-defined margins (moth-eaten appearance), with periosteal reaction (onion peel appearance) and associated soft tissue. Location may metaphyseal and/or diaphyseal. Pathologic fracture may be seen in 10–15%. CT delineates the disease extent better, but surgical planning may need MRI for relationship to neurovascular structures. Metastatic workup includes CT chest and bone scan. A stand-alone FDG-PET is sufficient for metastatic evaluation in standard-risk disease as the absence of marrow uptake on PET correlates well with a lack of marrow involvement [14, 15].

### 27.2.4 Lab Parameters

Investigations should include complete blood count, biochemistry including alkaline phosphatase, and LDH.

### 27.2.5 Biopsy

Principles remain the same as other sarcomas. Adequate tissue should be obtained for IHC and molecular profiling. Bone marrow aspirate and biopsy are recommended to rule out marrow involvement although studies are looking at whole body MRI or PET-CT for this goal.

### 27.2.6 Pathology

Pathology and molecular characteristics of ES have been discussed separately in another chapter.

### 27.2.7 Differential Diagnoses

Benign tumors such as eosinophilic granuloma and giant cell tumor of bone also present with lytic lesions. Malignant tumors such as osteosarcoma, primary bone lymphoma, undifferentiated high-grade pleomorphic sarcoma of bone, acute leukemia, and bony metastases from neuroblastoma may mimic ES. All small round blue cell tumors are the differentials on histology.

## 27.2.8 Staging

### 27.2.8.1 Prognosis

As in osteosarcoma, the presence of metastases is the most important adverse prognostic factor. Five-year survival drops from 70% to 33% with diagnosis of metastases. Site of metastatic disease also matters—those with lung metastases perform better than those with bone metastases or both. Patients with age >10 years, small tumors (volume <100 mL or size <8 cm), and extremity lesions fare better, possibly related to resectability with negative margins, as well as better local control with RT alone. Presence of fever, raised LDH, and anemia correlate with tumor bulk and adversely related with outcome. Response to systemic therapy and completeness of resection improve prognosis. Certain molecular alterations such as 1p deletion, p53 mutations, CDKN2A, and p16 deletions are linked to poor chemotherapy response and worse prognosis.

## 27.2.9 Treatment

### 27.2.9.1 Local Therapy

Surgery or radiation therapy or combination of both is essential for local control. Surgery is the preferred therapy unless it is not feasible with clear margins or the morbidity is expected to be considerable. The recommended timing for local therapy is after 12 weeks of induction chemotherapy. Survival may suffer considerably if local therapy is initiated beyond 16 weeks (10-year OS 70% vs. 57%) [16].

#### Surgery

Surgery is the preferred therapy if feasible due to potential avoidance of long-term effects of RT in children and for providing an estimate of prognosis with tumor response. Surgery, especially when feasible with wide margins, in limb lesions is the preferred local therapy option, while the difference in outcomes between surgery +/− radiotherapy and radiotherapy alone is not significant [17]. Dispensable bones (fibula and rib) can easily be tackled with surgery. Limb reconstruction techniques (grafts and metallic prosthesis) have improved the possibility of function preservation in extremity tumors (femur and tibia, distal humerus, and ulna). Although studies have reported better outcomes with surgery in pelvic tumors, resection is often difficult except for small tumors involving iliac wings, ischium, or pubic bones.

#### Radiation Therapy

ES is a radiosensitive tumor. Historical series report a decent local control but poor survival with RT alone, and over 90% tumors are now known to have micrometastases. With concerns of late morbidity of RT and improvement in surgery, the latter has become the preferred therapy although no randomized trials have compared the two modalities and large cooperative group trials have not shown a difference in outcomes in non-limb tumors [18].

Radiotherapy with curative intent is administered in two settings: (a) as adjuvant therapy when tumor volume is large (length >8 cm or volume >200 cc) or when surgical margins are involved or close (e.g., bulky pelvic tumors, hemithoracic irradiation in high risk chest wall tumors with R1/R2 resection, pleural effusion or infiltration preoperatively or contamination at surgery) to reduce the local recurrence rate with a possible (non-significant) survival gain, or (b) as radical therapy in centrally located tumors, sites with high surgical morbidity or unresectability even after induction chemotherapy or for function preservation (e.g., proximal humerus, upper scapula, skull bones, vertebral lesions, large pelvic tumors, acetabular lesions) [19].

Adjuvant hemithoracic RT improves event free survival with reduction in lung metastases in high-risk chest wall tumors [20].

When used in unresectable tumors, dose escalated RT may also improve local control with good functional outcomes [21].

In selected patients with metastatic disease (limited pulmonary metastases and good response to chemotherapy), local therapy may improve symptoms and delay progression or relapse. Small tumors may be considered for resection, while others may be considered for local RT [22]. Low-dose whole lung radiotherapy (15–20 Gy) improves event free survival even after complete response to systemic therapy or resection [23]. Even in patients with limited skeletal metastatic disease, RT to metastatic sites is recommended (45–50 Gy) [24, 25].

## Radiotherapy Planning

The preferred minimal technique is 3D conformal radiotherapy with CT-based planning. During the simulation process, limb position is decided based on planned beam orientation to avoid entry/exit through the other limb for extremity tumors. Biopsy/surgical scar sites are marked with radio-opaque markers. All baseline imaging including MRI is used for target delineation.

### Target Volume

Involved field radiation yields similar local control to whole bone radiation and is preferred [26]. Although external beam radiotherapy is most commonly used, selected patients with soft tissue disease may be suitable for brachytherapy either as adjuvant therapy or boost.

### Limb Tumors

For external beam radiotherapy, pre-chemotherapy gross tumor volume (bone and soft tissue) is expanded by 1 cm to yield a phase 1 clinical target volume (CTV1). When there is no anatomic compartmental violation, the CTV may be limited to the involved compartment. This volume is expanded for setup errors (0.5–1 cm) to yield the planning target volume (PTV1) that is prescribed a dose of 45 Gy in 25 fractions over 5 weeks (phase 1). CTV2 (phase 2) consists of post-chemotherapy soft tissue and initial bony extent with a margin of 1 cm. This volume, expanded with appropriate margin to PTV2, receives a further dose of 10.8 Gy in 6 fractions. For adjuvant therapy, PTV1 remains same, while those with microscopic positive disease receive

5.4 Gy/3 fractions and those with gross residual disease receive 10.8 Gy in 6 fractions in phase 2. Care is taken to avoid uninvolved epiphyseal growth plates in children and uninvolved joint spaces. Beam orientation is adjusted (with image guidance for daily setup error reduction as needed) to avoid circumferential irradiation of limbs and to avoid contralateral limb. Gonads are shielded using external shields when appropriate.

Pelvic Tumors
Even in phase 1, clinical target volume can be reduced to avoid uninvolved bowel/rectum/bladder/joint spaces. Bladder/rectal protocols should be followed in children capable of following instructions. Significant irradiation of bowel and bladder volume should be avoided to reduce risk of adhesions and hemorrhagic cystitis after ifosfamide. Ovaries/testes should be shielded wherever feasible.

Chest Wall Tumors
Ipsilateral hemithorax is given a dose of 15–20 Gy followed by remaining dose to involved site (total 45 Gy to involved site in adjuvant therapy for R0 resection, 50–55.8 Gy in R1/R2 resection based on same principles as limb tumors). Appropriate motion management techniques (breath hold, 4DCT, gating) should be used as available and feasible depending on the child's age.

While 3D conformal radiotherapy is preferred over open field treatments, further reduction in late morbidity may be achieved with utilization of IMRT, VMAT, or proton therapy as available. These techniques may also aid dose escalation in unresectable deep-seated tumors. Proton beam may potentially reduce the risk of second neoplasms by reducing integral radiotherapy doses [27, 28].

Figure 27.1 demonstrates the radiotherapy volumes and plans for various Ewing's tumors in definitive setting.

#### Radiation Fractionation
While conventional fractionation (1.8–2 Gy per fraction, 5 fractions per week) is standard, other schemes have been explored. Accelerated fractionation has not improved outcomes while hyperfractionation (55 Gy, 1.2 Gy twice daily) reduces long-term morbidity [29].

### 27.2.9.2 Systemic Therapy

#### Localized Disease
The present-day standard of care in localized Ewing's sarcoma involves a multipronged approach that involves chemotherapy, surgery, and radiotherapy.

The introduction of systemic therapy in the management of Ewing's sarcoma in the 1970s revolutionized outcomes that previously were abysmal with the use of surgery and radiotherapy.

The earliest trials established vincristine, cyclophosphamide, and actinomycin D as effective agents in the treatment of Ewing sarcoma. These were followed by several cooperative group trials that led to the establishment of the current regimens.

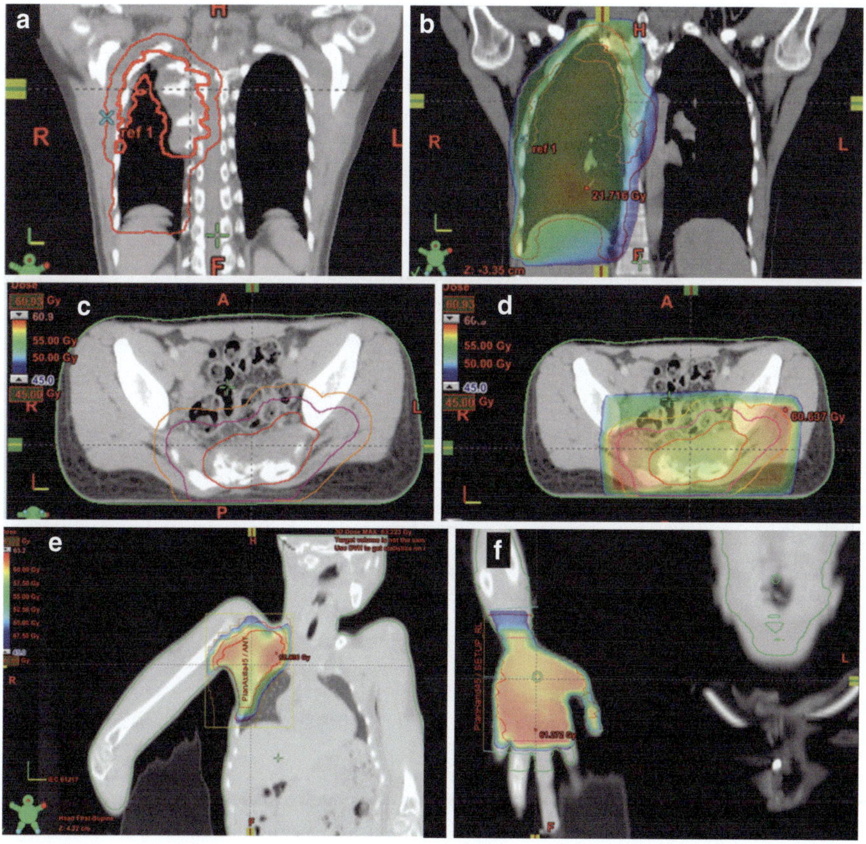


**Fig. 27.1** (**a**) Radiotherapy planning CT scan of a 14-year-old girl with high risk chest wall Ewing's sarcoma with lung invasion and extensive vertebral involvement after 4 cycles of VAC/IE chemotherapy with residual disease. Gross tumor volume (GTV) is marked in bright red, while planning target volume (PTV) for phase 1 is marked in light red encompassing the tumor as well as entire ipsilateral hemithorax. (**b**) Phase 1 plan for the patient where a dose of 19.8 gray (Gy) was planned at 1.8 Gy per fraction. Phase 2 plan (not shown) encompassed the GTV with appropriate margin and delivered a dose of 36 Gy in 20 fractions. (**c**) Radiotherapy planning CT scan of a 12-year-old boy with a large sacral Ewing's sarcoma with upfront surgical decompression, and post 4 cycles chemotherapy. Disease was deemed unresectable. GTV is marked in red and PTV in orange. (**d**) A dose of 55.8 Gy in 31 fractions was delivered to PTV. (**e**) Radiotherapy planning CT scan of a 13-year-old boy with Ewing's sarcoma of hand with axillary lymph node metastases. Disease was deemed inoperable since the hand would be rendered non-functional. After four-cycle chemotherapy, RT was planned for right axilla, and (**f**) right hand to a dose of 55.8 Gy in 31 fractions

IESS -1, the first cooperative trial in Ewing sarcoma, established VACA (Vincristine, Actinomycin D, Cyclophosphamide, Doxorubicin) as the regimen of choice [1]. The subsequent IESS-2 trial showed that an intermittent, high-dose, three-weekly administration of VACA is superior to a low-dose, continuous administration. The addition of adjuvant/neoadjuvant chemotherapy improved 5-year outcomes from less than 10% in the pre-chemotherapy era to about 50% with the VACA regimen [30].

The next set of cooperative trials aimed at improving these survival rates further by the addition of newer agents and by increasing the dose density of the effective agents. The INT-0091 trial compared the VAC (Vincristine, Adriamycin, Cyclophosphamide) regimen with a new regimen comprising of VAC alternating with ifosfamide-etoposide (IE). The study demonstrated a survival benefit with the alternating regimen in localized Ewing sarcoma and made VAC/IE the regimen of choice in this setting. The trial also capped the dose of doxorubicin at 375 mg /m2, following which it was replaced by dactinomycin [31].

Two landmark trials looked at the change in outcomes associated with dose intensification and interval compression. The INT-0154 trial intensified doses of the alkylator agents and compared a 30-week dose intense regimen with the conventional 42-week regimen. The cumulative alkylator exposure, however, in both arms remained the same. No benefit was seen with the intensification of doses, and the said trial failed to meet its endpoint [32]. The subsequent AEWS0031 trial reduced intervals between successive chemotherapy cycles from 3 weeks to 2 weeks (interval compressed). This strategy improved 6-year EFS rates from 65% to 73% and established the dose-dense/interval compressed VAC/IE regimen as the standard of care in localized Ewing's sarcoma [33].

### Metastatic Disease

The regimen of choice in metastatic Ewing's sarcomas is VAC, with the capping of doxorubicin at 375 mg/m$^2$ (Table 27.2).

**Table 27.2** Major trials in systemic therapy in Ewing sarcoma

| | Trial | Comparator arms | Outcomes | Major takeaways |
|---|---|---|---|---|
| 1 | IESS-2 | Continuous low dose VACA vs. intermittent high dose VACA | Five-year EFS better with intermittent chemotherapy (73% vs. 56%) | Intermittent, high-dose chemotherapy is better than continuous chemotherapy |
| 2 | INT-0091 | VAC VS. VAC/IE | Five-year EFS for localized Ewing—69% vs. 54% | Combination regimen is superior in localized disease; no benefit of combination in disseminated disease |
| 3 | INT-0154 | Dose intensification (30-week vs. 42-week regimen) | No difference in outcomes in the 2 arms | No survival benefit of dose intensification |
| 4 | AEWS0031 | Interval compression (2 weekly vs. 3 weekly) | 6 year EFS better in 2 weekly arm (73% vs. 65%) | Interval compression improves outcomes in localized disease |

*EFS* event free survival, *VAC* Vincristine, Adriamycin, Cyclophosphamide, *VACA* Vincristine, Actinomycin D, Cyclophosphamide, Adriamycin, *IE* Ifosfamide, Etoposide

#### Treatment of Ewing-Like Sarcomas

Given the recent identification and description of Ewing-like sarcomas, the optimal treatment modality and long-term outcomes associated with these tumors are not well established, and data on these tumors mostly comes from a few case series. BCOR rearranged sarcomas respond well to doxorubicin-based Ewing sarcoma treatment protocols and have outcomes comparable to classical Ewing sarcomas [34]. On the other hand, CIC fused sarcomas are believed to be relatively chemoresistant and are associated with poorer outcomes. Given their chemoresistance, upfront resection followed by adjuvant radiotherapy has been advocated as a better treatment option than upfront neoadjuvant chemotherapy, which might delay resections and hence, worsen outcomes [35]. Data with respect to NFAT2c fusion sarcomas is very limited, and their outcomes as compared to Ewing sarcomas are not currently clear [36].

### 27.2.9.3 Relapsed/Refractory Ewing Sarcoma

Despite the integration of multimodality treatment in Ewing sarcoma, up to 25% of patients with localized disease eventually relapse. This figure is as high as 75% for patients with metastatic disease at presentation. Up to two-thirds of relapses are distant, with the lungs being the most common sites of involvement followed by the skeletal system [37].

Disease relapses can be classified as early (< 2 years) or late (> 2 years) based on the time of relapse since the initial diagnosis. About 70% of all relapses are early relapses. The median time to relapse has been reported to be approximately 1.4 years for patients with localized disease and around 1 year for patients with metastatic disease. Median survival associated with relapsed disease is often dismal and is around 15% at 5 years [38].

#### Chemotherapy

Multiple cytotoxic regimens have been tried in the relapsed setting with varying degrees of success. The most commonly used regimens are high-dose ifosfamide, gemcitabine-docetaxel, temozolomide-irinotecan, and cyclophosphamide-topotecan. The response rates with these regimens vary between 29 and 47% [38]. Head-to-head comparison of the various regimens is scarce. The rEECur trial was the first trial that sought to answer this question, and included patients with relapsed Ewing sarcoma that were randomized to one of these four regimens. The design of the study included sequential elimination of the regimens that produce the lowest objective response rate, which is the primary endpoint of the Phase II portion of the study. Once two regimens have emerged, they will be compared in the Phase III portion of the study, which uses PFS as the primary endpoint. At the end of the first and second analyses, gemcitabine-docetaxel and temozolomide-irinotecan were excluded, respectively, based on the least response rates of 11.5% and 20% [39, 40]. The final analysis of the trial showed an EFS and OS benefit with Ifosfamide as compared to the temozolomide-irinotecan arm [41]. However, these results need to be interpreted with caution as the toxicity and discontinuation rates with ifosfamide were higher as compared to the other arms (25% vs. 0). The other criticisms of the trial include the lower response rates seen with the temozolomide-irinotecan arm as compared to those previously reported, and the higher median PFS and OS reported with temozolomide-irinotecan as compared to the topotecan-cyclophosphamide arm. To conclude, the best regimen in the relapsed setting, is yet unknown, and in the absence of definitive evidence, the choice of treatment should be individualized based on the performance status of the patient and the expected toxicities of each regimen. The rEECur trial is currently recruiting patients for two arms that were subsequently added to the trial—one arm with ifosfamide plus carboplatin and etoposide and the other with ifosfamide plus lenvatinib. The results of these two arms are awaited (Table 27.3).

## Role of Targeted Agents

Given the plateau in outcomes with cytotoxic agents in relapsed/refractory Ewing sarcoma, multiple targeted agents have been tried in these patients to improve outcomes. Foremost among these include the IGF-1R inhibitors, given the overexpression of IGF-1 in these tumors. However, suppression of the IGF-1 axis has not been seen to dramatically improve outcomes, as was anticipated earlier. Most trials have reported an ORR of around 10% with the addition of ganitumab, and IGF-1 inhibitor antibody [42]. The largest trial to target IGF-1, AEWS1221 has used the IGF-1 antibody ganitumab in metastatic disease with a back bone of VAC/IE. The results of this trial area waited [43].

The other pathways that have been targeted in Ewing sarcomas include the MET and VEGF pathways. The phase 2 trial CABONE evaluated cabozantinib in patients with relapsed disease and reported an ORR of 33% [44]. The multikinase inhibitors pazopanib and regorafenib too have been tried in relapsed Ewing sarcoma; however, the results have been modest at best with ORRs of about 10% [45]. Hence, cabozantinib is the only multikinase inhibitor that has proven to be of clinical benefit in relapsed and refractory Ewing sarcoma and can be used in the above setting.

## Role of Immunotherapy

Ewing sarcomas respond poorly to check point inhibition. No responses were noted in the SARC028 trial (pembrolizumab in advanced sarcomas) which included ten patients with Ewing sarcomas [46]. Similarly, responses to other CPIs like Nivolumab and Ipilimumab have been poor [47]. The possible explanation for these

**Table 27.3** rEECur trial: arms and outcomes

| | Median PFS (months) | Salient toxicity |
|---|---|---|
| Gemcitabine-docetaxel | 3 | – |
| Temozolomide-irinotecan | 4.7 | – |
| Topotecan-cyclophosphamide | 3.7 | – |
| Ifosfamide | 5.7 | Nephrotoxicity (8%), treatment discontinuation (25%) |

*PFS* progression-free survival

poor responses could be the low mutational burden and low level of infiltrating T-cells displayed by these tumors. Hence, check point inhibitors are not recommended for use in relapsed/refractory Ewing sarcomas.

#### 27.2.9.4 Role of HSCT in Ewing Sarcoma

The use of high-dose chemotherapy (HDCT) followed by stem cell rescue is based on the observation that outcome in chemosensitive malignancies is dependent on the dosage of chemotherapy used. The dose-response is often steep, and an increase in the drug dose administered can lead to a logarithmic increase in tumor cell killing. Using the same rationale, dose escalation with stem cell rescue has been utilized in Ewing sarcoma in both the upfront and relapsed settings.

##### Upfront Metastatic Setting

The data for HDCT in the upfront disseminated setting comes from two large prospective studies, i.e., the EURO EWING 99 study, and the EWING 2008 trials. In the EURO EWING 99 trial, patients with pleural/pulmonary deposits were randomized to six cycles of VIDE followed by one cycle of VAI and autologous stem cell transplantation (ASCT) with busulphan-melphalan (BuMel) or seven cycles of VAI followed by whole lung irradiation [48]. The EWING 2008 trial randomized patients with metastatic Ewing sarcoma (bone/lung) to six cycles of VIDE and eight cycles of VDC followed by ASCT with treosulphan-melphalan (TreoMel) or observation. Both trials showed no added benefit of ASCT in survival outcomes. A subset of patients aged less than 14 years were seen to benefit from ASCT in the EWING 2008 trial (3 year EFS 40% vs. 9%); however, the reason for this survival benefit in this subset could not be ascertained [49].

Hence, in the upfront setting, ASCT confers no additional benefit in metastatic Ewing sarcoma.

##### Relapsed Setting

In the relapsed setting, no prospective trials have studied the utility of high-dose chemotherapy with stem cell rescue. A large retrospective series on ASCT in the relapsed setting showed markedly improved outcomes with ASCT as compared to only conventional chemotherapy (median post-relapse survival (PRS) of 76 months with ASCT as compared to 10.5 months with no ASCT). The study stratified patients into risk groups based on clinical criteria, and patients with intermediate risk were seen to benefit the most from ASCT. The conditioning regimens used in the study were BuMel (60%) and TreoMel (23%), with better outcomes reported with the BuMel regimen [50]. Hence, patients who respond well to second-line chemotherapy may be offered the option of consolidation with ASCT to prevent relapses based on the improvement in survival reported from several case series [51] (Table 27.4).

**Table 27.4** Data on HSCT in Ewing sarcoma in the upfront setting

| Trial | Population | Arms | Conditioning | Outcome |
|---|---|---|---|---|
| EUROEWING 99 | Upfront metastatic | 6 VIDE+ 1<br>VAI + ASCT V/S 7<br>VAI + WLI | Bu-Mel | 3 year EFS 50.6% vs. 56.6%; no difference between 2 groups |
| EWING 2008 | Upfront metastatic | 6 VIDE +8<br>VDC +/– ASCT | Treo-Mel | 3 year EFS 20.9% vs. 19.2%; no benefit of ASCT |

*VIDE* Vincristine, Ifosfamide, Doxorubicin, Etoposide, *VAI* Vincristine, Adriamycin, Ifosfamide, *ASCT* Autologous Stem Cell Transplant, *WLI* whole lung irradiation, *Bu* Busulphan, *Mel* Melphalan, *Treo* Treosulphan, *EFS* event free survival

### 27.2.10 Follow-Up

Follow-up should be carried out every 3 months for first 2 years, then every 6 months for the next 3 years and annually after that. Each visit includes physical examination, CBC, CXR, and appropriate imaging for primary and distant metastases (PET-CECT, MRI, Bone scan, as appropriate).

## 27.3 Langerhans Cell Histiocytosis

Langerhans cell histiocytosis (LCH) is a rare condition and involves proliferation of Langerhans cell histiocytes and their precursors. It is not clear if it is an immune disorder or a neoplastic condition [52].

### 27.3.1 Epidemiology

The condition may involve a single or multiple bones, and rarely, extraskeletal sites such as lungs, bone marrow, liver, spleen, or central nervous system (including pituitary), and more commonly found in young children than older ages. There is a male preponderance, and it is more common in Whites than in Blacks. Except for association of pulmonary LCH with smoking in adults, there is no known environmental association. Familial clustering, association with other conditions such as Rosai-Dorfman disease or other histiocytic disorders, and SMAD6 gene single nucleotide polymorphism have been described.

### 27.3.2 Clinical Presentation

Symptoms are variable depending on location and number of disease sites. Single-system LCH (55% of children) is usually not associated with constitutional symptoms and can be unifocal or multifocal. Most common site is bone, though skin, lungs, pituitary and other CNS sites, and lymph nodes may be involved. Multisystem LCH involves two or more organs and may be low risk (involving bone, skin, nodes, pituitary, thymus, gastrointestinal tract) or high risk (involving lung, CNS, bone marrow, spleen, liver).

Bony lesions present with pain—most common sites are skull, femur, rib, and vertebrae in children. Skull lesions may manifest as jaw pain, loose dentition. Local swelling, seizures, recurrent middle ear infections, gum bleeds, or orbital swelling. Some lesions may be associated with central diabetes insipidus.

### 27.3.3 Imaging

Bony lesions may appear as large lytic lesions (eosinophilic granuloma) with variable surrounding sclerosis on X-ray or CT. CNS lesions with pituitary involvement may be seen as enhancing lesions on T1 contrast with T2 hyperintensity. Skeletal survey of all bones and X-ray chest or whole body PET-CECT is now being used to rule out involvement of multiple systems or multifocal disease. Bone scan is preferred in young infants to reduce amount of radiation exposure.

### 27.3.4 Lab Parameters

These are mostly normal. Depending on presence and degree of bone marrow involvement, cytopenias may be seen. If multiorgan or pituitary involvement is present, biochemical abnormalities including endocrinopathies may be noted.

### 27.3.5 Biopsy

Core biopsy is used to establish diagnosis once radiologic suspicion is raised. ICH may show CD1, CD207 (langerin), and S100 expression. Bone marrow biopsy may show anti-CD1a even if Langerhans cell are not apparent on histology. Molecular testing for *BRAF* V600E (present in 50%) can also aid diagnosis.

### 27.3.6 Differential Diagnoses

Differentials in pediatric age group may consist of Ewing's sarcoma (on imaging), other histiocytic disorders such as juvenile xanthogranuloma, hemophagocytic lymphohistiocytosis, and Rosai-Dorfman disease.

### 27.3.7 Treatment

Treatment is guided by age and extent of involvement. In children with single bony involvement, amenable to biopsy/curettage, the diagnostic modality may also be therapeutic. When there is involvement of multiple bones or CNS-risk skull bones or individual lesions are >5 cm or localized to weight bearing bones such as femur or vertebra, systemic therapy with vinblastine-prednisolone (~1 year) is used [53]. Although LCH is responsive to low dose radiotherapy (6–12 Gy in conventional fractionation), it is used only in adults or in sites where risk of fracture or neurologic deficit is high or when the disease is refractory to systemic therapy.

### 27.3.8 Follow-Up

Imaging with PET-CECT may be used periodically, although frequency and duration is not optimally defined. Late effects such as obesity, hormonal imbalance need to be watched and corrected.

## References


1. Flanagan AM, Blay JY, Bovée JVMG, Bredella A, Cool P, Nielsen GP, Yoshida A. 2020 Bone tumours: introduction. In: Lokuhetty D, White V, Cree I, editors. WHO classification of tumours, soft tissue and bone tumors. 5th ed. International Agency for Research on Cancer (IARC): Lyon Cedex; 2020. p. 340–4.
2. Wolf RE, Enneking WF. The staging and surgery of musculoskeletal neoplasms. Orthop Clin North Am. 1996;27(3):473–81.
3. Kneisl JS, Rosenberg AE, Anderson PM, et al. Bone. In: Amin MB, editor. AJCC Cancer Staging Manual. 8th ed. Chicago: AJCC; 2017. p. 471.
4. Bacci G, Bertoni F, Longhi A, Ferrari S, Forni C, Biagini R, Bacchini P, Donati D, Manfrini M, Bernini G, Lari S. Neoadjuvant chemotherapy for high-grade central osteosarcoma of the extremity. Histologic response to preoperative chemotherapy correlates with histologic subtype of the tumor. Cancer. 2003;97(12):3068–75.
5. Anninga JK, Gelderblom H, Fiocco M, Kroep JR, Taminiau AH, Hogendoorn PC, Egeler RM. Chemotherapeutic adjuvant treatment for osteosarcoma: where do we stand? Eur J Cancer. 2011;47(16):2431–45.
6. Goorin AM, Schwartzentruber DJ, Devidas M, Gebhardt MC, Ayala AG, Harris MB, Helman LJ, Grier HE, Link MP, Pediatric Oncology Group. Presurgical chemotherapy compared with immediate surgery and adjuvant chemotherapy for nonmetastatic osteosarcoma: pediatric oncology group study POG-8651. J Clin Oncol. 2003;21(8):1574–80.
7. Suárez-Mattos A, Arroyave F, Infante AM, Narváez C, Soto C, Gómez L, Amaya-Nieto J. Response to neoadjuvant chemotherapy and survival of children and adolescents with high-grade osteosarcoma treated based on the EURAMOS-1 protocol. Bol Med Hosp Infant Mex. 2022;79(1):17–25.
8. Machak GN, Tkachev SI, Solovyev YN, Sinyukov PA, Ivanov SM, Kochergina NV, Ryjkov AD, Tepliakov VV, Bokhian BY, Glebovskaya VV. Neoadjuvant chemotherapy and local radiotherapy for high-grade osteosarcoma of the extremities. Mayo Clin Proc. 2003;78(2):147–55.

9. Matsunobu A, Imai R, Kamada T, Imaizumi T, Tsuji H, Tsujii H, Shioyama Y, Honda H, Tatezaki S, Working Group for Bone and Soft Tissue Sarcomas. Impact of carbon ion radiotherapy for unresectable osteosarcoma of the trunk. Cancer. 2012;118(18):4555–63.
10. Cederberg KB, Iyer RS, Chaturvedi A, McCarville MB, McDaniel JD, Sandberg JK, Shammas A, Sharp SE, Nadel HR. Imaging of pediatric bone tumors: a COG Diagnostic Imaging Committee/SPR Oncology Committee White paper. Pediatr Blood Cancer. 2023;70(Suppl 4):e30000.
11. Gaspar N, Hawkins DS, Dirksen U, Lewis IJ, Ferrari S, Le Deley MC, et al. Ewing sarcoma: current management and future approaches through collaboration. J Clin Oncol. 2015;33(27):3036–46.
12. Jawad MU, Cheung MC, Min ES, Schneiderbauer MM, Koniaris LG, Scully SP. Ewing sarcoma demonstrates racial disparities in incidence-related and sex-related differences in outcome: an analysis of 1631 cases from the SEER database, 1973–2005. Cancer. 2009;115(15):3526–36.
13. Choi JH, Ro JY. The 2020 WHO Classification of tumors of soft tissue: selected changes and new entities. Adv Anat Pathol. 2021;28(1):44–58.
14. Kopp LM, Hu C, Rozo B, White-Collins A, Huh WW, Yarborough A, et al. Utility of bone marrow aspiration and biopsy in initial staging of Ewing sarcoma. Pediatr Blood Cancer. 2015;62(1):12–5.
15. Newman EN, Jones RL, Hawkins DS. An evaluation of [F-18]-fluoro deoxy-D-glucose positron emission tomography, bone scan, and bone marrow aspiration/biopsy as staging investigations in Ewing sarcoma. Pediatr Blood Cancer. 2013;60(7):1113–7.
16. Lin TA, Ludmir EB, Liao KP, McAleer MF, Grosshans DR, McGovern SL, Bishop AJ, Woodhouse KD, Paulino AC, Yeboa DN. Timing of local therapy affects survival in Ewing sarcoma. Int J Radiat Oncol Biol Phys. 2019;104(1):127–36.
17. Bacci G, Longhi A, Briccoli A, Bertoni F, Versari M, Picci P. The role of surgical margins in treatment of Ewing's sarcoma family tumors: experience of a single institution with 512 patients treated with adjuvant and neoadjuvant chemotherapy. Int J Radiat Oncol Biol Phys. 2006;65(3):766–72.
18. DuBois SG, Krailo MD, Gebhardt MC, Donaldson SS, Marcus KJ, Dormans J, Shamberger RC, Sailer S, Nicholas RW, Healey JH, Tarbell NJ, Randall RL, Devidas M, Meyer JS, Granowetter L, Womer RB, Bernstein M, Marina N, Grier HE. Comparative evaluation of local control strategies in localized Ewing sarcoma of bone: a report from the Children's Oncology Group. Cancer. 2015;121(3):467–75.
19. Foulon S, Brennan B, Gaspar N, Dirksen U, Jeys L, Cassoni A, Claude L, Seddon B, Marec-Berard P, Whelan J, Paulussen M, Streitbuerger A, Oberlin O, Juergens H, Grimer R, Le Deley MC. Can postoperative radiotherapy be omitted in localised standard-risk Ewing sarcoma? An observational study of the Euro-E.W.I.N.G group. Eur J Cancer. 2016;61:128–36.
20. Schuck A, Ahrens S, Konarzewska A, Paulussen M, Fröhlich B, Könemann S, Rübe C, Rübe CE, Dunst J, Willich N, Jürgens H. Hemithorax irradiation for Ewing tumors of the chest wall. Int J Radiat Oncol Biol Phys. 2002;54(3):830–8.
21. Laskar S, Sinha S, Chatterjee A, Khanna N, Manjali JJ, Puri A, Gulia A, Nayak P, Vora T, Chinnaswamy G, Prasad M, Bajpai J, Juvekar S, Desai S, Janu A, Rangarajan V, Purandare N, Shah S, Rekhi B, Jambhekar N, Muckaden MA, Kurkure P. Radiation therapy dose escalation in unresectable Ewing sarcoma: final results of a phase 3 randomized controlled trial. Int J Radiat Oncol Biol Phys. 2022;113(5):996–1002.
22. Sandoval C, Meyer WH, Parham DM, Kun LE, Hustu HO, Luo X, Pratt CB. Outcome in 43 children presenting with metastatic Ewing sarcoma: the St. Jude Children's Research Hospital experience, 1962 to 1992. Med Pediatr Oncol. 1996;26(3):180–5.
23. Paulussen M, Ahrens S, Craft AW, Dunst J, Fröhlich B, Jabar S, Rübe C, Winkelmann W, Wissing S, Zoubek A, Jürgens H. Ewing's tumors with primary lung metastases: survival analysis of 114 (European intergroup) cooperative Ewing's sarcoma studies patients. J Clin Oncol. 1998;16(9):3044–52.

24. Liu AK, Stinauer M, Albano E, Greffe B, Tello T, Maloney K. Local control of metastatic sites with radiation therapy in metastatic Ewing sarcoma and rhabdomyosarcoma. Pediatr Blood Cancer. 2011;57(1):169–71.
25. Khanna N, Pandey A, Bajpai J. Metastatic Ewing's sarcoma: revisiting the "evidence on the fence". Indian J Med Paediatr Oncol. 2017;38(2):173–81.
26. Donaldson SS, Torrey M, Link MP, Glicksman A, Gilula L, Laurie F, Manning J, Neff J, Reinus W, Thompson E, Shuster JJ. A multidisciplinary study investigating radiotherapy in Ewing's sarcoma: end results of POG #8346. Pediatric Oncology Group. Int J Radiat Oncol Biol Phys. 1998;42(1):125–35.
27. Isacsson U, Hagberg H, Johansson KA, Montelius A, Jung B, Glimelius B. Potential advantages of protons over conventional radiation beams for para spinal tumours. Radiother Oncol. 1997;45(1):63–70.
28. Miralbell R, Lomax A, Cella L, Schneider U. Potential reduction of the incidence of radiation-induced second cancers by using proton beams in the treatment of pediatric tumors. Int J Radiat Oncol Biol Phys. 2002;54(3):824–9.
29. Indelicato DJ, Keole SR, Shahlaee AH, Shi W, Morris CG, Marcus RB Jr. Definitive radiotherapy for Ewing tumors of extremities and pelvis: long-term disease control, limb function, and treatment toxicity. Int J Radiat Oncol Biol Phys. 2008;72(3):871–7.
30. Burgert EO, Nesbit ME, Garnsey LA, Gehan EA, Herrmann J, Vietti TJ, et al. Multimodal therapy for the management of nonpelvic, localized Ewing's sarcoma of bone: intergroup study IESS-II. J Clin Oncol. 1990;8(9):1514–24.
31. Grier HE, Krailo MD, Tarbell NJ, Link MP, Fryer CJ, Pritchard DJ, Gebhardt MC, Dickman PS, Perlman EJ, Meyers PA, Donaldson SS, Moore S, Rausen AR, Vietti TJ, Miser JS. Addition of ifosfamide and etoposide to standard chemotherapy for Ewing's sarcoma and primitive neuroectodermal tumor of bone. N Engl J Med. 2003;348(8):694–701.
32. Granowetter L, Womer R, Devidas M, Krailo M, Wang C, Bernstein M, et al. Dose-intensified compared with standard chemotherapy for non metastatic Ewing sarcoma family of tumors: a Children's Oncology Group Study. J Clin Oncol. 2009;27(15):2536–41.
33. Womer RB, West DC, Krailo MD, Dickman PS, Pawel BR, Grier HE, Marcus K, Sailer S, Healey JH, Dormans JP, Weiss AR. Randomized controlled trial of interval-compressed chemotherapy for the treatment of localized Ewing sarcoma: a report from the Children's Oncology Group. J Clin Oncol. 2012;30(33):4148–54.
34. Kyriazoglou A, Bagos P. Meta-analysis of BCOR rearranged sarcomas: challenging the therapeutic approach. Acta Oncol. 2021;60(6):721–6.
35. Connolly EA, Bhadri VA, Wake J, Ingley KM, Lewin J, Bae S, et al. Systemic treatments and outcomes in CIC-rearranged sarcoma: a national multi-centre clinicopathological series and literature review. Cancer Med. 2022;11(8):1805–16.
36. Szuhai K, IJszenga M, de Jong D, Karseladze A, Tanke HJ, Hogendoorn PCW. The NFATc2 gene is involved in a novel cloned translocation in a Ewing sarcoma variant that couples its function in immunology to oncology. Clin Cancer Res. 2009;15(7):2259–68.
37. Grünewald TGP, Cidre-Aranaz F, Surdez D, Tomazou EM, de Álava E, Kovar H, et al. Ewing sarcoma. Nat Rev Dis Primers. 2018;4(1):1–22.
38. Van Mater D, Wagner L. Management of recurrent Ewing sarcoma: challenges and approaches. Onco Targets Ther. 2019;12:2279–88.
39. McCabe MG, Moroz V, Khan M, Dirksen U, Evans A, Fenwick N, et al. Results of the first interim assessment of rEECur, an international randomized controlled trial of chemotherapy for the treatment of recurrent and primary refractory Ewing sarcoma. J Clin Oncol. 2019;37(15_suppl):11007.
40. McCabe MG, Kirton L, Khan M, Fenwick N, Dirksen U, Gaspar N, et al. Results of the second interim assessment of rEECur, an International randomized controlled trial of chemotherapy for the treatment of recurrent and primary refractory Ewing sarcoma (RR-ES). J Clin Oncol. 2020;38(suppl 15):11502. https://doi.org/10.1200/JCO.2020.38.15_suppl.11502.
41. McCabe M, Kirton L, Khan M, et al. Phase III assessment of topotecan and cyclophosphamide and high-dose ifosfamide in rEECur: An international randomized controlled trial of chemo-

therapy for the treatment of recurrent and primary refractory Ewing sarcoma (RR-ES). J Clin Oncol. 2022;40(17_suppl):LBA2.
42. Tap WD, Demetri G, Barnette P, Desai J, Kavan P, Tozer R, et al. Phase II study of ganitumab, a fully human anti-type-1 insulin-like growth factor receptor antibody, in patients with metastatic Ewing family tumors or desmoplastic small round cell tumors. J Clin Oncol. 2012;30(15):1849–56.
43. National Cancer Institute (NCI). Randomized phase 3 trial evaluating the addition of the IGF-1R monoclonal antibody Ganitumab (AMG 479, NSC# 750008) to multiagent chemotherapy for patients with newly diagnosed metastatic Ewing sarcoma [internet]. clinicaltrials.gov; 2022. Report No.: NCT02306161. https://clinicaltrials.gov/ct2/show/NCT02306161. Accessed 13 Sep 2022.
44. Italiano A, Mir O, Mathoulin-Pelissier S, Penel N, Piperno-Neumann S, Bompas E, Chevreau C, Duffaud F, Entz-Werlé N, Saada E, Ray-Coquard I, Lervat C, Gaspar N, Marec-Berard P, Pacquement H, Wright J, Toulmonde M, Bessede A, Crombe A, Kind M, Bellera C, Blay JY. Cabozantinib in patients with advanced Ewing sarcoma or osteosarcoma (CABONE): a multicentre, single-arm, phase 2 trial. Lancet Oncol. 2020;21(3):446–55.
45. Attia S, Bolejack V, Ganjoo KN, George S, Agulnik M, Rushing DA, et al. A phase II trial of regorafenib (REGO) in patients (pts) with advanced Ewing sarcoma and related tumors (EWS) of soft tissue and bone: SARC024 trial results. J Clin Oncol. 2017;35(15_suppl):11005.
46. Tawbi HA, Burgess M, Bolejack V, Van Tine BA, Schuetze SM, Hu J, D'Angelo S, Attia S, Riedel RF, Priebat DA, Movva S, Davis LE, Okuno SH, Reed DR, Crowley J, Butterfield LH, Salazar R, Rodriguez-Canales J, Lazar AJ, Wistuba II, Baker LH, Maki RG, Reinke D, Patel S. Pembrolizumab in advanced soft-tissue sarcoma and bone sarcoma (SARC028): a multicentre, two-cohort, single-arm, open-label, phase 2 trial. Lancet Oncol. 2017;18(11):1493–501.
47. D'Angelo SP, Mahoney MR, Van Tine BA, Atkins J, Milhem MM, Jahagirdar BN, et al. A non-comparative multi-center randomized phase II study of nivolumab +/− ipilimumab for patients with metastatic sarcoma (Alliance A091401). Lancet Oncol. 2018;19(3):416–26.
48. Ladenstein R, Pötschger U, Le Deley MC, Whelan J, Paulussen M, Oberlin O, et al. Primary disseminated multifocal EWING sarcoma: results of the Euro-EWING 99 trial. J Clin Oncol. 2010;28(20):3284–91.
49. Dirksen U, Brennan B, Le Deley MC, Cozic N, van den Berg H, Bhadri V, et al. High-dose chemotherapy compared with standard chemotherapy and lung radiation in Ewing sarcoma with pulmonary metastases: results of the European Ewing tumour working initiative of National Groups, 99 trial and EWING 2008. J Clin Oncol. 2019;37(34):3192–202.
50. Windsor R, Hamilton A, McTiernan A, Dileo P, Michelagnoli M, Seddon B, et al. Survival after high-dose chemotherapy for refractory and recurrent Ewing sarcoma. Eur J Cancer. 1990;2022(170):131–9.
51. Rasper M, Jabar S, Ranft A, Jürgens H, Amler S, Dirksen U. The value of high-dose chemotherapy in patients with first relapsed Ewing sarcoma. Pediatr Blood Cancer. 2014;61(8):1382–6.
52. Allen CE, Merad M, McClain KL. Langerhans-cell histiocytosis. N Engl J Med. 2018;379(9):856–68.
53. Gadner H, Minkov M, Grois N, Pötschger U, Thiem E, Aricò M, Astigarraga I, Braier J, Donadieu J, Henter JI, Janka-Schaub G, McClain KL, Weitzman S, Windebank K, Ladisch S, Histiocyte Society. Therapy prolongation improves outcome in multisystem Langerhans cell histiocytosis. Blood. 2013;121(25):5006–14.

# 28 Retinoblastoma

Renu Madan, Neiwete Lomi, Safal Muhammed, and Narendra Kumar

## 28.1 Introduction

Retinoblastoma (RB) is the commonest intraocular malignancy in children, with the incidence of 1:15,000 to 1:18,000 children [1]. The average age of diagnosis is 18 months, and it present bilaterally in about 25 to 35% of cases without any gender or racial predisposition [2]. It is caused by mutation in a tumor suppressor gene, *RB1* gene which is located at chromosome 13q14.2n. Both copies are required to lost or mutated for development of retinoblastoma. Knudson proposed the two-hit hypothesis in 1971 and stated that mutations in both copies of *RB1* gene are required for the development of retinoblastoma [3]. Only 6% of the newly diagnosed RB cases are familial, while the rest are sporadic [2]. High-income countries have better outcome of RB, with survival rate of approx. 95%, as compared to developing countries or low-/middle-income countries (LMIC) [4]. Causes of high mortality in developing countries are delayed presentation, late diagnosis, unaffordable treatment facilities, cultural taboo for enucleation, and poor compliance to treatment and treatment abandonment [5].

R. Madan (✉) · N. Kumar
Department of Radiotherapy and Oncology, Postgraduate Institute of Medical Education and Research, Chandigarh, India

N. Lomi
Department of Ophthalmology, Dr. Rajendra Prasad Centre for Ophthalmic Sciences, AIIMS, New Delhi, Delhi, India

S. Muhammed
Department of Pediatrics, Indian Naval Hospital Ship Asvini, Mumbai, Maharashtra, India



R. Madan et al. (eds.), *Evidence Based Practice in Pediatric Radiation Oncology*, https://doi.org/10.1007/978-981-96-4872-6_28

### 28.1.1 Clinical Presentation

Leukocoria, also known as, white reflex is the most common symptom of retinoblastoma. Other clinical presentation includes strabismus, red eye, painful blind eye, decrease in vision, orbital cellulitis, hyphemia, and phthisis bulbi.

### 28.1.2 Diagnostic Workup

A dilated fundus examination with indirect ophthalmoscopy, particularly examination under anesthesia, can diagnose >90% of cases [6]. Wide-angle fundus camera or Retcam can help in treatment response assessment. Ultrasound B-scan is an important tool in diagnosing RB which typically shows an irregular or well defined intraocular mass with intra-lesional calcification which is represented by high internal reflectivity. Ultrasound biomicroscopy (UBM) is another important tool for diagnosing and staging intraocular retinoblastoma which also helps in visualization of anterior segment, ciliary body, and anterior retina.

### 28.1.3 Metastatic Workup

Metastatic workup is indicated in extraocular retinoblastoma (EORB). Contrast enhanced fats suppressed MRI of brain and orbit should be performed to look for any intracranial lesion. As compared to vitreous, retinoblastomas are hypointense on T2-weighted images and slightly hyperintense on T1-weighted images. On contrast administration, these tumors show a moderate enhancement (Fig. 28.1).

CT scans of the brain and orbit, though commonly used in LMIC because of ease of availability and affordability, can miss out on some extraocular spread. Bone marrow aspiration and biopsy, lumbar puncture, and bone scan are required to look for metastatic disease. Staging workup with whole-body 18-fluorodeoxyglucose

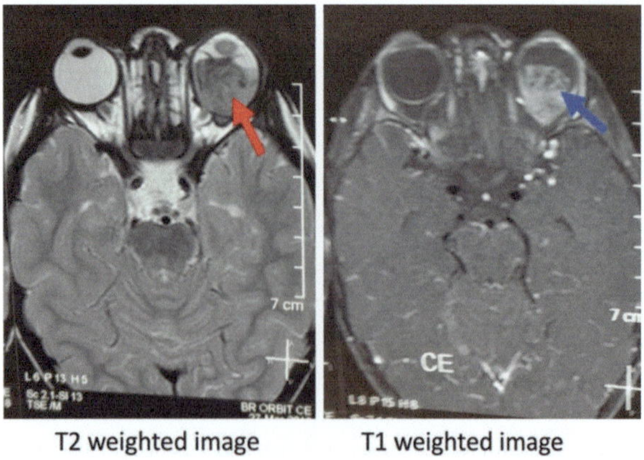


**Fig. 28.1** MRI brain and orbit showing left eye intraocular mass with hypointense on T2-weighted image (red arrow) and hyperintense on T1-weighted image (blue arrow) with posterior scleral breach and optic nerve involvement in a case of extraocular retinoblastoma

(18-FDG) positron emission tomography with computed tomography (PET/CT) is optional [7].

## 28.2 Classification of Retinoblastoma

Table 28.1 provides new International Classification of Intraocular Retinoblastoma (ICRB) which correlates well with the outcomes of various grades of tumors with the newer therapeutic modalities [8]. Table 28.2 provides International Retinoblastoma Staging System (IRSS) of retinoblastoma [9].

## 28.3 Treatment

The goals of the therapy have evolved with time. In the era, when effective chemotherapy and local therapy were not available, the treatment was aimed at saving the patients' life by doing enucleation and administration of external beam radiotherapy

**Table 28.1** International classification of intraocular retinoblastoma [8]

| | |
|---|---|
| Group A | Small intraretinal tumors away from foveola and disc<br>• All tumors are 3 mm or smaller in greatest dimension, confined to the retina<br>• All tumors are located further than 3 mm from the foveola and 1.5 mm from the optic disc |
| Group B | All remaining discrete tumors confined to the retina<br>• All other tumors confined to the retina not in group A<br>• Tumor-associated subretinal fluid less than 3 mm from the tumor with no subretinal seeding |
| Group C | Discrete local disease with minimal subretinal or vitreous seeding<br>• Tumor(s) are discrete<br>• Subretinal fluid, present or past, without seeding involving up to one-fourth of retina<br>• Local fine vitreous seeding may be present close to discrete tumor<br>• Local subretinal seeding less than 3 mm from the tumor |
| Group D | Diffuse disease with significant vitreous or subretinal seeding<br>• Tumor(s) may be massive or diffuse<br>• Subretinal fluid present or past without seeding, involving up to total retinal detachment<br>• Diffuse or massive vitreous disease may include "greasy" seeds or avascular tumor masses<br>• Diffuse subretinal seeding may include subretinal plaques or tumor nodules |
| Group E | Presence of any one or more of these poor prognosis features<br>• Tumor touching the lens<br>• Tumor anterior to anterior vitreous face involving ciliary body or anterior segment<br>• Diffuse infiltrating retinoblastoma<br>• Neovascular glaucoma<br>• Opaque media from hemorrhage<br>• Tumor necrosis with aseptic orbital cellulites<br>• Phthisis bulbi |

**Table 28.2** International Retinoblastoma Staging System (IRSS) [9]

| IRSS stage | Clinical description |
|---|---|
| 0 | Child treated conservatively |
| I | Eye enucleated, completely resected histolopathogically |
| II | Eye enucleated, microscopic residual tumor |
| III | Locoregional extension present |
| a | Overt orbital disease (clinical or radiological) |
| b | Preauricular or cervical lymph node extension |
| IV | Metastatic disease |
| a | Hematogenous metastasis (without central nervous system involvement)<br>1. Single lesion<br>2. Multiple lesions |
| b | Central nervous system extension (with or without any other site of regional or metastatic disease)<br>1. Prechiasmatic lesion<br>2. Central nervous system disease<br>3. Leptomeningeal and cerebrospinal fluid spread |

(EBRT). However, currently globe salvage has become possible in most of the intraocular retinoblastoma patients. Advances in local therapeutics and increasing availability and use of intra-arterial chemotherapy have marginalized the role of systemic therapy in resource-rich settings. Thus, in the modern era, the primary goal of treatment is to save the life, secondary is globe salvage, and tertiary goal is to save the vision along with minimizing both the acute toxicity and late squeal from treatment, particularly second malignancies. The rate of globe salvage depends upon the International Classification of Retinoblastoma (ICRB) grouping; 93% globe salvage in group B eyes, 90% group C eyes, and the much lower rate of 47% group D eyes. All group A eyes can be salvaged without chemotherapy [10]. The standard treatment protocol depends on the stage, laterality, and locations of tumors (Fig. 28.2).

### 28.3.1 Chemotherapy

Chemotherapeutic agents may be administered systematically by intravenous route or locally by selective intra-arterial, intra-vitreal, periocular, and intra-cameral routes.

#### 28.3.1.1 Intra-Arterial Chemotherapy (IAC)

Though first described by Reese et al. in 1950, the techniques of intra-arterial chemotherapy (IAC) were refined and were subsequently popularized by the work done by Yamane et al. and Abramson et al. in 2000s. Since IAC shuns the adverse effects of intravenous chemotherapy, it has replaced systemic chemotherapy as the first line of treatment for globe salvage of advanced intraocular retinoblastoma in most high-income countries and many tertiary centers of LMIC. It provides a selective catheterization of the ophthalmic artery, thereby providing high intraocular drugs

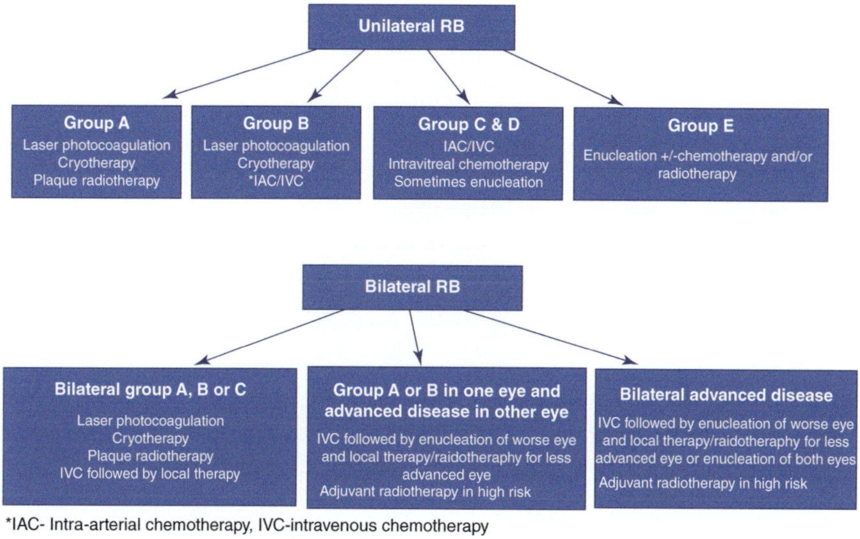


**Fig. 28.2** Treatment algorithm of retinoblastoma

concentration without systemic adverse events [11]. Arterial access is achieved with 4F pediatric guide catheter through the femoral artery, and the microcatheter is navigated till the origin of ophthalmic artery from where the drug is injected. IAC is commonly indicated for group B, C, and D retinoblastoma. IAC results in 30-fold increase in the concentration of drug at the tumor site. On an average, 3 cycles at 4 weekly cycles are required for adequate reduction in the tumor size. Melphalan (3–7.5 mg) is the most commonly used agent [12]. It can be used alone or in combination with topotecan (1–2 mg) or carboplatin (15–50 mg). Local adverse effects of IAC include retinal detachment, vitreous hemorrhage, and retinal or choroidal ischemia. Systemic complications are rare and include vasospasm, nausea, vomiting, neutropenia, and fever.

#### 28.3.1.2 Intra-Vitreal Chemotherapy

Treatment of vitreous seeds is one of the most challenging in retinoblastoma. Intra-vitreal chemotherapy helps to achieve maximum drug concentration close to the tumor with lowest systemic drug toxicity. Melphalan is a common intra-vitreal drug used to treat vitreous seeds in retinoblastoma. It is a cytotoxic nitrogen mustard derivative alkylating agent that inhibits both DNA and RNA synthesis. It is given intra-vitreal in the dose of 20–30 μg/mL in 0.1 mL.

Another drug is topotecan hydrochloride used in a dose of 30 μg/mL in 0.1 mL with lesser side effect comparing to melphalan [13].

#### 28.3.1.3 Periocular Chemotherapy

Recurrence of vitreous and subretinal seeds due to limited drug penetrations in systemic chemotherapy advocates the use of periocular chemotherapy, which helps in delivering higher doses at tumor site along with limiting the adverse effects of systemic therapy. Periocular carboplatin is widely used in group C and D retinoblastoma; however, it may lead to local side effects like orbital fat necrosis, ocular motility changes, preseptal chemosis, and cellulitis [14]. Topotecan is another drug used periocular with lesser side effects.

#### 28.3.1.4 Intra-Cameral Chemotherapy

Anterior chamber seeding has been shown to be a poor prognostic factor due to the limited drug penetration to the site and is considered for absolute indication for enucleation. Intra-cameral melphalan injection is a novel technique used safely to eradicate aqueous seedings [15].

#### 28.3.1.5 Systemic or Intravenous Chemotherapy (IVC)

Traditionally, chemotherapy did not have a major role for the treatment of intraocular retinoblastoma. With the identification of effective chemotherapy regimens and local treatment like laser/thermo–/cryotherapy and intra-vitreal chemotherapy, globe salvage became an achievable goal in most patients with intraocular retinoblastoma. Systemic chemotherapy in retinoblastoma may be used in three different contexts.

1. *To enable globe salvage in intraocular retinoblastoma*: Over the last three decades, aggressive local treatment along with systemic chemotherapy (chemoreduction) has resulted in the salvage of eyes in most cases of advanced intraocular retinoblastoma. In addition to the accompanying vision salvage in most cases and cosmetic benefits in all cases, this approach has also virtually eliminated the use of external beam radiotherapy (EBRT) in such patients, thus avoiding its long-term adverse effects. Chemoreduction plus local treatment can result in 60 to 85% globe salvage rates [16]. Reassessment for local treatment is usually done after two cycles of chemotherapy as the response noted is maximum at this time.
2. *Successful management of extraocular and metastatic disease*: Extraocular retinoblastoma requires more intensive systemic therapy with more courses of systemic chemotherapy. Treatment outcome of locoregional disease restricted to orbit is excellent with the current therapies. However, systemic metastasis particularly to central nervous system (CNS) remains dismal.
3. *Adjuvant therapy after enucleation*: Enucleation achieves a cure rate of approximately 85–90% of the patients with intraocular retinoblastoma [16], though upfront enucleation has been increasingly restricted to group E disease where there are no realistic hopes of salvaging vision and/or globe. However, when enucleation is performed upfront and the histopathological examination reveals high-risk pathology such as massive choroidal invasion of ≥3 mm and post-laminar optic nerve involvement (PLONI) without cut end positivity, adjuvant chemotherapy must be offered.

#### 28.3.1.6 IVC Regimens

The combination CEV (carboplatin, etoposide, and vincristine) is the most commonly employed chemoreduction regimen in the management of retinoblastoma (Table 28.3). These drugs are administered 3–4 weekly. While six cycles are administered for intraocular disease, 12 cycles are required for the management of extraocular or locoregional disease (orbital retinoblastoma or histopathology demonstrating high-risk features). The other drugs which are sparingly used in the management of intraocular and locoregional disease include cyclophosphamide, doxorubicin, and topotecan. Cyclophosphamide was earlier used commonly by German groups has now been eliminated from their newer regimens. Topotecan is highly active against retinoblastoma and can be used though all routes, namely, systemic, intra-arterial and intra-vitreal.

### 28.3.2 Focal Consolidative Therapy

#### 28.3.2.1 Transpupillary Thermotherapy (TTT)

In this technique, the heat is generated from a semiconductor diode laser in range of 40-60 °C which is applied at the tumor to produce apoptosis [17]. This heat is applied at the sub-photocoagulation threshold level. The large spot size of 1300 μm is delivered though the indirect ophthalmoscopic delivery system. TTT produces a satisfactory regression in tumor thickness 2–3 mm. Retinal serious detachment, retinal hole, and traction may occurs following heavy thermotherapy.

#### 28.3.2.2 Cryotherapy

Triple freeze-thaw cryotherapy is used for small peripheral lesions of size approximately 4 mm diameter and 2 mm thickness [2]. The therapy is repeated at every 4–6 weeks interval until tumor regression. Post therapy complications can lead to retinal detachment (RD) or tear, rarely scleral necrosis.

#### 28.3.2.3 Laser Photocoagulation

Laser photocoagulation is used to hamper the blood supply to the lesions, situated posteriorly. It can be used for the lesions of size <4 mm in diameter and 2 mm in thickness [2]. Complications include decrease visual field if tumor located in juxtapapillary area, transient RD, retinal hole, traction and vascular occlusion, and

**28.3** CEV regimen for retinoblastoma

| CEV regimen | | |
|---|---|---|
| Vincristine | 1.5 mg/m$^2$ on day 1 (0.05 mg/kg for children below 36 months of age) | Maximum allowable dose: 2 mg |
| Etoposide | 150 mg/m$^2$ on day 1 and 2 (5 mg/kg for children below 36 months of age) | |
| Carboplatin | 560 mg/m$^2$ on day 1 (18.6 mg/kg for children below 36 months of age) | Calvert approach can be used to further improve the dosing accuracy |

preretinal fibrosis. Since it restricts the tumoral blood supply, it is not used in those on active chemotherapy.

#### 28.3.2.4 Plaque Brachytherapy

In this technique, radioactive plaque is placed over the sclera aligned with the tumor base; hence, it provides maximum radiation to the tumor and limits the exposure to normal structures. The common radioactive isotopes used are Iodine-125 and Ruthenium-106. Following criteria should be met for primary brachytherapy: (1) The lesion should be unilateral and anterior, (2) there should be no vitreous seeding, (3) the tumor should be situated at least 3 mm from optic disc, and (4) tumor dimension should be <15 mm in diameter and <10 mm in thickness [18]. It is contraindicated in tumor associated with diffuse active vitreous seeds. Complications may include radiation papillopathy, maculopathy, and cataract.

#### 28.3.2.5 Enucleation

Primary enucleation is the standard treatment for unilateral advanced intraocular tumors along with neovascular glaucoma. Minimal manipulation and obtaining of more than 10 mm optic nerve stump is mandatory to prevent tumor recurrences [19]. The enucleated eye should be examined for any extraocular extension and optic nerve involvement and sent for histopathological examination.

#### 28.3.2.6 Exenteration

Exenteration involves removal of eyeball, eyelids, muscle, optic nerve, and orbital fats. It is indicated in orbital retinoblastoma involving the conjunctival fornix, eyelids, and adjacent orbital adnexa tissue. Detailed metastasis workup is indicated in such patients and prognosis is usually poor.

### 28.3.3 External Beam Radiotherapy (EBRT)

Traditionally radiation therapy/radiotherapy (RT) was the primary treatment for all retinoblastoma owing to their high radiosensitivity. Various series have shown variable long-term eye preservation rates [20]. However, the role of RT has been diminished in the present era due to increased risk of subsequent malignant neoplasm (SMN) and availability of other eye salvage modalities. Currently, radiation therapy is used for advanced or recurrent intraocular RB, EORB, and metastatic RB. Postoperative RT in uniformly indicated in all EORB and in presence of high-risk features (on MRI or histopathology) such as tumor present at cut end of optic nerve, scleral breech, or orbital disease [21]. It should ideally be started within 4–6 weeks of surgery [22]. RT is not recommended in children younger than 12 months of age due to increased risk of side effects such as orbital hypoplasia and subsequent malignant neoplasm [23].

### 28.3.4 Radiotherapy Dose and Target Volume

#### 28.3.4.1 Post Enucleation

Any gross disease, if present should be delineated as gross tumor volume (GTV). Clinical target volume (CTV) includes the gross disease and entire orbit. Though there is no strong evidence, few centers advocate extension of CTV till optic chiasma in case of positive optic nerve resection margin [24]. Planning target volume (PTV) margin is given according to institute protocols and is usually 3–5 mm. A dose of 40–45 Gy in 1.8 to 2 Gy per fraction should be prescribed to PTV [25]. RT can also be planned in two phases: 36 Gy in 1.8 to 2 Gy per fraction to the entire orbit followed by a boost of 9–10 Gy to the area of gross/microscopic disease such as remainder of optic nerve and chiasma [26]. Figure 28.3 provides radiotherapy planning of group E RB. Both three-dimensional conformal radiotherapy (3DCRT) and volumetric modulated arc therapy (VMAT) plans were generated for the patient, but finally the patient was treated with 3DCRT plan.

#### 28.3.4.2 Salvage Settings

RT in this setting should only be considered when other local modalities fail and facility of plaque brachytherapy is not available. Any residual disease should be delineated as GTV. Subsequent expansion of 5 mm and 3–5 mm is given for CTV and PTV, respectively. A total dose of 36–45 Gy in 1.8–2 Gy per fraction should be prescribed to the PTV.

#### 28.3.4.3 Management of Metastatic Disease

CNS, bone, and bone marrow are the most common sites of distant metastasis. The management in these patients remains challenging.

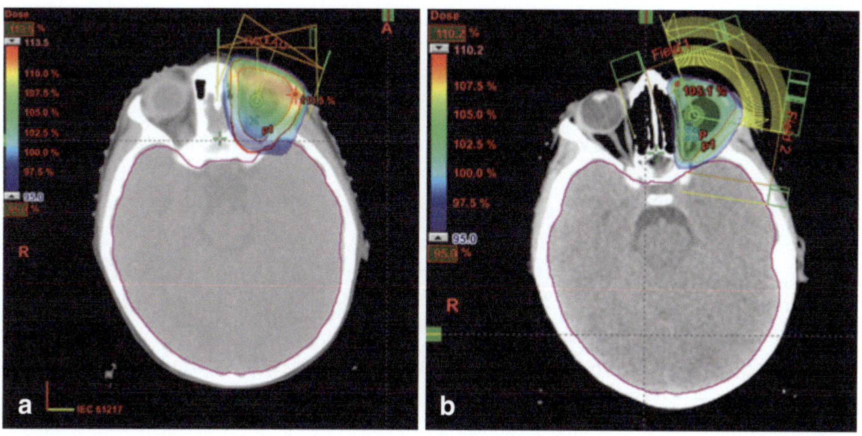


**Fig. 28.3** Radiotherapy planning for group E retinoblastoma. (**a**) 3DCRT technique and (**b**) VMAT technique

#### 28.3.4.4 RT in Metastatic Disease

The role of radiation in metastatic disease is not well defined. Often it is used to palliate the symptoms due to ulcerative growth, bleeding, pain, and in case of extensive CNS or leptomeningeal disease [27]. For intracranial metastasis, whole brain RT (WBRT) to a dose of 8 Gy in 1# or 20 Gy in 5 # or 30 Gy in 10 # fractions can be planned. For spinal metastasis or positive CSF cytology, craniospinal irradiation (CSI) can be planned to a dose of 23.4 Gy (3–5 years) or 36 Gy (>5 years). RT to primary site in metastatic setting can also be considered if there is a good response to chemotherapy at metastatic sites.

### 28.3.5 Chemotherapy in Metastatic Disease

The two commonly described regimens are cyclophosphamide, carboplatin, etoposide, and vincristine (CCEV); cisplatin, cyclophosphamide, etoposide, and vincristine (PCEV). High-dose chemotherapy followed by autologous stem cell transplantation (ASCT) has shown to improve outcome in selected patients. The conditioning regimens include Busulfan/Melphalan, Melphalan/Thiotepa/Cyclophosphamide, and Carboplatin/Etposide/Melphalan [28]. In addition, CNS-directed treatment is employed for CNS metastasis, though these have not resulted in improved survival. CNS-directed therapies include intrathecal drug administration (methotrexate, cytarabine, and dexamethasone) and cranial or craniospinal irradiation. However, the outcome still remains poor particularly in CNS metastasis.

### 28.3.6 Trilateral RB

Trilateral RB (TRB) is seen in 3–4% patients of RB and consists of histologically similar intracranial tumor in the pineal gland, supra-sellar or parasellar locations, along with bilateral retinoblastoma [29]. The overall prognosis in these patients remains poor.

### 28.3.7 Survivorship Concerns

1. Subsequent malignant neoplasms (SMN): Both radiotherapy and chemotherapy increase the risk of SMNs, which are the commonest cause of death in RB. Incidence of SMNs is higher in hereditary RB. In one study, cumulative incidence of SMN was 18–35% and 2% at 40 years in hereditary and nonhereditary cohorts, respectively [30]. Among SMNs, sarcoma and melanoma are the more common in hereditary RB, while carcinomas are the more common in nonhereditary RB [30].
2. Bone abnormality: RB survivors are at increased risk of bony deformities due to enucleation and RT [31].

3. Others: Diminished vision, short stature, hearing loss, poor school performance, and impaired overall quality of life.

## 28.4 Conclusion

Retinoblastoma is the most common malignant intraocular tumor in children. Despite the therapeutic advancement, outcome in LMIC remains poor due to late diagnosis, unaffordable heath care facilities, culture taboo, and noncompliance to the treatment. Life-long supportive care should be provided to meet the survivorship issues.

## References


1. Bishop JO, Madsen EC. Retinoblastoma. Review of current status. Surv Ophthalmol. 1975;19:342–66.
2. Shields JA, Shields CL. Intraocular tumors—a text and atlas. Philadelphia, PA: WB Saunders; 1992.
3. Knudson AG Jr. Mutation and cancer: statistical study of retinoblastoma. Proc Natl Acad Sci U S A. 1971;68(4):820–3.
4. Chawla B, Hasan F, Azad R, Seth R, Upadhyay AD, Pathy S, et al. Clinical presentation and survival of retinoblastoma in Indian children. Br J Ophthalmol. 2016;100:172–8.
5. Bakhshi S, Gupta S, Gogia V, et al. Compliance in retinoblastoma. Indian J Pediatr. 2010;77:535–40.
6. Vemuganti G, Honavar SG, John R. Clinicopathological profile of retinoblastoma in Asian Indians. Invest Ophthalmol Vis Sci. 2000;41(S):790.
7. Bakhshi S, Meel R, Kashyap S, Sharma S. Bone marrow aspirations and lumbar punctures in retinoblastoma at diagnosis. J Pediatr Hematol Oncol. 2011;33(5):e182–5.
8. Linn MA. Intraocular retinoblastoma: the case for a new group classification. Ophthalmol Clin North Am. 2005;18:41–53.
9. Chantada G, Doz F, Antoneli CB, Grundy R, Clare Stannard FF, Dunkel IJ, et al. A proposal for an international retinoblastoma staging system. Pediatr Blood Cancer. 2006;47:801–5.
10. Shields CL, Mashayekhi A, Au AK, Czyz C, Leahey A, Meadows AT, et al. The international classification of retinoblastoma predicts chemoreduction success. Ophthalmology. 2006;113:2276–80.
11. Yamane T, Kaneko A, Mohri M. The technique of ophthalmic arterial infusion therapy for patients with intraocular retinoblastoma. Int J Clin Oncol. 2004;9:6973.
12. Chen Q, Zhang B, Dong Y, Mo X, Zhang L, Huang W, et al. Comparison between intravenous chemotherapy and intra-arterial chemotherapy for retinoblastoma: a meta-analysis. BMC Cancer. 2018;18(1):486.
13. Rao R, Honavar SG, Sharma V, Reddy VAP. Intravitreal topotecan in the management of refractory and recurrent vitreous seeds in retinoblastoma. Br J Ophthalmol. 2018;102(4):490–5.
14. Mulvihill A, Budning A, Jay V, Vandenhoven C, Heon E, Gallie B, et al. Ocular motility changes after sub-tenon carboplatin chemotherapy for retinoblastoma. Arch Ophthalmol. 2003;121:1120–4.
15. Munier FL, Gaillard M-C, Decembrini S, Bongiovanni M, Beck-Popovic M. Ocul Oncol Pathol. 2017;3:149–55.
16. Rodriguez-Galindo C, Orbach DB, Vander Veen D. Retinoblastoma. Pediatr Clin North Am. 2015;62:201–23.

17. Shields CL, Santos MC, Diniz W, et al. Thermotherapy for retinoblastoma. Arch Ophthalmol. 1999;117:885–93.
18. American Brachytherapy Society. The American brachytherapy society consensus guidelines for plaque brachytherapy of uveal melanoma andretinoblastoma. Brachytherapy. 2014;13:1–14.
19. Honavar SG, Singh AD. Management of advanced retinoblastoma. Ophthalmol Clin North Am. 2005;18:65–73.
20. Abramson DH, Beaverson KL, Chang ST, et al. Outcome following initial external beam radiotherapy in patients with Reese-Ellsworth group Vb retinoblastoma. Arch Ophthalmol. 2004;122(9):1316–23.
21. Chantada GL, Dunkel IJ, de Dávila MT, et al. Retinoblastoma patients with high risk ocular pathological features: who needs adjuvant therapy? Br J Ophthalmol. 2004;88(8):1069–73.
22. Singh U, Katoch D, Kaur S, et al. Retinoblastoma: a sixteen-year review of the presentation, treatment, and outcome from a Tertiary Care Institute in Northern India. Ocul Oncol Pathol. 2017;4(1):23–32.
23. Abramson DH, Frank CM. Second nonocular tumors in survivors of bilateral retinoblastoma: a possible age effect on radiation-related risk. Ophthalmology. 1998;105:573–9.
24. Pérez V, Sampor C, Rey G, et al. Treatment of nonmetastatic unilateral retinoblastoma in children. JAMA Ophthalmol. 2018;136(7):747–52.
25. Chantada G, Fandiño A, Casak S, et al. Treatment of overt extraocular retinoblastoma. Med Pediatr Oncol. 2003;40:158–61.
26. Aerts I, Sastre-Garau X, Savignoni A, et al. Results of a multicenter prospective study on the postoperative treatment of unilateral retinoblastoma after primary enucleation. J Clin Oncol. 2013;31(11):1458–63.
27. Rao AD, Chen Q, Ermoian RP, et al. Practice patterns of palliative radiation therapy in pediatric oncology patients in an international pediatric research consortium. Pediatr Blood Cancer. 2017;64(11).
28. Yasui N, Kawamoto H, Fujiwara M, Aihara Y, Ogawa C, Hosono A, et al. High-dose chemotherapy for high-risk retinoblastoma: clinical course and outcome of 14 cases in the National Cancer Center, Japan. Bone Marrow Transplant. 2015;50:221–4.
29. Kivelä T. Trilateral retinoblastoma: a meta-analysis of hereditary retinoblastoma associated with primary ectopic intracranial retinoblastoma. J Clin Oncol. 1999;17(6):1829–37.
30. Marees T, Moll AC, Imhof SM, et al. Risk of second malignancies in survivors of retinoblastoma: more than 40 years of follow-up. J Natl Cancer Inst. 2008;100(24):1771–9.
31. Kaste SC, Chen G, Fontanesi J, et al. Orbital development in long-term survivors of retinoblastoma. J Clin Oncol. 1997;15(03):1183–9.

# Management of Neuroblastoma

# 29

Nehal Khanna, Nitin Peters, Saswati Behera, and Vamsi Krishna

## 29.1 Introduction

Neuroblastoma (NBL) is the most common malignancy in infants and the most common extracranial solid tumor in children [1]. The outcome is very good in low and intermediate risk disease. However, in high-risk disease, cure rates are below 50% despite aggressive treatment. Neuroblastoma is said to arise from primitive adrenergic neuroblasts of the neural crest cells primarily in the sympathetic ganglion. On light microscopy, it is classically described as a small round blue cell tumor with Homer Wright pseudo rosettes, necrosis, calcification, hyperchromatic nuclei, and scant cytoplasm.

The Shimada system was a popular histological classification of NBL into good and poor prognostic groups based on the stromal abundance, differentiation, Mitosis Karyorrhexis Index (MKI) and Age. The International Neuroblastoma Pathology Committee (INPC) classification is the current classification system in use [2]. It incorporates the Shimada system and tumor subtypes to classify NBL into favorable and unfavorable histology. MYCN gene amplifications are seen in about a fifth of patients and are said to correlate with aggressive stage, unfavorable histology, and overall worse outcome. It forms an important part of various risk stratification models in NBL [3].

N. Khanna
Department of Radiation Oncology, TMH, Mumbai, Maharashtra, India

N. Peters (✉)
Department of Pediatric Surgery, PGIMER, Chandigarh, India

S. Behera
Department of Pediatric Surgery, AIIMS, Bhatinda, Punjab, India

V. Krishna
Department of Radiotherapy, PGIMER, Chandigarh, India


R. Madan et al. (eds.), *Evidence Based Practice in Pediatric Radiation Oncology*, https://doi.org/10.1007/978-981-96-4872-6_29

## 29.2 Diagnostic Workup

NBL can arise anywhere throughout the sympathetic nervous system. The adrenal gland is the most common site followed by abdomen, thorax, neck, and pelvis [4]. About 70% of the patients present with metastasis at diagnosis with lymph nodes, liver, bone marrow, cortical bone, and skin being the common sites. The tumor is metabolically active with production of catecholamines and other vasoactive peptides resulting in hypertension, diarrhea, or myoclonic syndromes [5].

The diagnosis is established by biopsy of the suspected mass followed by microscopic examination. In recent years, image-guided core needle biopsy (CNB) techniques have replaced the classical open surgical biopsy (OSB) in most centers worldwide. Apart from providing adequate tumor tissue, CNB has reduced complications rate like tumor bleeding, injury to surrounding structures, need for blood transfusion, and post-procedure hospital stays. Being a heterogeneous tumor, image-guided biopsy helps to harvest solid tumor tissue and prevent false negative results.

Immunohistochemistry helps in the further characterization of small round cell tumors. The biopsy specimen should also be subjected to MYC amplification testing by Fluorescence in situ hybridization (FISH) whenever available. In patients whom a tumor biopsy is difficult to obtain, a bone marrow trephine biopsy showing infiltration by neuroblastoma cells supplemented by elevated urine/serum homovanillic (HVA) or vanillylmandelic acid (VMA) levels can also establish the diagnosis [6, 7]. Local contrast-enhanced CT scan is recommended for the primary tumor extent. Bone marrow biopsy must be done for all patients. MRI is helpful in cases of paraspinal masses with suspected cord compression. For distant metastatic workup, metaiodobenzylguanidine (mIBG) scan is the most sensitive investigation to pick up soft tissue or skeletal lesions [8]. In 10% cases of neuroblastomas which are not MIBG avid (with $I^{131 \text{ or } 123}$), PET/CT with DOTA-conjugated peptides such as $^{68}$Ga-DOTATATE could be extremely helpful. Reports have suggested that Ga-DOTATATE scans could pick up progressive disease earlier than MIBG scans and play a vital role in detecting unsuspected metastasis, restaging, and further management [9]. A Tc-99 bone scan and FDG-PET CT are other alternatives. Routine hematological, biochemical, and coagulation workup must be done. In centers where MYC testing are not available, some guidelines have proposed the use of elevated serum LDH $\geq$750 IU/L and ferritin $\geq$120 ng/mL as alternative high-risk markers [7]. If MYC status is not available in patients otherwise classified as low risk, they are still classified as low risk.

## 29.3 Staging and Risk Stratification

The International Neuroblastoma Staging system (INSS) was a traditional staging system designed for NBL and is based on surgical staging and lymph node sampling (Table 29.1) [10]. The INSS staging requires a thorough surgical evaluation. After the advent of effective systemic therapy, patients who were considered not operable

**Table 29.1** International Neuroblastoma Staging system (INSS)

| Stage | Description |
|---|---|
| Stage 1 | Localized tumor confined to the area of origin; complete gross excision, with or without microscopic residual disease; identifiable ipsilateral and contralateral lymph nodes negative microscopically |
| Stage 2A | Unilateral tumor with incomplete gross excision; identifiable ipsilateral and contralateral lymph nodes negative microscopically |
| Stage 2B | Unilateral tumor with complete or incomplete gross excision; with positive ipsilateral regional lymph nodes; identifiable contralateral lymph nodes negative microscopically |
| Stage 3 | Tumor infiltrating across the midline with or without regional lymph node involvement; or, unilateral tumor with contralateral regional lymph node involvement; or, midline tumor with bilateral regional lymph node involvement |
| Stage 4 | Dissemination of tumor to distant lymph nodes, bone, bone marrow, liver, and/or other organs (except as defined in stage 4S) |
| Stage 4S | Localized primary tumor as defined for stage 1 or 2 with dissemination limited to liver, skin, and/or bone marrow |

on initial radiological evaluation were taken for neoadjuvant chemotherapy. To identify and predict operability several image-defined risk factors (IDRFs) were identified. Various IDRFs have been shown in Table 29.2 [11]. Based on these IDRFs, the International Neuroblastoma Risk Group staging system was devised (INRG) [12]. Table 29.3 shows International Neuroblastoma Risk Group staging system. INRG system includes age, stage, histology, differentiation, MYC amplification status, chromosomal aberrations, and DNA ploidy to determine the risk group [13]. Table 29.4 shows INRG-based pretreatment risk stratification.

## 29.4 Risk-Adapted Treatment and Chemotherapy Protocols

Small adrenal masses detected in infants younger than 6 months or in antenatal period can be observed for spontaneous regression. Localized low-risk disease has excellent outcomes after surgery alone with EFS rates >95% [7]. Children under 18 months with low-risk localized unresectable disease can be kept under observation if asymptomatic. Chemotherapy is indicated in this group if there are life-threatening symptoms. Carboplatin and Etoposide for 2–4 cycles is the first choice in low-risk patients with life-threatening conditions, while Cyclophosphamide, Vincristine, and Adriamycin are the second line option [14]. Chemotherapy regimen for low- and intermediate-risk NB consists of either Carboplatin and Etoposide or CADO (Cyclophophamide, Vincristine, and Doxorubicin) [14]. Infants with INRG stage MS but low risk must be given chemotherapy even if asymptomatic [1].

Intermediate-risk disease consists of infants with metastatic disease (INRG:M) and children with localized unresectable disease. Four to eight cycles of neoadjuvant chemotherapy followed by assessment for maximal safe resection is the approach of choice. Imaging is done after 4 cycles to assess extent of debulking and metastatic remission. Carboplatin and Etoposide is the first-line regimen.

**Table 29.2** Image-defined risk factors (IDRFs)

| Anatomical region | Description |
|---|---|
| Multiple body compartments | • Ipsilateral tumor extension within two body compartments (e.g., neck and chest, chest and abdomen, or abdomen and pelvis) |
| Neck | • Tumor encasing carotid artery, vertebral artery, and/ or internal jugular vein<br>• Tumor extending to skull base<br>• Tumor compressing trachea |
| Cervicothoracic region | • Tumor encasing brachial plexus roots<br>• Tumor encasing subclavian vessels, vertebral artery, and/ or carotid artery<br>• Tumor compressing trachea |
| Thorax | • Tumor encasing aorta and/or major branches<br>• Tumor compressing trachea and/or principle bronchi<br>• Lower mediastinal tumor infiltrating costovertebral junction between T9 and T12 vertebral levels |
| Thoracoabdominal junction | • Tumor encasing aorta and/or vena cava |
| Abdomen and pelvis | • Tumor infiltrating porta hepatis and/or hepatoduodenal ligament<br>• Tumor encasing branches of superior mesenteric artery at mesenteric root<br>• Tumor encasing origin of celiac axis and/ or origin of superior mesenteric artery<br>• Tumor invading one or both renal pedicles<br>• Tumor encasing aorta and/or vena cava<br>• Tumor encasing iliac vessels<br>• Pelvic tumor crossing sciatic notch |
| Intraspinal tumor extension | • Intraspinal tumor extension (above L2) provided that (any of the following):<br>• More than one-third of spinal canal in axial plane invaded<br>• Perimedullary leptomeningeal spaces not visible<br>• Spinal cord signal intensity is abnormal |
| Infiltration of adjacent organs and structures | • Pericardium<br>• Diaphragm<br>• Kidney<br>• Liver<br>• Duodenopancreatic block<br>• Mesentery |

**Table 29.3** International Neuroblastoma Risk Group staging system

| Stage | Description |
|---|---|
| Stage L1 | Localized tumor not involving vital structures as defined by the list of image-defined risk factors and confined to one body compartment |
| Stage L2 | Locoregional tumor with presence of one or more image-defined risk factors |
| Stage M | Distant metastatic disease (except stage MS) |
| Stage MS | Metastatic disease in children younger than 18 months with metastases confined to skin, liver, and/or bone marrow |

**Table 29.4** INRG-based pretreatment risk stratification

| INRG stage | Age (months) | Histologic category | Tumor differentiation | *MYCN* | 11q Aberration | Ploidy | Pretreatment risk group |
|---|---|---|---|---|---|---|---|
| L1/L2 | Any | GN maturing, GNB intermixed | | | | | A (Very low) |
| L1 | Any | Any, except GN maturing or GNB intermixed | | NA | | | B (Very low) |
| | | | | Amplified | | | K (High) |
| L2 | <18 | Any, except GN maturing or GNB intermixed | | NA | No | | D (Low) |
| | | | | | Yes | | G (Intermediate) |
| L2 | ≥18 | GNB nodular neuroblastoma | Differentiating | NA | No | | E (Low) |
| | | | | | Yes | | H (Intermediate) |
| L2 | ≥18 | Any | Poorly differentiated or undifferentiated | NA | | | H (Intermediate) |
| | | | | Amplified | | | N (High) |
| M | <18 | Any | | NA | | Hyperdiploid | F (Low) |
| M | <12 | Any | | NA | | Diploid | I (Intermediate) |
| M | 12 to <18 | Any | | NA | | Diploid | J (Intermediate) |
| M | <18 | Any | | Amplified | | | O (High) |
| M | ≥18 | Any | | | | | P (High) |
| MS | <18 | Any | | NA | No | | C (Very low) |
| | | | | | Yes | | Q (High) |
| | | | | Amplified | | | R (High) |

*GN* ganglioneuroma, *GNB* ganglioneuroblastoma, *INRG* International Neuroblastoma Risk Group, *NA* not amplified

Cyclophosphamide, Vincristine, and Adriamycin (CADO) is the second-line option and is resorted to in cases of unsatisfactory response to first-line agents [1, 7].

High-risk disease is treated in five phases—induction therapy, surgery, high-dose myeloablative chemotherapy followed by stem cell transplantation, radiotherapy, and biological therapy. If facilities for autologous stem cell transplantation are not available, upfront palliative care can be offered with optional oral metronomic cyclophosphamide or etoposide. The objective of induction therapy is to produce maximal metastatic remission and reduction in tumor bulk. Various protocols such as SIOP-PODC regimen, POG 9341 regimen, and SIOPEN Rapid COJEC regimen are used for induction. Cisplatin, etoposide, Vincristine, Cyclophosphamide, doxorubicin, Ifosfamide, and Carboplatin are used in various induction protocols. Surgery after induction chemotherapy should follow the principles of organ preservation and maximal safe resection. Various studies have demonstrated survival benefit after near gross total resection (at least 90% resection) in high-risk NBL [1, 7, 15, 16].

## 29.5 ASCT in High-Risk NBL

ASCT is a crucial part of curative intent treatment for high-risk NBL [17]. The first step is the harvest of peripheral blood stem cells (PBSCs) during induction chemotherapy. The exact timing depends on the induction protocol used. Earlier harvest tends to lead to higher stem cell yield. These PBSCs must be cryopreserved up to the time of transplantation. Stem cell harvest may be delayed and be done closer to conditioning if cryopreservation facilities are not available. Melphalan and Buslphan (Bu-Mel) is the most common conditioning regimen used to ablate the bone marrow.

Stem cell apheresis is done on days 4–5. G-CSF is given to mobilize the stem cells. ASCT must ideally be performed in a dedicated bone marrow transplant unit. Prevention of hospital-acquired infection is crucial. Hand hygiene must be strictly followed. Other infection control measures include avoidance of indwelling catheters, use of oral over intravenous drugs, and promotion of enteral feeds whenever possible. Cis-Retinoic acid is used as post consolidation biological therapy [18].

## 29.6 Role of Surgery

### 29.6.1 Surgical Strategies

As per the current treatment protocols, diagnostic tissue biopsy is performed at initial presentation, and primary resection is delayed until three to five cycles of neoadjuvant chemotherapy except in cases of obvious metastatic diseases. However, the optimal timing of definitive surgery is still debatable and often individualized.

Many studies have demonstrated a higher rate of surgical complications in tumors operated shortly after the time of diagnosis. However, the overall survival is similar between these patients as explained by Shamberger et al. [19]. The decreased rate of morbidity seen in delayed surgery can be explained with the fact that there is a significant decrease in volume of primary tumor during induction chemotherapy which is maximum after first two cycles. Some studies have shown improved overall survival after 4 cycles of neoadjuvant chemotherapy as compared to 2 cycles in high-risk neuroblastoma patients [20]. In addition to that, there is a reduction of IDRFs during the induction therapy which again correlates with reduced surgical complications due to many factors like lesser duration of tumor dissection, reduced intraoperative hemorrhage, and thus lesser duration of surgery and anesthesia exposure [21].

### 29.6.2 The Extent of Resection in Neuroblastoma

Operative notes should consist of the following: no operation or **biopsy** removing less than 50% of tumor tissue; **incomplete resection** of 50% to less than 90% of tumor volume present at the time of surgery; **gross total resection** removing more than 90% of the tumor; or **complete resection** without macroscopic postoperative tumor residuals. It was not possible to include the category of microscopic complete resection because neuroblastomas are rarely removed in toto, and therefore, microscopic complete resection is usually impossible.

### 29.6.3 Preoperative Preparations

Identification of IDRFs and other intraoperative challenges should be anticipated well before surgery. Written informed consent is always an integral part and should never be missed. Parents should be informed about possible postoperative sequelae in special cases like Horner syndrome and intraspinal extension.

The anesthesia team with expertise for difficult cases should be available. The need for single lung ventilation, intraoperative blood products transfusion, and risk of both hypotension and hypertension crisis due to catecholamines release should be kept in mind.

### 29.6.4 Cervical Neuroblastoma

Cervical NB is generally picked up early and has favorable tumor biology.

The patient is laid supine with neck extended and head rotated to the contralateral side to improve exposure. A shoulder roll and head ring are secured to maintain stability. The entire neck and upper chest are exposed as per the requirement. Under aseptic precautions, a transverse incision is given along Langer's line. Care should be taken to avoid injury to the greater auricular nerve along the anterior border of sternocleidomastoid muscle (SCM) and spinal accessory nerve in the field. Large lesions might require the division of SCM for better exposure. In case of gross cervical lymphadenopathy, a formal neck dissection is performed involving lymphadenectomy.

### 29.6.5 Cervicothoracic Neuroblastoma

Due to the presence of complex neurovascular structures of thoracic inlet and mediastinal components, operating in this area is a surgical challenge. Generally, approaches like trans-manubrial and trap door thoracotomy (anterior thoracotomy) are used to access most of the tumor mass.

After careful dissection from encased mediastinal neurovascular structures, the tumor is often resected in piecemeal. The anterior and lateral divisions of the phrenic nerve are carefully identified and preserved. Thoracic duct injury is most likely near the right hemidiaphragm or just posterior to the carina. Any visible lymphatic injury should be sealed during surgery to prevent future chylothorax.

These incisions and approaches are often modified according to the site and extent of the tumor mass. Larger lesions occupying most of the mediastinum and reaching both thoracic cavities might require bilateral anterior thoracotomy (Clamshell thoracotomy). Newer approaches like cervical-parasternal thoracotomy incisions are also explained to access tumors reaching posterior costovertebral spaces [22].

### 29.6.6 Thoracoabdominal Neuroblastoma

The majority of abdominal NBs arise from the adrenal gland or sympathetic ganglia in the upper abdomen covering retroperitoneum. In such cases, thoracoabdominal approaches are favorable. Thoracoabdominal incisions provide excellent visualization of encased vessels and involved lymph nodes (Figs. 29.1 and 29.2). The incision is given starting from the chest at posterior axillary line along the eighth intercostal space in left and ninth interspace in the right. The incision is extended medially toward midline in the upper abdomen and further inferiorly as required. Surgeons should not risk extensive resection and loss of vital organs or major vessels in case of tumors with favorable biology.

After complete resection, hemostasis is achieved, and the incision is closed in layers. Diaphragm is primarily approximated using non-absorbable monofilament sutures and chest is closed after securing appropriately sized chest tubes.

### 29.6.7 Pelvic Neuroblastoma

Neuroblastomas arising in the pelvis are difficult to handle due to encasement of iliac vessels, lumbosacral trunk, and variable degree of bowel and bladder involvement. However, primary pelvic tumors present early without metastasis and usually have favorable biology and respond well even after gross macroscopic resection.

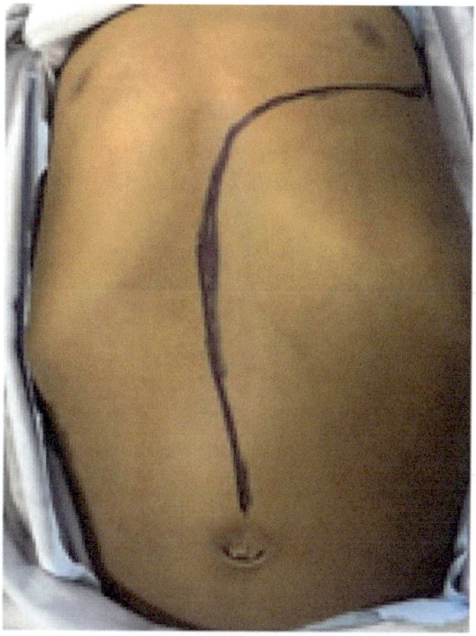

**Fig. 29.1** Cervical neuroblastoma excision

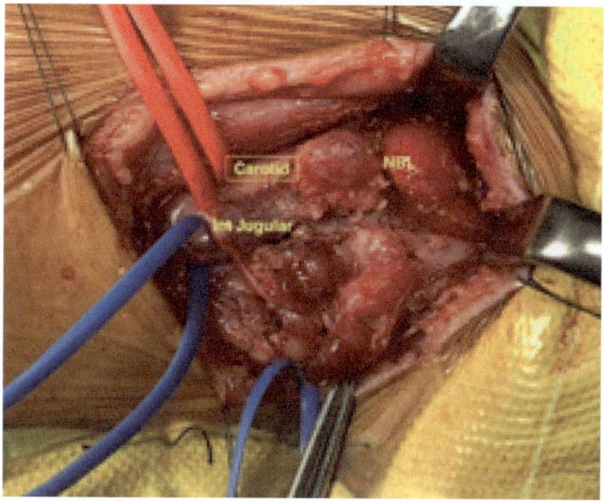


**Fig. 29.2** Thoraco-abdominal excision

Wherever required, procedures like cystoscopy, urodynamics, and rectal manometry are useful. Vascular controls should be ensured beforehand to prevent injury to major vessels like aortic bifurcation and iliac complex. Nerve stimulation is useful intraoperatively to delineate lumbosacral trunk and pelvic complex. At times, preoperative stenting of the ureters may be required for ease of dissection of the tumor from the lateral pelvic walls.

Postoperative morbidity like foot drop, due to injury of pelvic nerves, should be explained beforehand. Other complications due to neurologic impairment include neuropathic bladder, partial cauda equina syndrome, and variable degrees of fecal and urinary incontinence.

Alternative approach to pelvis have been described such as retropubic, transperineal, and other approaches used for common pelvic tumors like rhabdomyosarcomas and congenital anomalies like anorectal malformations. However, outcomes are comparable in all the above described approaches and should be planned according to the scenario [23].

### 29.6.8 Minimal Invasive Approach

Operative strategies of minimal invasive surgery (MIS) must consider individual case profiles. There are no strict guidelines on MIS; however, some studies have preferred well-confined smaller tumors without IDRFs or involvement of major vessels [24].

Gabra et al. have suggested that MIS is a secure approach for NB allowing more than 95% absolute contradictions. Conversion to open surgery is quite low; however, complication rates are higher in case of larger tumors with volume more than 75 mL [25].

The indications, risk factors, possible complications, and mode of surgery should be discussed beforehand in the tumor board for each and every case.

Factors like pneumatic pressure, tissue handling, hemostasis, and extent of resection should be anticipated. Conversion to open surgery is always a safer alternative in certain situations and should be explained to the parents before surgery.

The extent of lymph node sampling using MIS is variable as per the surgical expertise and often the most common, deviation from principles of oncological surgery. The impact of lymph node sampling on survival and disease outcome is still debatable in literature; however, various reports emphasize on poor lymph node retrieval with the MIS approach. Thus, MIS in neuroblastoma are developing with each passing day.

## 29.7 Special Considerations

### 29.7.1 Vascular Dissection

Major vessels like aorta and its branches are often found encased while attempting resection of tumors arising in the abdomino-pelvic region. It is vital to trace the course and origin of these vessels which is followed by finding an appropriate plane between tumor mass and the adventitia of the vessel. This maneuver is carefully done using the "bivalving technique" with a gently curved dissector after taking prior vascular control. Energy sources like bipolar cautery or harmonic scalpel are utilized to dissect out the tumor parenchyma from the vessel in toto or in piece meals. In cases where the periadventitial plane is obliterated, the sub-adventitial vascular plane is accessed [26]. This approach can weaken the vessel under dissection and makes it vulnerable to rupture or avulse due to traction during surgery. It is advisable to leave a small portion of the adhered tumor tissue rather than jeopardizing major vessels.

Special care should be taken while dissecting veins like the vena cava and its tributaries which are thin walled and fragile as compared to aorta and can bleed profusely if avulsed during surgery.

### 29.7.2 Radiotherapy in Neuroblastoma

#### 29.7.2.1 Role of Radiation in Non-High-Risk Neuroblastoma

Multiple studies including the latest COG ANBL00B1 has reported very good outcomes in children with low-risk and intermediate-risk neuroblastoma with treatment options ranging from observation to surgery and chemotherapy without the use of radiation [27]. Thus, the role of radiation is limited in this group of patients. However, radiation is a useful option when used in children with tumor progression despite surgery and chemotherapy, or unresectable primary after chemotherapy having unfavorable biology or with symptomatic life- or organ-threatening conditions [28]. Radiation can be lifesaving in children with respiratory compromise due to hepatomegaly because of extensive hepatic metasatses in a 4S neuroblastoma [28]. Lower and easily tolerable dose of radiation is delivered to partial liver (3–6 Gy) in fractionated doses for symptom relief. Another indication of radiation could be for spinal cord compression in children who do not respond to chemotherapy [29]. As surgery and radiation lead to late orthopedic sequelae in young children albeit with good oncological outcomes, chemotherapy is the most preferred initial treatment in this clinical situation.

#### 29.7.2.2 Role of Radiotherapy in High-Risk Neuroblastoma

Radiation therapy in an integral part of the multimodal management protocol in high-risk neuroblastoma. A randomized controlled trial published in 1991 showed a benefit of adding radiation to the tumor bed as well as the lymph nodal region as it provides superior initial and long-term disease control compared with chemotherapy alone [30]. This study established the role of adjuvant radiation after surgical resection in high-risk disease. Adjuvant radiation to the tumor bed is generally sequenced after myeloablative therapy and stem cell transplant, and before immunotherapy/differentiating agent as a standard therapy for optimum outcomes [27].

Although distant relapse is the main obstacle to cure in these patients, local failure remains a significant problem. Late local recurrences are seen even in aggressively treated cases, some more than 5 years after completion of therapy. Thus, it is important to optimize local control with the addition of radiation to the tumor bed.

In a study from the Joint Center for Radiation Therapy/Dana-Farber Cancer Institute/Children's Hospital, 118 children who had undergone complete or near complete remission after chemotherapy and surgery and received adjuvant radiation experienced better local control than when radiation was not delivered [31].

This study emphasizes the importance of adjuvant RT even when only microscopic disease is left behind after surgery. Data from St Jude Children's Research Hospital displayed that the addition of RT to the therapy of a group of patients with more residual locoregional disease appeared to improve the local failure rate to approximately that of patients with less residual disease [32].

Both these studies show that use of radiation leads to better outcomes irrespective of the extent of residual disease post chemotherapy and surgery. As extensive lymph node irradiation has not shown benefit in terms of local progression or overall survival, it is generally not considered [33].

Multiple studies have reported local control outcomes of more than 90% with doses ranging from 20 Gy to 24 Gy at 1.5 to 1.8 Gy per fraction [34, 35]. Kushner et al. reported similar results with hyper fractionation, i.e., 21 Gy in 1.5 Gy twice-daily fractions regardless of the resection status [36], It has been understood that gross residual disease may mandate dose escalation of adjuvant radiation. However, in the Children's Oncology Group (COG) ANBL0532 phase III study, children received 21.6 Gy to the preoperative primary tumor volume and an additional boost of 14.4 Gy to the gross residual disease if any and the outcomes were compared with the COG A3973 historical cohort [37]. It was seen that the boost radiation to residual disease did not improve the incidence of local progression. Radiation target volumes are often irregular and close to critical normal structures. Though the doses are moderate, late sequelae are a concern in young children. Thus, the use of conformal radiation has an edge above conventional therapy [38, 39]. Panandikar et al. reported that ICRU 62-compliant IMRT with image guidance is a safe and effective method of achieving excellent locoregional control while respecting normal tissue tolerances [38]. Oshiro et al. in their study evaluating 21 sites mentioned that proton beam therapy can be may be conducted safely for patients with neuroblastoma that is difficult to manage using photon beams [40]. Hill-Kayser et al. proposed that proton therapy offers optimal combination of target coverage and organ sparing as compared to photon therapy in most of the cases [41]. However, they also recommended a customized approach with careful evaluation of renal dosimetry and mentioned that IMRT may be preferred in select cases.

#### 29.7.2.3 Role of Radiotherapy in Metastatic High-Risk Neuroblastoma

It has been observed in multiple reports that metastatic sites identified at the diagnosis experience higher relapse rates as compared to metastatic sites that have received radiation [42–44]. As many children present with extensive metastatic disease at the time of diagnosis, it is not feasible to treat all the metastatic sites. Hence, the sites that do not respond to systemic therapy and show residual disease on MIBG scan are considered for focal radiation as per the current treatment paradigm. Mazloom et al. consider 24 Gy to the avid residual metastatic sites along with radiation to the primary and achieved excellent local control at the metastatic sites [44]. They also mentioned that the number of MIBG-avid sites present after induction therapy was predictive of poor outcomes.

### 29.7.2.4 Long-Term Side Effects of Radiation in Children Treated with Neuroblastoma

As the survival of neuroblastoma is improving, it is important to understand the long-term side effects of radiation. However, with the current use of conformal radiation, the doses to the critical normal tissues can be limited and the long-term effects are expected to reduce. The late effects related to radiation could be renal, musculoskeletal, neurologic, endocrine, and second cancers [45, 46]. Long-term follow-up of children treated in clinical trials NB 90 and 94 showed that late effects occurred in 73% of the children and within the radiation fields in 50% of the children [47]. The most common late effect was musculoskeletal, and the threshold of its occurrence was 31 Gy. Results of a study from Memorial Sloan Kettering Cancer center, evaluating 276 children with high-risk neuroblastoma, found no evidence of chronic renal damage with modern radiation delivery techniques [48]. They also suggested mean kidney doses of 15 Gy to the more exposed kidney and 11 Gy to the less exposed kidney.

## References


1. Brodeur GM, Hogarty MD, Mosse YP, et al. Neuroblastoma. In: Pizzo PA, Poplack DG, editors. Principles and practice of pediatric oncology. 6th ed. Philadelphia: Williams and Wilkins; 2011. p. 886–922.
2. Shimada H, Ambros IM, Dehner LP, et al. The International Neuroblastoma Pathology Classification (the Shimada System). Cancer. 1999;86(2):364–72.
3. Dzieran J, Rodriguez Garcia A, Westermark UK, et al. *MYCN*-amplified neuroblastoma maintains an aggressive and undifferentiated phenotype by deregulation of estrogen and NGF signaling. Proc Natl Acad Sci USA. 2018;115(6):E1229–38.
4. Goodman MT, Gurney JG, Smith MA, Olshan AF. Sympathetic nervous system tumors. In: Ries LA, Smith MA, Gurney JG, et al., editors. Cancer incidence and survival among children and adolescents: United States SEER program, 1975–1995. Bethesda, MD: National Cancer Institute; 1999. p. 35.
5. Dinh T, Truong B, Matthay KK, DuBois SG. Comparison of clinical features and outcomes in patients with bilateral versus unilateral adrenal neuroblastoma. J Pediatr Hematol Oncol. 2017;39(2):108–13.
6. Barco S, Gennai I, Reggiardo G, Galleni B, Barbagallo L, Maffia A, et al. Urinary homovanillic and vanillylmandelic acid in the diagnosis of neuroblastoma: report from the Italian Cooperative Group for Neuroblastoma. Clin Biochem. 2014;47(9):848–52.
7. Parikh NS, Howard SC, Chantada G, Israels T, Khattab M, Alcasabas P, et al. SIOP-PODC adapted risk stratification and treatment guidelines: recommendations for neuroblastoma in low- and middle-income settings. Pediatr Blood Cancer. 2015;62(8):1305–16.
8. Vik TA, Pfluger T, Kadota R, Castel V, Tulchinsky M, Farto JC, et al. (123)I-mIBG scintigraphy in patients with known or suspected neuroblastoma: results from a prospective multicenter trial. Pediatr Blood Cancer. 2009;52(7):784–90.
9. Telli T, Lay Ergün E, Volkan Salanci B, Özgen KP. The complementary role of 68Ga-DOTATATE PET/CT in neuroblastoma. Clin Nucl Med. 2020;45(4):326–9.
10. Brodeur GM, Seeger RC, Barrett A, Berthold F, Castleberry RP, D'Angio G, et al. International criteria for diagnosis, staging, and response to treatment in patients with neuroblastoma. J Clin Oncol. 1988;6(12):1874–81.

11. Parhar D, Joharifard S, Lo AC, Schlosser MP, Daodu OO. How well do image-defined risk factors (IDRFs) predict surgical outcomes and survival in patients with neuroblastoma? A systematic review and meta-analysis. Pediatr Surg Int. 2020;36(8):897–907.
12. Monclair T, Brodeur GM, Ambros PF, Brisse HJ, Cecchetto G, Holmes K, et al. The international neuroblastoma risk group (INRG) staging system: an INRG task force report. J Clin Oncol. 2009;27(2):298–303.
13. Cohn SL, Pearson ADJ, London WB, Monclair T, Ambros PF, Brodeur GM, et al. The international neuroblastoma risk group (INRG) classification system: an INRG task force report. J Clin Oncol. 2009;27(2):289–97.
14. Treatment of patients with low/intermediate risk neuroblastoma. Children's Cancer and Leukaemia Group (CCLG). Neuroblastoma special interest group. 2015. http://www.cclg.org.uk/clinical-information/treatment-guidelines. Accessed 30 Nov 2016.
15. Zage PE, Kletzel M, Murray K, Marcus R, Castleberry R, Zhang Y, et al. Outcomes of the POG 9340/9341/9342 trials for children with high-risk neuroblastoma: a report from the children's oncology group. Pediatr Blood Cancer. 2008;51(6):747–53.
16. von Allmen D, Davidoff AM, London WB, Van Ryn C, Haas-Kogan DA, Kreissman SG, et al. Impact of extent of resection on local control and survival in patients from the COG A3973 study with high-risk neuroblastoma. J Clin Oncol. 2017;35(2):208–16.
17. Park JR, Kreissman SG, London WB, Naranjo A, Cohn SL, Hogarty MD, et al. Effect of tandem autologous stem cell transplant vs single transplant on event-free survival in patients with high-risk neuroblastoma: a randomized clinical trial. JAMA. 2019;322(8):746–55.
18. Matthay KK, Villablanca JG, Seeger RC, Stram DO, Harris RE, Ramsay NK, et al. Treatment of high-risk neuroblastoma with intensive chemotherapy, radiotherapy, autologous bone marrow transplantation, and 13-cis-retinoic acid. Children's cancer group. N Engl J Med. 1999;341(16):1165–73.
19. Shamberger RC, Allarde-Segundo A, Kozakewich HP, Grier HE. Surgical management of stage III and IV neuroblastoma: resection before or after chemotherapy? J Pediatr Surg. 1991;26(9):1113–8.
20. Rojas Y, Jaramillo S, Lyons K, et al. The optimal timing of surgical resection in high-risk neuroblastoma. J Pediatr Surg. 2016;51(10):1665–9.
21. Mansfield SA, McCarville MB, Lucas JT Jr, et al. Impact of neoadjuvant chemotherapy on image-defined risk factors in high-risk neuroblastoma. Ann Surg Oncol. 2022;29(1):661–70.
22. Martucciello G, Fati F, Avanzini S, Senes FM, Paraboschi I. The cervico-parasternal thoracotomy (CPT): a new surgical approach for the resection of cervicothoracic neuroblastomas. Children. 2021;8(3):229.
23. Fati F, Pulvirenti R, Paraboschi I, Martucciello G. Surgical approaches to neuroblastoma: review of the operative techniques. Children. 2021;8(6):446.
24. Galazka P, Czyzewski K, Marjanska A, Daniluk-Matras I, Styczynski J. Minimally invasive surgery in pediatric oncology: proposal of guidelines. Anticancer Res. 2019;39(11):5853–9.
25. Gabra HO, Irtan S, Cross K, et al. Minimally invasive surgery for neuroblastic tumours: a SIOPEN multicentre study: proposal for guidelines. Eur J Surg Oncol. 2022;48(1):283–91.
26. Warmann SW, Seitz G, Schaefer JF, Scheel-Walter HG, Leuschner I, Fuchs J. Vascular encasement as element of risk stratification in abdominal neuroblastoma. Surg Oncol. 2011;20(4):231–5.
27. Irwin MS, Naranjo A, Zhang FF, Cohn SL, London WB, Gastier-Foster JM, et al. Revised neuroblastoma risk classification system: a report from the Children's Oncology Group. J Clin Oncol. 2021;39(29):3229–41.
28. Doré M, Mahé MA, Corradini N, Demoor-Goldschmidt C. Neuroblastome néonatal, compliqué d'une hépatomégalie tumorale menaçante, traité par irradiation: absence de séquelle 20ans après [Neonatal neuroblastoma complicated with a threatening tumoral hepatomegaly treated by irradiation: No sequel 20 years later]. Cancer Radiother. 2015;19(8):749–51.
29. Bernardi BD, Quaglietta L, Haupt R, Castellano A, Tirtei E, Luksch R, et al. Neuroblastoma with symptomatic epidural compression in the infant: the AIEOP experience. Pediatr Blood Cancer. 2014;61:1369–75.

30. Castleberry RP, Kun LE, Shuster JJ, Altshuler G, Smith IE, Nitschke R, Wharam M, McWilliams N, Joshi V, Hayes FA. Radiotherapy improves the outlook for patients older than 1 year with pediatric oncology group stage C neuroblastoma. J Clin Oncol. 1991;9(5):789–95.
31. Rosen EM, Cassady JR, Kretschmar C, Levey R, Sallan SE. Neuroblastoma: the Joint Center for Radiation Therapy/Dana-Farber Cancer Institute/Children's Hospital experience. J Clin Oncol. 1984;2(7):719–32.
32. Robbins JR, Krasin MJ, Atmaram S, Panandiker P, Watkins A, Wuc J, et al. Radiation therapy as part of local control of metastatic neuroblastoma: the St Jude children's research hospital experience. J Pediatr Surg. 2010;45:678–86.
33. Braunstein SE, London WB, Kreissman SG, et al. Role of the extent of prophylactic regional lymph node radiotherapy on survival in high-risk neuroblastoma: a report from the COG A3973 study. Pediatr Blood Cancer. 2019;66(7):e27736.
34. Bradfield SM, Douglas JG, Hawkins DS, et al. Fractionated low-dose radiotherapy after myeloablative stem cell transplantation for local control in patients with high-risk neuroblastoma. Cancer. 2004;100:1268–75.
35. Gatcombe HG, Marcus RB, Katzensrein HM, Tighiouart M, Esiashvili N. Excellent local control from radiation therapy for high risk neuroblastoma. Int J Radiat Oncol Biol Phys. 2009;74(5):1549–54.
36. Kushner BH, Wolden S, LaQuaglia MP, et al. Hyperfractionated low-dose radiotherapy for high-risk neuroblastoma after intensive chemotherapy and surgery. J Clin Oncol. 2001;19:2821–8.
37. Liu KX, Naranjo A, Zhang FF, DuBois SG, Braunstein SE, Voss SD, et al. Prospective evaluation of radiation dose escalation in patients with high-risk neuroblastoma and gross residual disease after surgery: a report from the children's oncology group ANBL0532 study. J Clin Oncol. 2020;38(24):2741–52.
38. Panandiker ASP, Beltran C, Billups CA, McGregor LM, Furman WL, Davidoff AM. Intensity modulated radiation therapy provides excellent local control in high-risk abdominal neuroblastoma. Pediatr Blood Cancer. 2013;60:761–5.
39. Paulino AC, Ferenci MS, Chiang KY, Nowlan AW, Marcus RB Jr. Comparison of conventional to intensity modulated radiation therapy for abdominal neuroblastoma. Pediatr Blood Cancer. 2006;46:739–44.
40. Oshiro Y, Mizumoto M, Okumura T, Sugahara S, Fukushima T, Ishikawa H, et al. Clinical results of proton beam therapy for advanced neuroblastoma. Radiat Oncol. 2013;8:142.
41. Hill-Kayser C, Tochner Z, Both S, Lustig R, Reilly A, Balamuth N, et al. Proton versus photon radiation therapy for patients with high-risk neuroblastoma: the need for a customized approach. Pediatr Blood Cancer. 2013;60:1606–11.
42. Polishchuk AL, Li R, Hill-Kayser C, et al. Likelihood of bone recurrence in prior sites of metastasis in patients with high-risk neuroblastoma. Int J Radiat Oncol Biol Phys. 2014;89(4):839–45.
43. Li R, Polishchuk A, DuBois S, et al. Patterns of relapse in high-risk neuroblastoma patients treated with and without total body irradiation. Int J Radiat Oncol Biol Phys. 2017;97(2):270–7.
44. Mazloom A, Louis CU, Nuchtern J, et al. Radiation therapy to the primary and postinduction chemotherapy MIBG-avid sites in high-risk neuroblastoma. Int J Radiat Oncol Biol Phys. 2014;90(4):858–62.
45. Laverdière C, Liu Q, Yasui Y, et al. Long-term outcomes in survivors of neuroblastoma: a report from the childhood cancer survivor study. J Natl Cancer Inst. 2009;101:1131–11340.
46. Paulino AC, Mayr N, Simon JH, et al. Locoregional control in infants with neuroblastoma: role of radiation therapy and late toxicity. Int J Radiat Oncol Biol Phys. 2002;52:1025–31.
47. Ducassou A, Gambart M, Munzer C, et al. On behalf of the neuroblastoma study group and radiotherapy group of the French Society of Children with cancer (SFCE). Long-term side effects of radiotherapy for pediatric localized neuroblastoma results from clinical trials NB90 and NB94. Strahlenther Onkol. 2015;191:604–12.
48. Beckham TH, LaQuaglia MP, Kushner BH, Modak S, Wolden S. Renal function outcomes of high-risk neuroblastoma patients undergoing radiation therapy. Int J Radiat Oncol Biol Phys. 2017;99(2):486–93.

# Management of Pediatric Hodgkin Lymphoma

30

Divyesh Kumar, Pritam Singha Roy, and Harmandeep Singh

## 30.1 Introduction

Hodgkin's lymphoma (HL) is a clonal malignancy of the lymphatic system that arises from B cells of germinal and post-germinal centers. The disease has a bimodal age distribution, the first is observed between 15 and 30 years old and the second in the over 55 years old age group. Broadly, it is classified into classical and nodular lymphocyte-predominant HL. Classical HL is further subclassified into nodular sclerosis, lymphocyte rich, lymphocyte depleted, and mixed cellularity. The history of HL dates back to the year 1832 when the abnormalities in the lymph nodes were studied by English pathologist, Sir Thomas Hodgkin and was later named after him [1]. It is believed that the earliest mention of this disease was probably provided by Malpighi in the year 1666.

### 30.1.1 Clinical Assessment

The initial evaluation of a child with suspected Hodgkin lymphoma (HL) aims to exclude the other clinical differentials and assess the extent of the disease grossly. The differentials of pediatric Hodgkin lymphoma (PHL) include tuberculosis, reactive adenopathy, and indolent non-Hodgkin lymphoma such as anaplastic large cell lymphoma. The clinical assessment focuses on the distribution of lymphadenopathy, Waldeyer's ring, B-symptoms, bulky node(s), organomegaly, and signs of

D. Kumar (✉)
Department of Radiotherapy, PGIMER, Chandigarh, India

P. Singha Roy
Pediatric Hematology-Oncology, Medica Superspecialty Hospital, Kolkata, India

H. Singh
Department of Nuclear Medicine, PGIMER, Chandigarh, India



R. Madan et al. (eds.), *Evidence Based Practice in Pediatric Radiation Oncology*,
https://doi.org/10.1007/978-981-96-4872-6_30

superior mediastinal syndrome. The B-symptoms include any of unintentional weight loss of ≥10% within the preceding 6 months, drenching sweats on ≥3 nights, or unexplained recurrent fever ≥38 °C [2].

### 30.1.2 Initial Laboratory Evaluation

The preliminary investigations encompass a complete blood count with erythrocyte sedimentation rate (ESR), serum chemistry, ultrasound of the abdomen, and a chest radiograph. The blood work confirms adequate organ function, supports subsequent chemotherapy, and provides certain prognostic information, such as hemoglobin, ESR, and serum albumin.

### 30.1.3 Confirmation of Diagnosis and Staging

Excision biopsy of an enlarged superficial lymph node is the preferred diagnostic modality. In the absence of superficial lymphadenopathy, an image-guided needle biopsy from a deep-seated node is the alternative. An $^{18}$F-fluorodeoxyglucose positron-emission tomography (FDG-PET) coupled with computed tomography (CT) or magnetic resonance imaging of the neck, thorax, abdomen, and pelvis is the staging evaluation of choice. Excellent sensitivity and negative predictive value of PET/CT in detecting bone marrow infiltration obviates the need for marrow aspiration/biopsy in PHL [3, 4].

## 30.2 Imaging (18F-FDG PET-CT)

2-deoxy-2-[fluorine-18] Fluoro-D-glucose positron-emission tomography-computed tomography (18F-FDG PET-CT) is a hybrid imaging technique, providing both functional and anatomical information. FDG is a glucose analogue, which is transported into and phosphorylated by proliferating cells having high rate of glycolysis, as in tumors, e.g., Hodgkin lymphoma. Due to high sensitivity and impact on management in pediatric HL clinical trials, 18F-FDG PET-CT has gained acceptance as a recommended imaging modality for staging and response assessment in pediatric HL. The radiation dose from PET-CT needs optimization in pediatric population to minimize risks associated with radiation. PETMRI, if available, can eliminate radiation exposure due to CT. The nuclear medicine physician and team need to have optimal training and experience to perform procedures safely in children and interpret them.

### 30.2.1 Patient Preparation for FDG PET

Patients need to fast for 4–6 h prior to the procedure and avoid strenuous physical activity in the last 24 h. After intravenous cannulation, the child should be warm and relaxed for 15 min before 18F-FDG injection. The dose of 18F-FDG needs to be adjusted according to body weight (100 kBq/kg, minimum 37 MBq). PET with diagnostic CT scan is done 45–60 min after tracer injection. If the scan is done for interim response assessment, study should be planned immediately before next cycle of chemotherapy (2 weeks gap after last cycle). However, the final response assessment with PET scan needs to be planned after 4 weeks of the last chemotherapy cycle and 3 months after the radiotherapy completion, to avoid false positive results.

### 30.2.2 Role of PET-CT in Pediatric HL

1. *Staging*: 18F-FDG PET with diagnostic contrast-enhanced CT is a recommended imaging modality to stage pediatric HL, as per latest NCCN guidelines (v.1, 2022) [5]. PET-CT is a tool for risk- and response-adapted approach to manage pediatric HL [6]. PET and CT complement each other to provide comprehensive assessment of disease involvement. Following findings are considered PET+ for HL involvement at baseline: PET+ lymph node with long axis ≥1 cm, PET+ splenic lesion seen on morphological imaging (only splenomegaly and diffuse uptake are considered negative), subcentimetric PET+ lung lesions if no other etiology is expected, focal PET+ liver lesions, >3 sites of focal FDG uptake in bone marrow without changes on CT are considered definitive and marrow biopsy is not advised to confirm this finding (diffuse bone marrow uptake on PET is non-specific), PET+ cortical bone lesion. Bulky disease is defined differently according to European (≥200 mL volume) or US (>6 cm contiguous extra-mediastinal nodal mass or tumor involving >1/third of thoracic diameter on X-ray) guidelines (Fig. 30.1).
2. *Response assessment*: Interim response assessment after 2–3 chemotherapy cycles using PET-CT is recommended in intermediate-high risk disease, whereas end-treatment PET is recommended in all risk categories.

   Deauville scoring system is used for interim and end-treatment response assessment. The metabolic activity in the most active residual lesion is compared with physiological liver and blood activity in the images to arrive at the score: 1 (no uptake), 2 (uptake ≤ mediastinal blood pool), 3 (uptake > blood pool but ≤ liver), 4 (uptake moderately higher than liver), 5 (uptake markedly higher than liver), and X (uptake sites unlikely related to lymphoma). Deauville 1–3 at interim PET and 1–2 at end-treatment PET are considered as PET negative (complete response), whereas higher scores are considered as PET positive. PET-positive lesions at end treatment need to be re-biopsied to confirm residual disease before further treatment. Deauville scoring has been validated

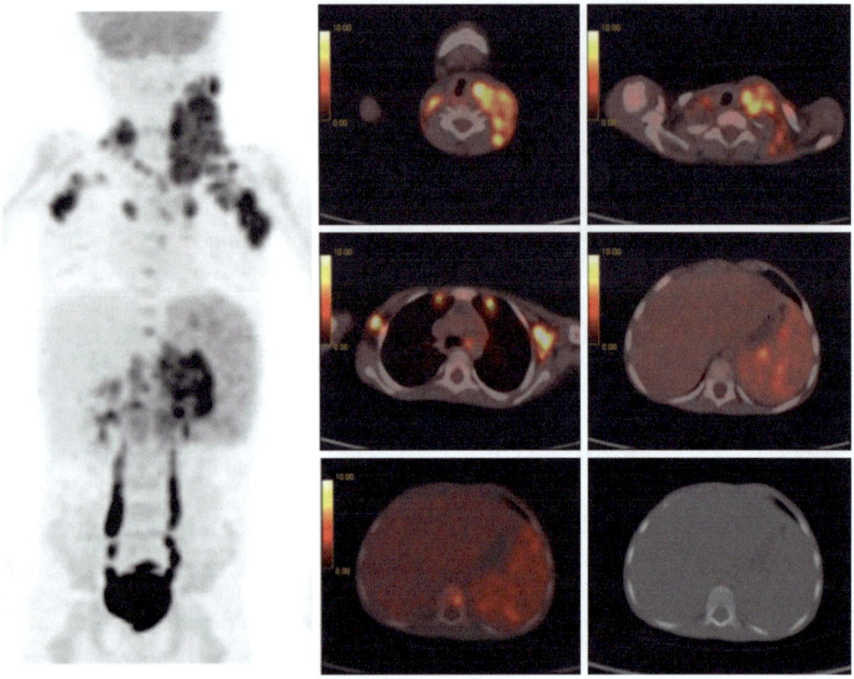

**Fig. 30.1** A 5-year male presented with history of fever, loss of weight and swelling in neck and axillae for 6 months. Biopsy from cervical lymph node revealed Hodgkin's lymphoma. Maximum intensity projection and axial fused PET-CT images of 18F-FDG PET-CT done for staging revealed metabolically active enlarged lymph nodes on both sides of diaphragm, splenic and marrow lesions (stage IV disease)

in clinical trials and incorporated in decision management algorithms for Pediatric HL (Fig. 30.2).

3. *Restaging*: PET-CT is not recommended for routine surveillance after completion of therapy and no residual disease. However, it is recommended when relapse is suspected clinically and recurrence need to be confirmed with histopathology. In addition to HL lesions, high glucose metabolism and resultant FDG uptake can be seen normally in some organs such as brain and liver as well as physiological processes such as adrenergic brown fat activation seen frequently in children in response to cold temperature. Inflammatory cells accumulated at sites of infection or inflammation can provide information about site of infection, in pyrexia of unknown origin cases. But it can lead to false positive interpretation in cases undergoing imaging for tumor localization, as in HL. Correlation with CT findings is needed for accurate interpretation of PET-CT, especially in cases with involvement of unexpected sites. Histopathological confirmation is advised in cases of discordant PET and CT findings and positive end-treatment PET before re-treatment.

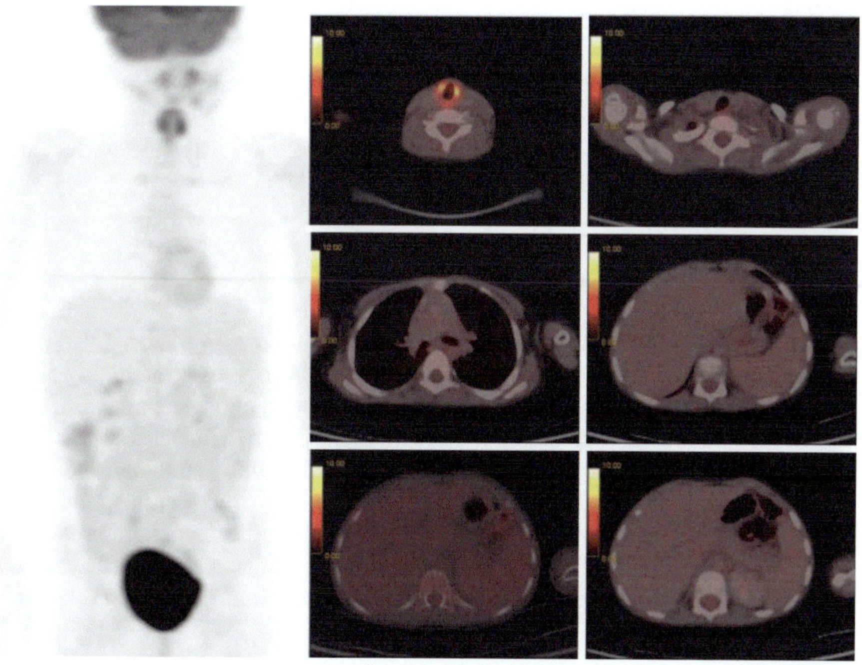

**Fig. 30.2** The patient underwent interim 18F-FDG PET-CT after 2 cycles of ABVD chemotherapy. Maximum intensity projection and axial fused PET-CT images of interim 18F-FDG PET-CT revealed metabolically inactive cervical lymph nodes with reduction in size and number of lesions (Deauville 1)

### 30.2.3 Prognostic Factors

An advanced stage, presence of B-symptoms, and bulky disease are conspicuous poor prognostic markers. The "bulky disease" is defined differently across the study groups, as either a diameter >1/3rd of the thoracic diameter on an upright anterior-posterior chest radiograph or extramediastinal nodal aggregate >6 cm in the longest transverse diameter on axial CT (Children's Oncology Group; COG) [7] or a contiguous tumor volume ≥200 mL (European Network of Pediatric Hodgkin's Lymphoma group; EuroNet-PHL) [8].

In addition, an elevated ESR (≥30 mm/h) is known to confer inferior event-free survival (EFS) for patients with limited-stage disease [8].

Childhood Hodgkin International Prognostic Score (CHIPS), a novel prognostic scoring system proposed by COG, carries reasonable value in predicting EFS. CHIPS incorporates four adverse prognostic markers: bulky mediastinal adenopathy, stage IV disease, hypoalbuminemia (<3.5 g/L), and fever [9]. A retrospective analysis by COG demonstrated adolescent age to confer a worse EFS than young children [10]. Finally, the response to induction chemotherapy carries immense prognostic relevance and is utilized for titrating the intensity of post-induction treatment, particularly radiotherapy.

### 30.2.4 Risk Stratification

Risk-stratified therapy is the standard of care for PHL. The risk-stratification systems differ subtly across the cooperative groups, albeit based on similar fundamental principles. The risk-stratification strategies followed by the COG and EuroNet-PHL are summarized in Table 30.1 [8, 11].

### 30.2.5 Systemic Therapy

#### 30.2.5.1 Principles of Chemotherapy and the Active Agents

The cardinal principle of chemotherapy combines non-cross-resistant, highly effective agents lacking overlapping toxicity. The amelioration of the late effects of chemotherapy is a crucial consideration and is the crux of the clinical trials on PHL over the last two decades. The late effects include infertility, pulmonary toxicity, cardiovascular diseases, and second malignancy [12]. Corticosteroids, anthracyclines, alkylating agents, vinca alkaloids, etoposide, and bleomycin are proven by the cooperative group studies to have promising activity against PHL. The chemotherapy regimens commonly used to treat PHL are summarized in Table 30.2 [13, 14].

#### 30.2.5.2 The Chemotherapy Regimens for Pediatric Classical Hodgkin Lymphoma

**The EuroNet-PHL-C1 Protocol**

The EuroNet-PHL, a multinational collaboration of five European pediatric oncology groups, has been instrumental in the evolution of PHL treatment. A low cumulative dose of anthracycline and replacing procarbazine with dacarbazine helped lessen the burden of cardiotoxicity and gonadal dysfunction, respectively. The

**Table 30.1** Risk stratification of pediatric Hodgkin lymphoma [8]

| EuroNet-PHL Group | | Children's Oncology Group | |
|---|---|---|---|
| TL-1 | Stage I, IIA | Low risk | Stage IA, IIA |
| TL-2 | Stage I, IIA with bulky disease[a] or ESR $\geq$30 mm/h or extranodal disease | Intermediate risk | Stage IA, IIA with extranodal disease or bulky disease[b] |
| | Stage IIB, IIIA | | Stage IB, IIB, IIIA, IVA |
| TL-3 | Stage IIB, IIIA with extranodal disease | High risk | Stage IIIB, IVB |
| | Stage IIIB, IV | | |

*CT* computed tomography, *ESR* erythrocyte sedimentation rate, *EuroNet-PHL* European Network on Pediatric Hodgkin's Lymphoma, *TL* treatment level

[a]Contiguous tumor volume $\geq$200 mL

[b]Mediastinal mass with a diameter >1/3rd of the thoracic diameter on an upright anterior-posterior chest radiograph or extramediastinal nodal aggregate >6 cm in the longest transverse diameter on axial CT

**Table 30.2** Chemotherapy protocols for pediatric Hodgkin lymphoma

| Name of the chemotherapy protocol | | Details of the chemotherapy regimen | Number of cycles administered |
|---|---|---|---|
| EuroNet-PHL [5]; OEPA/COPDac | | Induction therapy (OEPA): Vincristine 1.5 mg/$m^2$; days 1, 8, and 15, etoposide125 mg/$m^2$; days 1–5, prednisolone 60 mg/$m^2$/day; days 1–14, doxorubicin 40 mg/$m^2$; days 1 and 15<br>Consolidation therapy (COPDac): Cyclophosphamide 500 mg/$m^2$; days 1 and 8, vincristine 1.5 mg/$m^2$; days 1 and 8, prednisolone 40 mg/$m^2$; days 1–15, dacarbazine 250 mg/$m^2$; days 1–3 | Induction: 2 cycles for any TL<br>Consolidation: 1, 2, or 4 cycles for TL-1, TL-2 or TL-3, respectively |
| COG [8] | Low risk: AVPC | Doxorubicin 25 mg/ $m^2$; days 1 and 2, vincristine 1.4 mg/$m^2$; days 1 and 8, prednisone 40 mg/$m^2$; days 1–7, cyclophosphamide 600 mg/$m^2$; days 1 and 2 | 3 cycles[a] |
| | Intermediate or high risk: ABVE-PC | Doxorubicin: 30 mg/$m^2$; days 0 and 1, bleomycin 5 mg/$m^2$ (day 0) and 10 mg/$m^2$ (day 7), vincristine 1.5 mg/$m^2$; days 0 and 7, etoposide 75 mg/$m^2$; days 0–4, prednisolone 40 mg/$m^2$; days 0–7, cyclophosphamide 800 (intermediate risk) or 1200 mg/$m^2$ (high risk); day 0 | 4 (Intermediate risk) or 5 (high risk) cycles[b] |
| ABVD [11, 14] | | Doxorubicin 25 mg/$m^2$, bleomycin 15 mg/$m^2$, vinblastine 6 mg/$m^2$, dacarbazine: 375 mg/$m^2$ (each drug administered on day 1 and 15) | Stage I, IIA: 4 cycles; stage IIB or higher: 6 cycles |

*COG* Children's Oncology Group, *EuroNet-PHL* European Network for Pediatric Hodgkin's Lymphoma, *PET* positron-emission tomography, *TL* treatment level

[a]COG lacks a consensus on the chemotherapy strategy for low-risk disease. 3 cycles of AVPC may not be optimal for patients with nodular sclerosis histology, a high erythrocyte sedimentation rate, or positive PET after cycle 1 of chemotherapy

[b]Consolidation for slow early responders is augmented with 2 additional blocks DECA (dexamethasone, etoposide, cisplatin, cytarabine) or IV (ifosfamide, vinorelbine) for intermediate- or high-risk diseases, respectively. Patients with CHIPS score ≥2 also merit intensification of treatment

induction chemotherapy consists of two cycles of oncovin, etoposide, prednisolone, and adriamycin (OEPA). The induction therapy translates to an adequate response on the early reassessment PET, defined as ≥partial remission and PET-negativity, in 40% of patients, sparing them from radiotherapy [8].

The consolidation therapy combines cyclophosphamide, oncovin, prednisolone, and dacarbazine (COPDac). The number of consolidation blocks is adjusted on the risk stratification: low-, intermediate-, or high-risk disease receives 1, 2, or 4 cycles, respectively (Table 30.2). The ongoing EuroNet-PHL-C2 trial intensifies the consolidation therapy to curtail radiotherapy in a larger proportion of patients with intermediate or high-risk diseases [15].

### COG Protocols

The COG adopts a strategy of risk-stratified chemotherapy and early PET-based response assessment, similar to the European approach [11]. The chemotherapy regimens are inspired by the ABVD (adriamycin, bleomycin, vinblastine, dacarbazine) protocol, widely used for treating HL in adults. The two noticeable adaptations introduced by COG to the ABVD backbone include the replacement of dacarbazine and vinblastine with etoposide and vincristine, respectively. Patients with the low-risk disease received 3 cycles of chemotherapy. Radiotherapy is restricted to the patients failing to achieve a complete response following 3 cycles of chemotherapy. Patients with intermediate- or high-risk diseases receive 2 cycles of induction therapy followed by 2–4 cycles of consolidation (Table 30.2). Prospective COG trials have demonstrated a beneficial role in intensifying the consolidation treatment for the slow early responder group of patients [7, 16]. Brentuximab vedotin, a CD30-targeted antibody-drug conjugate, is currently being explored by COG in the frontline treatment of high-risk PHL [17, 18].

### The ABVD Protocol

The ABVD is a time-tested, highly effective chemotherapy regimen for adult HL. However, an apprehension of cardiomyopathy due to higher cumulative doses of anthracycline and bleomycin-induced pulmonary toxicity has precluded ABVD from gaining popularity in pediatric oncology. Nevertheless, low cost, ease of administration, fewer hematological toxicities, and lesser requirement of supportive care make the regimen an attractive alternative in the low-and middle-income countries (LMICs). Limited literature, predominantly from the LMICs, demonstrates excellent outcomes with ABVD regimen, both for limited or advanced-stage PHL. Patients with early (stage I, IIA) or advanced (≥stage IIB) disease are treated with 4 or 6 cycles of chemotherapy, respectively. Radiotherapy is restricted to patients with bulky disease or inadequate response to the initial two cycles of chemotherapy [14, 19, 20].

## 30.3 Role of Radiotherapy in Pediatric Hodgkin Lymphoma

Initially thought of as an incurable disease but ever since the discovery of X-rays, RT is useful for managing patients with HL. The earliest response to it with RT was first described by Pusey [21]. Later on, the work was carried forward by Gilbert who extended the radiation fields into the adjacent clinically uninvolved areas [22]. In 1950, Veterans ad colleagues published their findings where they found complete response (CR) with the usage of RT in patients of HL [23]. Subsequently in 1962, Kaplan published his findings of the usage of extended field radiation therapy (EFRT), where he found 5-year survival for a limited stage to be 70% [24]. Although RT improves survival in HL, the indications of RT in PHL are limited owing to the fear of late toxicities, particularly radiation-induced secondary malignancies (RISM). It also led to the field reduction from EFRT to more confined involved field radiation therapy (IFRT), and nowadays with further field reductions to involved

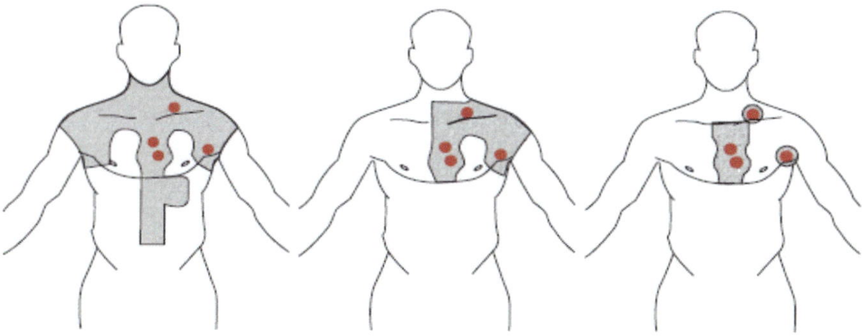

**Fig. 30.3** Figures depicting various RT fields (From left to right, i.e., Mantle field, IFRT, and INRT)

nodal radiation therapy (INRT) and involved site radiation therapy (ISRT) status (Fig. 30.3).

### 30.3.1 Journey from RT Alone to Its Use in Combined Modality Treatment (CMT) or Stage-Based Approach

RT alone remained the pillar of curative treatment for HL in the past; however, the cure was confined to patients whose entire extent of the disease could be included within radiation fields. More extensive fields carried the risk of RT-induced toxicities and thus, to manage the more extensive disease and overcome the effect of RT-induced late toxicities; researchers started their work on chemotherapy (CT) either alone or in combination with RT and over time, the role of CT has dominated over RT because of its excellent response. Hence, currently a risk-adapted CMT approach is used for PHL, and RT is given to those with inadequate response to CT or patients with poor prognostic factors.

### 30.3.2 Evaluation of RT Techniques in HL

RT techniques and field arrangements has been modified over time for managing patients of HL. In the prechemotherapy era, EFRT remained the primary modality of treatment. EFRT included the mantle field and the inverted Y field. Lymphatic regions included in the mantle field were the cervical, the mid-chest, and the axillary lymph nodes, whereas in the inverted Y field or the para-aortic fields were the regions below the diaphragm, i.e., all para-aortic, iliacal, and inguinal lymph nodes as well as upper femoral nodes. REPLY-As EFRT has its long-term consequences, slowly and gradually field reduction was tried and RT only to the involved sites was given, thus IFRT evolved as a part of CMT. In one study, HD-8 trial, EFRT and IFRT was compared [25]. The authors did not find any statistically significant differences in the outcome. As expected, fewer toxicities and late side effects were observed with IFRT. Further, not only field reduction but also dose reduction was sought subsequently. EORTC/GELA group advocated for further reduction in the RT field, also called involved nodal radiation therapy, where only lymph nodes that remained enlarged after CT was proposed. A small study in support of it was done by T. Girinsky et al. and it was found that there was a significant decrease in the RT dose to the cardiac and breast region [26]. Campbell et al. in their comparative study between EFRT/IFRT and INRT found a total of 12 relapses, i.e., four after EFRT (3%), five after IFRT (5%), and three after INRT (3%). Overall, no increase in relapses with INRT was observed when compared to EFRT/IFRT and also no recurrence after INRT in lymph nodes (size <5 cm) was observed [27].

Techniques such as intensity-modulated radiation therapy (IMRT) and volume-modulated arc therapy (VMAT) have gradually evolved which help in sparing organs at risk [28]. Techniques such as deep-inspiration breath-hold radiotherapy (DIBH) help in minimizing the dose to heart and lung in mediastinal lymphoma [29].

### 30.3.3 Indications of RT/Dose and Target Volume in the Present Era

RT indications and dosages vary with the risk category as shown in Fig. 30.4. According to EuroNet-PHL-C1 protocol, the decision of RT in all treatment groups (TG 1–3) depends on the response assessment after 2 cycles of chemotherapy as assessed by CT/MRI supplemented by PET scan. Those with adequate response to chemotherapy will not receive RT, while those with inadequate response will receive RT [8].

RT dose prescription varies with the intensity and regimen of chemotherapy before RT. Typically, RT doses as low as 15 to 25 Gy are used, and doses rarely

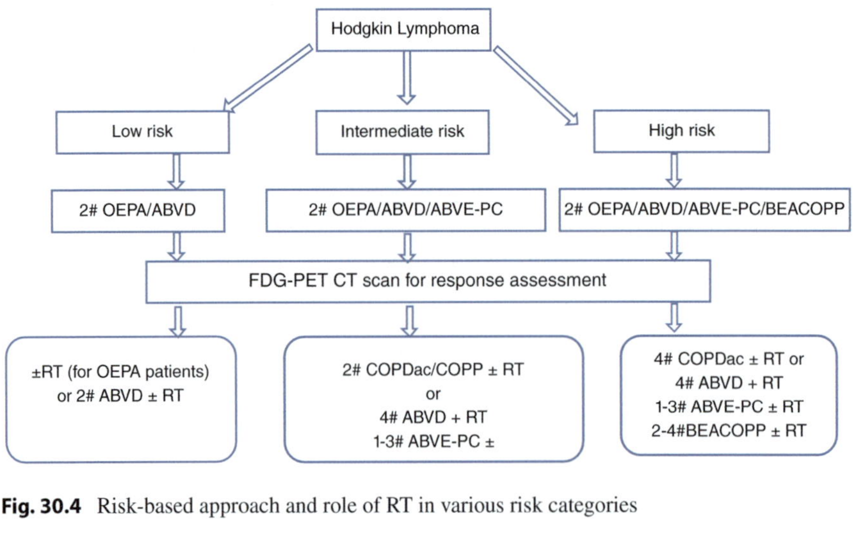


**Fig. 30.4** Risk-based approach and role of RT in various risk categories

exceeding 25 Gy are used in the pediatric setting [30]. A dose of 21 Gy in 14 fractions is used by the American Children's Oncology group [7]. According to EuroNet-PHL-C1 protocol, all initially involved lymph nodes with a margin of 1–2 cm should receive RT to a dose of 19.8 Gy/11 fractions. Those with poor response to chemotherapy (any site showing <75% response and >5 $cm^3$ or any residual site of disease >100 $cm^3$) or bulky disease should receive a boost to residual disease (+1–2 cm margin) to a dose of 10 Gy/5 fractions.

Detailed information on radiotherapy indications and target delineation is described in EuroNet-PHL-C1 protocol [8].

### 30.3.4 Proton Therapy in HL

With the advancement in technology, there is a huge interest in treating patients with proton therapy (PT). The PT carries the advantage of delivering a high dose of RT precisely with a steep cut off the dose after the peak attained (Brag peak), hence gives were little radiation to normal structures. Although very few organ toxicities have been found with the usage of PT, more studies are still required for confirming the findings [31]. Concerning second malignancies, PT carries a relatively lesser risk of developing carcinoma and sarcoma in comparison to other techniques. A study done by S. Lautenschlaeger et al. proposed using intensity-modulated proton therapy (IMPT) in younger patients (<30 years), especially for mediastinal lymphoma [32]. For pediatric HL patients, a study done by Tringale et al. found that PT resulted in marked dose sparing of organ at risk (OARs) with low rates of toxicity, no marginal failures, and excellent 5-year survival [33].

### 30.3.5 RT in Relapsed/Recurrent Cases

Despite excellent outcomes and good prognosis, relapse/recurrence is experienced in 10–15% of patients with HL disease. EuroNet group has discussed the detailed management of relapse/refractory HL [34].

## 30.4 Toxicities of Chemotherapy

Neutropenic sepsis is the most feared acute toxicity. Hematological toxicities are more frequent with the OEPA induction therapy than with ABVD, necessitating greater vigilance while using the EuroNet-PHL protocol [35]. Bleomycin-induced pulmonary toxicity is relatively rare in children than in adults. Late toxicities include anthracycline-related cardiomyopathy, alkylator-induced infertility, and second malignancy.

## 30.5 Supportive Care

Amelioration of chemotoxicities is pivotal in optimizing the survival in PHL. Episodes of febrile neutropenia warrant prompt antimicrobial therapy. Assessment of cardiac function at diagnosis and serially thereafter is performed to screen for anthracycline cardiotoxicity. A pulmonary function test is necessary before instituting a bleomycin-containing regimen. The option of fertility preservation should be offered to adolescents/ young adults.

## 30.6 Management of Nodular Lymphocyte-Predominant Hodgkin Lymphoma (NLPHL)

NLPHL is a biologically distinct form of HL, having a unique immunohistochemical (CD20 +, CD15/CD30 dual-negative) and molecular landscape. The disease often presents at a limited stage, restricted to the peripheral nodes. For stage IA disease, an excellent disease-free survival can be achieved with complete surgical excision of the involved node, barring adjuvant therapy. Incompletely resected stage IA or stage II diseases are conventionally treated with low-intensity chemotherapy. A combination of cyclophosphamide, vinblastine, and prednisolone (CVP) is most commonly utilized in this setting. Advanced-stage disease merits intensive chemotherapy. In the absence of uniform guidelines, the advanced-stage NLPHL is treated in line with the childhood classical HL or even mature B-non-Hodgkin lymphoma employing ABVD, OEPA/COPDac, or CHOP regimen with the incorporation of rituximab [36]. RT in the form of ISRT to the dose of 21Gy is given after 3 cycles of chemotherapy regimen if CR is not achieved [37].

## 30.7 Challenges in the LMICs

Late referral to the healthcare facility is rampant in the LMICs with a high prevalence of tuberculosis. Empirical antitubercular therapy in patients with lymphadenopathy leads to untoward delay in referral [38]. Delayed diagnosis results in advanced stage and a greater bulk of disease, malnutrition, and a higher burden of treatment-related toxicities. A high prevalence of treatment abandonment, incomplete staging evaluation due to limited access to radiology or nuclear imaging facilities, a lack of multidisciplinary coordination, and restricted availability of radiotherapy services are additional challenges in the developing world [39].

## References

1. Hodgkin T. On some morbid appearances of the absorbent glands and spleen. Med Chir Trans. 1832;17:68–114.

2. Shanbhag S, Ambinder RF. Hodgkin lymphoma: a review and update on recent progress. CA Cancer J Clin. 2018;68:116–32.
3. Hassan A, Siddique M, Bashir H, et al. 18F-FDG PET-CT imaging versus bone marrow biopsy in pediatric Hodgkin's lymphoma: a quantitative assessment of marrow uptake and novel insights into clinical implications of marrow involvement. Eur J Nucl Med Mol Imaging. 2017;44:1198–206.
4. Li Z, Li C, Chen B, et al. FDG-PET/CT versus bone marrow biopsy in bone marrow involvement in newly diagnosed paediatric lymphoma: a systematic review and meta-analysis. J Orthop Surg. 2021;16:482.
5. National Comprehensive Cancer Network. Pediatric Hodgkin Lymphoma (Version 1.2022). https://www.nccn.org/login?ReturnURL=https://www.nccn.org/professionals/physician_gls/pdf/ped_hodgkin.pdf. Accessed 16 Jun 2022.
6. Kluge R, Kurch L, Georgi T, Metzger M. Current role of FDG-PET in pediatric Hodgkin's lymphoma. Semin Nucl Med. 2017;47(3):242–57. Epub 2017 Mar 6. https://doi.org/10.1053/j.semnuclmed.2017.01.001.
7. Friedman DL, Chen L, Wolden S, et al. Dose-intensive response-based chemotherapy and radiation therapy for children and adolescents with newly diagnosed intermediate-risk Hodgkin lymphoma: a report from the Children's Oncology Group Study AHOD0031. J Clin Oncol. 2014;32:3651–8.
8. Mauz-Körholz C, Landman-Parker J, Balwierz W, et al. Response-adapted omission of radiotherapy and comparison of consolidation chemotherapy in children and adolescents with intermediate-stage and advanced-stage classical Hodgkin lymphoma (EuroNet-PHL-C1): a titration study with an open-label, embedded, multinational, non-inferiority, randomised controlled trial. Lancet Oncol. 2022;23:125–37.
9. Schwartz CL, Chen L, McCarten K, et al. Childhood Hodgkin international prognostic score (CHIPS) predicts event-free survival in Hodgkin lymphoma: a report from the children's oncology group. Pediatr Blood Cancer. 2017;64:e26278.
10. Kahn JM, Pei Q, Friedman DL, et al. Survival by age in paediatric and adolescent patients with Hodgkin lymphoma: a retrospective pooled analysis of children's oncology group trials. Lancet Haematol. 2022;9:e49–57.
11. Lo AC, Dieckmann K, Pelz T, et al. Pediatric classical Hodgkin lymphoma. Pediatr Blood Cancer. 2021;68(Suppl 2):e28562.
12. Ehrhardt MJ, Flerlage JE, Armenian SH, Castellino SM, Hodgson DC, Hudson MM. Integration of pediatric Hodgkin lymphoma treatment and late effects guidelines: seeing the Forest beyond the trees. J Natl Compr Cancer Netw. 2021;19:755–64.
13. Keller FG, Castellino SM, Chen L, et al. Results of the AHOD0431 trial of response adapted therapy and a salvage strategy for limited-stage classical Hodgkin lymphoma: a report from the children's oncology group. Cancer. 2018;124:3210–9.
14. Mahajan A, Singh M, Bakhshi S, et al. Treating early-stage Hodgkin lymphoma in resource-limited settings: InPOG-HL-15-01 experience. Pediatr Blood Cancer. 2021;68:e29219.
15. University of Giessen. European Network-Paediatric Hodgkin lymphoma study group (EuroNet-PHL) second international inter-group study for classical Hodgkin lymphoma in children and adolescents. clinicaltrialsgov; 2021. https://clinicaltrials.gov/ct2/show/NCT02684708.
16. Kelly KM, Cole PD, Pei Q, et al. Response-adapted therapy for the treatment of children with newly diagnosed high risk Hodgkin lymphoma (AHOD0831): a report from the Children's Oncology Group. Br J Haematol. 2019;187:39–48.
17. National Cancer Institute (NCI). A randomized phase 3 study of Brentuximab Vedotin (SGN-35) for newly diagnosed high-risk classical Hodgkin Lymphoma (CHL) in children and young adults. clinicaltrials.gov; 2022. https://clinicaltrials.gov/ct2/show/NCT02166463.
18. Metzger ML, Link MP, Billett AL, et al. Excellent outcome for pediatric patients with high-risk Hodgkin lymphoma treated with Brentuximab Vedotin and risk-adapted residual node radiation. J Clin Oncol. 2021;39:2276–83.

19. Jain S, Bakhshi S, Seth R, et al. Risk based and response adapted radiation therapy for children and adolescents with newly diagnosed advanced stage Hodgkin lymphoma treated with ABVD chemotherapy: a report from the Indian pediatric oncology group study InPOG-HL-15-01. Leuk Lymphoma. 2022;63:1111–8.
20. Sherief LM, Elsafy UR, Abdelkhalek ER, et al. Hodgkin lymphoma in childhood: clinicopathological features and therapy outcome at 2 centers from a developing country. Medicine (Baltimore). 2015;94(15):e670.
21. Pusey WA. Cases of sarcoma and Hodgkin's disease treated by exposure to X-rays: preliminary report. J Am Med Assoc. 1902;38:166–9.
22. Gilbert R. Notre methode de roentgentherapie de la lymphomagranulomatose (Hodgkin's): resultats eloignes. Acta Radiol. 1931;12:523.
23. Petres MA. A study of survival in Hodgkin's disease treated radiologically. Am J Roentgenol. 1950;63:299–311.
24. Kaplan H. The radical radiotherapy of regionally localized Hodgkin's disease. Radiology. 1962;78:553–61.
25. Weber DC, Peguret N, Dipasquale G, Cozzi L. Involved node and involved-field volumetric modulated arc vs. fixed beam intensity-modulated radiotherapy for female patients with early-stage supra-diaphragmatic Hodgkin's lymphoma: a comparative planning study. International Journal of Radiation Oncology Biology Physics. 2009;75(5):1578–86.
26. Girinsky T, Pichenot C, Beaudre A, Ghalibafian M, Lefkopoulos D. Is intensity-modulated radiotherapy better than conventional radiation treatment and three-dimensional conformal radiotherapy for mediastinal masses in patients with Hodgkin's disease, and is there a role for beam orientation optimization and dose constraints assigned to virtual volumes? Int J Radiat Oncol Biol Phys. 64(1):218.
27. Campbell BA, Voss N, Pickles T, et al. Involved-nodal radiation therapy as a component of combination therapy for limited-stage Hodgkin's lymphoma: a question of field size. J Clin Oncol. 2008;26(32):5170–4.
28. Goodman KA, Toner S, Hunt M, et al. Intensity-modulated radiotherapy for lymphoma involving the mediastinum. Int J Radiat Oncol Biol Phys. 2005;62:198–206.
29. Paumier A, Ghalibafian M, Gilmore J, et al. Dosimetric benefits of intensity-modulated radiotherapy combined with the deep-inspiration breath hold technique in patients with mediastinal Hodgkin's lymphoma. Int J Radiat Oncol Biol Phys. 2012;82(4):1522–7.
30. Hunger SP, Link MP, Donaldson SS. ABVD/MOPP and low-dose involvedfield radiotherapy in pediatric Hodgkin's disease: the Stanford experience. J Clin Oncol. 1994;12(10):2160–6.
31. Newhauser WD, Fontenot JD, Mahajan A, et al. The risk of developing a second cancer after receiving craniospinal proton irradiation. Phys Med Biol. 2009;54(8):2277–91.
32. Lautenschlaeger S, Iancu G, Flatten V, Baumann K, Thiemer M, Dumke C, Zink K, Hauswald H, Vordermark D, Mauz-Körholz C, Engenhart-Cabillic R, Eberle F. Advantage of proton-radiotherapy for pediatric patients and adolescents with Hodgkin's disease. Radiat Oncol. 2019;14(1):157.
33. Tringale KR, Modlin LA, Sine K, Forlenza CJ, Cahlon O, Wolden SL. Vital organ sparing with proton therapy for pediatric Hodgkin lymphoma: toxicity and outcomes in 50 patients. Radiother Oncol. 2022;168:46–52.
34. Daw S, Hasenclever D, Mascarin M, et al. Risk and response adapted treatment guidelines for managing first relapsed and refractory classical Hodgkin lymphoma in children and young people. Recommendations from the EuroNet Pediatric Hodgkin Lymphoma Group. Hemasphere. 2020;4(1):e329.
35. Palayullakandi A, Trehan A, Jain R, et al. Retrospective single-center experience with OEPA/COPDAC and PET-CT based strategy for pediatric Hodgkin lymphoma in a LMIC setting. Pediatr Hematol Oncol. 2022;39:587.
36. Mauz-Körholz C, Lange T, Hasenclever D, et al. Pediatric nodular lymphocyte-predominant Hodgkin lymphoma: treatment recommendations of the GPOH-HD study group. Klin Padiatr. 2015;227:314–21.

37. Appel BE, Chen L, Buxton AB, Hutchison RE, Hodgson DC, Ehrlich PF, Constine LS, Schwartz CL. Minimal treatment of low-risk, pediatric lymphocyte-predominant Hodgkin lymphoma: a report from the Children's Oncology Group. J Clin Oncol. 2016;34(20):2372–9.
38. Mahajan A, Bakhshi S, Singh M, et al. Empirical antitubercular treatment for lymphadenopathy: are we missing lymphoma? Indian J Pediatr. 2022;90:761.
39. Hessissen L, Khtar R, Madani A, et al. Improving the prognosis of pediatric Hodgkin lymphoma in developing countries: a Moroccan Society of Pediatric Hematology and Oncology study. Pediatr Blood Cancer. 2013;60:1464–9.

# Total Body Irradiation and Role of RT in Leukemia

# 31

Soumya Sarkar, Prateek Mehra, and Deepak Gupta

## 31.1 Introduction

Hematopoietic stem cell transplantation is the technique through which a patient's hematopoietic system is reconstituted to ensure that the incoming stem cells are able to colonize the bone marrow. This requires the usage of high-dose chemotherapy and/or total body irradiation (TBI). TBI takes advantage of the fact that hematopoietic cells are exquisitely sensitive to irradiation. Hematopoietic stem cell transplantation can be of two types—autologous or allogeneic. Autologous transplant involves administration of high-dose chemotherapy and/or TBI to ablate the cancer cells and the hematopoietic system of the patient. Allogeneic transplantation, however, involves a graft-versus-tumor effect in addition to the cytotoxicity by medication or radiotherapy. Autologous transplantation is usually indicated in diseases such as multiple myeloma, relapsed Hodgkin's lymphoma, and relapsed diffuse large B cell lymphoma. Allogeneic transplantation is indicated in high risk/relapsed acute myeloblastic leukemia (AML) and acute lymphoblastic leukemia (ALL).

Conditioning is the process of using high-dose chemotherapy or TBI to overcome tumor resistance in autologous stem cell transplant. However, in an allogeneic stem cell transplant, conditioning serves to cause immunosuppression to prevent graft rejection, to provide space in the bone marrow for donor stem cells, and to achieve maximal cytoreduction before transplant is carried out. These regimens can vary in several ways, depending on the type of transplant, whether it is myeloablative or non-myeloablative, the disease type and status, and the expected tolerance of the patient.

Many dose regimens have been tried for TBI. A randomized trial compared 12 gray (Gy) versus 15.75 Gy in AML patients [1].While relapse-free survival

S. Sarkar · P. Mehra · D. Gupta (✉)
Division of Radiation Oncology, Medanta Cancer Institute, Medanta The Medicity, Gurgaon, Haryana, India





R. Madan et al. (eds.), *Evidence Based Practice in Pediatric Radiation Oncology*, https://doi.org/10.1007/978-981-96-4872-6_31

increased in the 15.75 Gy group, it came at the cost of increased transplant-related mortality and no difference in overall survival was observed. Trials comparing single fraction regimens, e.g., 9.2 Gy or 10 Gy in one fraction, against 12 Gy in 6 fractions have found higher incidence of pneumonitis in single fraction regimens [2]. A Parisian study compared single fraction and multi-fraction regimens with varying dose rates and found no significant differences between the regimens [3]. Most data support the usage of fractionated regimens with a low-dose rate approach.

When considering the role of chemotherapy, one must keep in mind that the choice of chemotherapy agent depends on the underlying disease. Usually, high-dose cyclophosphamide is used; however, other options include etoposide, melphalan, or fludarabine combined with TBI. Chemotherapy can be given either before or after TBI. However, concurrent usage is discouraged because of possibility of increased toxicity. TBI given before chemotherapy allows for the patient to tolerate TBI more easily because the side effects of chemotherapy have not manifested yet, however, TBI after chemotherapy allows for the stem cell transplant to occur immediately afterward, hence decreasing the neutropenic period after TBI. Chemotherapy-alone regimens are used in institutes where TBI may not be available. The more common regimens include busulfan and cyclophosphamide or busulfan and fludarabine [4, 5]. Hodgkin's and non-Hodgkin's lymphoma patients can be treated with BEAM protocol (carmustine, etoposide, cytosine arabinoside, and melphalan) [6]. Comparisons have been made between TBI-based and chemotherapy-alone-based regimens. However, because of inclusion of multiple leukemia subtypes and usage of older TBI or chemotherapy regimens, there is difficulty in reaching strong conclusions. The general trend of the data indicates that TBI appears to be an important part of the regimen in ALL, but in AML, a combination of TBI with cyclophosphamide is preferable.

Toxicity of the conditioning regimens must be kept in mind before beginning any treatment. It is important to assess what the patient will be able to tolerate before commencing conditioning. The side effects include nausea, vomiting, fatigue, effects due to myelosuppression, such as neutropenia, anemia, and thrombocytopenia, and drug-specific adverse events. When TBI is administered, an important toxicity to be kept in mind is pneumonitis. Assessment of pulmonary function should be carried out before TBI is considered. Other major adverse events of TBI include cataracts and endocrine deficiencies.

## 31.2 Treatment Techniques

Historically, TBI was delivered with a relatively homogenous dose throughout the whole body as leukemias are systemically distributed. Higher photon energies more than 20 megavolts (MV) have been used to deliver higher doses to the marrow, because of increased pair production and higher bone absorption [7]. Beam spoilers are used to correct skin-sparing effects of megavoltage irradiation. Increased doses of radiation can be delivered to brain in patients with central nervous system (CNS) involvement or to the testes in males with ALL. Because of large variations in body structure and tissue density between patients, it is recommended that the dose homogeneity remain within ±10% of the prescribed dose, though commonly ±5% is attainable.

### 31.2.1 Linear Accelerator-Based TBI

Linear accelerator-based TBI commonly uses large radiation fields than the maximum field size (40 by 40 cm) available at standard source-to-surface distance (SSD) by treating patients at extended SSDs of 200 to 600 cm. In treatment rooms capable of accommodating an SSD of 5 m or more, a single square field with maximum collimator opening is sufficient to accommodate typical sized patients placed along the diagonal of the field. At shorter SSDs, multiple abutting fields are used, and irradiation of the whole body is achieved by translating the radiation field [8] or the patient [9] or by sweeping the radiation field over a stationary patient [10]. Using multiple fields leads to dosimetric complications at the junctions. But this also raises the possibility that with the sequential delivery of abutting fields, the cells circulating through the body may receive a lower dose (Fig. 31.1).

There has been significant improvement in treatment delivery with the advent of intensity-modulated radiation therapy (IMRT) and other advanced delivery systems like volumetric-modulated arc therapy (VMAT) and Tomotherapy. These techniques help in delivering customized dose distributions throughout the whole body. These

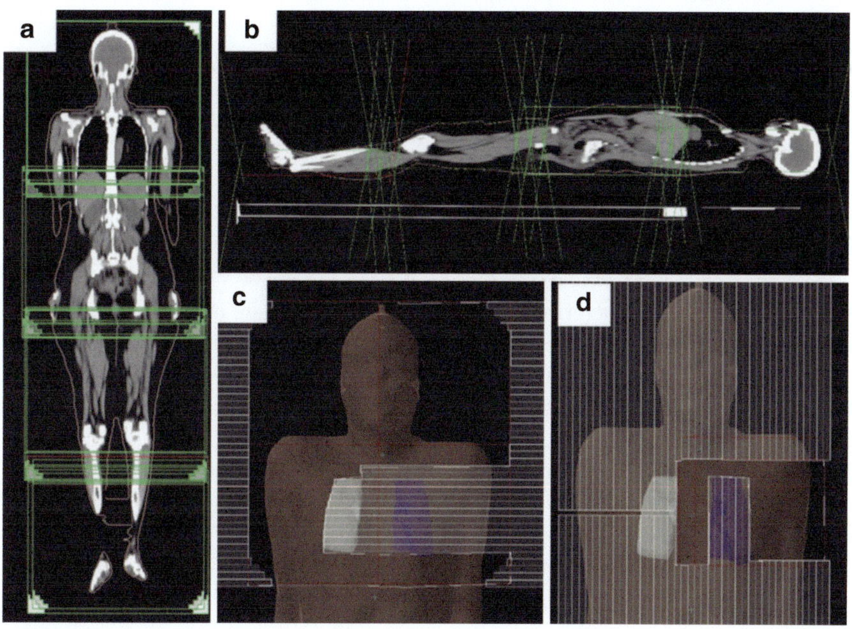


**Fig. 31.1** Treatment plan showing shifting field technique (**a** and **b**), lung shield (**c**), boost field (**d**) in Linac-based TBI

**Table 31.1** Comparison of TBI on conventional Linac versus Tomotherapy

| Characteristics | Linac | Tomotherapy |
|---|---|---|
| Patient position | Standing, supine, bilateral, prone | Only supine |
| Electron boost | Available | Not available |
| Lung shielding | Required | Not required |
| No of junctions | 3 or more | Only one |
| Patient comfort | Less | Is more |
| Rotational correction | Manual | Automatic |
| Overall dose distribution | Good | Excellent |

techniques increase the therapeutic ratio of TBI by delivering integrated boost dose to total marrow or the lymphatic system while reducing the dose to critical organs.

### 31.2.2 Tomotherapy-Based TBI

Tomotherapy allows better dose distribution and homogeneity with selective dose reduction to organs at risk (Table 31.1). TBI planning includes 2 radiation planning scans [head-first scan (HFS) and feet-first scan (FFS)] if patient length exceeds 120 cm. A radio-opaque marker is placed on the anterior surface of thigh, corresponding to the junction area. A margin of 2 cm is given for the planning target volume (PTV). In case of HFS and FFS scan, the PTV is divided into upper and lower PTV. A gap of 7 cm between the PTVs accounts for the junction dose. During planning, about 7 PTVs are contoured between upper and lower PTV and graduated lower doses are prescribed to it. Thus, a homogeneous prescription dose can be achieved at the junction after plan summation. For single-fraction TBI, Tomo-direct plan can be made. But if patient separation is >40 cm, helical Tomotherapy is the only option.

## 31.3 Dose Characterization of TBI

Careful dosimetric characterization is necessary for accurate treatment planning.

The American Association of Physicists in Medicine (AAPM) task group 29 (TG-29) report on the physical aspects of TBI provides a comprehensive guideline on dosimetry and techniques specific to large-field TBI [11]. After an irradiation technique has been chosen and commissioned for clinical use, an in vivo dosimetry check should be performed. Doses should be measured for actual treatment given by placing thermoluminescent dosimeter (TLD) capsules or chips on patient's skin, surrounded by suitable build-up bolus. TLD results must be compared with exit doses by summing entrance and exit doses at the location of TLDs and considering the thickness variation, compensation, and off-axis ratios at the depth of TLDs. A variation of ±5% between calculated and measured doses is acceptable. Most treatment protocols allows for an overall dose uniformity of ±10%.

AAPM task group 17 (TG 17) recommends that TBI should be delivered at a low-dose rate of 5–10 cGy/min. The clinical outcome after TBI depends on the dose rate [12]. Field sizes with long axis more than 1.8 m is required to adequately cover the body size of an adult. In conventional radiotherapy, skin sparing is typically planned when using megavoltage irradiation. However, it is important for the skin surface to receive nearly the full prescribed dose, as leukemia can circulate through the skin. When indicated, the skin dose can be increased by applying a bolus directly on the skin surface or by using a beam spoiler placed between the radiation source and the patient [13]. The beam spoiler generates scattered electrons as the TBI photons pass through it, which deposit most of their energy at shallow depths near the skin surface.

### 31.3.1 Dose Specification

As different centers use different treatment techniques for TBI, there can be significant variations in dose distributions depending on the treatment methods employed. AAPM TG 17 reports various methods for prescribing the dose for TBI:

1. Calculation of the integral dose to determine the average dose.
2. Calculation of limited average that includes areas of high and low dose.
3. Minimum tumor dose at the midpoint of the maximum separation.
4. Single-point prescription which specifies acceptable dose limits for the highest and lowest doses at any point throughout the body.

### 31.3.2 Dose Attenuation for Lung and Other Organs

Lung shielding has been used in many transplant centers to reduce the risk of pneumonitis (Fig. 31.2).

However, overcompensation carries a risk of leukemia recurrence. A study analyzing patients receiving 10 Gy as a single fraction of TBI reported increased leukemia recurrences whose lung dose was reduced to 6 Gy with lung blocks compared with 8 Gy [14]. Different techniques have been used to attenuate lung doses like lead filters and brass compensators depending on the treatment technique. Some institutes have used partial transmission blocks to the liver and kidneys to reduce the risk of hepatic veno-occlusive disease or nephropathy [15, 16]. When TBI is used for non-neoplastic conditions, such as aplastic anemia, where the primary goal is immunosuppression, radiosensitive structures such as the gonads or eyes can be shielded to reduce their radiation exposure [17].

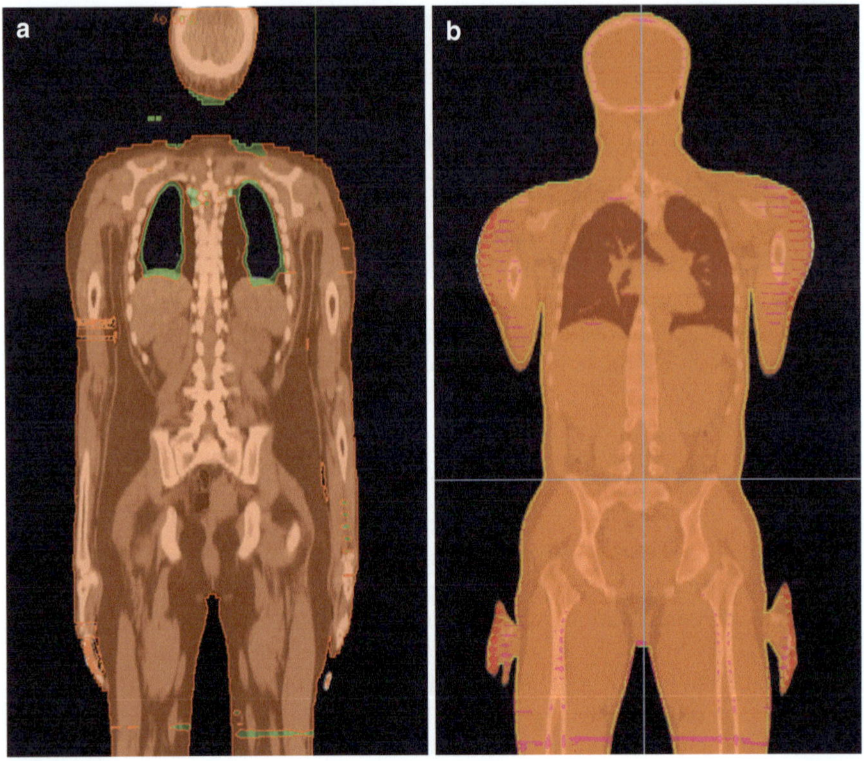

**Fig. 31.2** TBI plan on tomotherapy with lung shield (**a**) and without lung shield (**b**)

## 31.4 Boosting of Selected Organs with TBI

Theoretically, regions of the body where there is a higher burden of disease at the time of transplant can be boosted along with TBI. This is particularly important when treating diseases with a propensity to involve the CNS or testes. In patients with ALL, CNS-preventative therapy may include cranial irradiation. Increased cumulative dose upto 18 Gy may be delivered to the CNS. Similarly, the testes in males with ALL may be boosted to a cumulative dose of approximately 16–18 Gy. As the risk of toxicity with testicular irradiation is low regardless of fraction size, and testicular relapses have not observed after TBI, dose prescriptions for testicular boosting may vary from 0 to 4 Gy.

### 31.4.1 Acute and Late Toxicities of TBI

Toxicity from TBI can be due to various factors, including the total dose, fractionation, the type of disease being treated, the use of concurrent chemotherapy with radiotherapy, and individual patient characteristics [18]. Isolation of toxicities related to TBI alone is complicated.

#### 31.4.1.1 Acute Toxicity

Nausea, vomiting, and diarrhea are the common early side effects encountered in single fraction 8 to 10 Gy TBI. Xerostomia, headaches, fevers, and hypertension have been reported in roughly half of patients receiving single-fraction TBI [19]. The use of fractionated dose in TBI reduces the incidence and severity of these side effects [20, 21]. Patients can develop xerostomia, dry eye, and mucositis within 10 days. Complete reversible alopecia develops at 2 weeks in all patients [22]. Parotiditis usually occurs after the first day of irradiation and usually subsides over 2–3 days. It is unique to TBI and is very common with single-fraction RT but occurs in <10% of cases with fractionated regimens [20].

#### 31.4.1.2 Late Toxicity

##### Lung

Interstitial pneumonitis is the major dose-limiting toxicity associated with TBI. The lung-sparing effect of fractionation has been shown to be beneficial down to approximately 1 Gy [23]. Travis et al. examined the rate of lung repair between fractions and identified two repair phases: a fast repair half-time of 0.40 h and a slow repair half-time of 4.01 h [24]. The slow repair phase is particularly important when designing TBI schedules that involve 2 or 3 fractions per day. In a randomized controlled trial by Deeg et al. comparing single-fraction TBI (9.2 or 10 Gy) with fractionated TBI (12 Gy in 6 fractions over 3 days) for patients with AML in first remission, the risk of interstitial pneumonitis was reduced from 26% to 15% with fractionation [2].

Another strategy to reduce the risk of interstitial pneumonitis is to decrease the radiation dose rate. In fractionated TBI, dose rates ranging from 5 to 20 cGy/min are commonly used, typically determined by the available output of linear accelerators at extended treatment distances. A small study comparing dose rates of 7.5 cGy/min versus 15 cGy/min in TBI with a prescribed dose of 12 Gy in 6 fractions found a pneumonitis risk of 13% versus 43%, respectively, though the study had several confounding factors [25]. Additionally, a study by Sagus Sampath et al. concluded that the total lung dose is a more critical factor in determining the risk of pneumonitis [26].

##### Lens

The Seattle marrow transplant team reported >75% patients developing cataract 5 years or more after single-fraction TBI. The risk of cataract gets reduced with fractionation. Ozhasin et al. reported a significant difference in the 5-year estimated cataract incidence between single-fraction TBI (39%) and fractionated TBI (13%). Another study showed that the probability of cataract surgery was 85% after single-fraction TBI and 20% after fractionated TBI [27]. Seattle long-term analysis reported the risk of cataracts to be 85%, 50%, 34%, and 19% after 10-Gy single-fraction TBI, >12-Gy fractionated TBI, 12-Gy fractionated TBI, and no TBI, respectively [28]. Steroid therapy is an independent risk factor for cataract formation after bone marrow transplantation, even in the absence of TBI. Lens shielding in TBI is not done to avoid the risk of retro-ocular relapse of leukemia, but can be considered in aplastic anemia and other non-neoplastic disease managed with stem cell transplant (SCT).

### Growth and Endocrine Effects

Decreased growth velocity is reported in children undergoing bone marrow transplantation with TBI, although the incidence is less with fractionated TBI compared to single-fraction TBI. Growth hormone deficiency has been reported in approximately 34% of adults who received TBI in their childhood. Other endocrine effects include Leydig cell dysfunction in 23% and primary hypothyroidism in 34% [29]. High-dose TBI produces primary gonadal failure in almost all patients, but recovery may occur in females [30]. Thyroid dysfunction has been reported in as many as 43% of patients after TBI [31, 32].

### Liver

Hepatic veno-occlusive disease (VOD), also referred as sinusoidal obstructive syndrome (SOS), is seen in myeloablative transplants. This hepatocyte injury and hepatic thrombosis are secondary late effects [33–35]. This syndrome is associated with high morbidity and mortality in high-dose transplant regimens and is characterized by hepatomegaly, ascites, jaundice, encephalopathy, and weight gain in 10 to 40% of patients [20, 36]. Fractionated TBI and keeping total dose below 13.2 Gy reduces incidence of VOD/SOS. Barrett et al. showed a decrease in the incidence of VOD/SOS with a lower dose rate [37]. Administration of low molecular weight heparins and ursodiol is used as prevention strategies to reduce VOD/SOS [35].

### Kidney

Recent studies report the risk of renal toxicity at 17% in patients receiving TBI, immunosuppressive agents, and in presence of significant graft-versus-host disease (GVHD) [38]. As patients undergoing transplant receive various nephrotoxic drugs, the contribution of TBI to renal dysfunction is not well established [39]. A study by Helenglass et al. compared cyclophosphamide-TBI with melphalan-TBI and reported that the benefit of melphalan in reducing the relapse rate was offset by its nephrotoxic effect. Some studies have suggested that kidney doses over 12 Gy are associated with increased risk of nephropathy [16].

### Secondary Cancers

The risk of secondary malignancy in patients receiving TBI is approximately 4 times higher than the general population [40]. Rochelle Curtis et al. analyzed 19,229 patients who received transplants and reported 80 new solid tumors with an observed to expected (O/E) ratio of 2.7 ($p < 0.001$). The cumulative incidence rate was 2.2% at 10 years and 6.7% at 15 years. The risk was significantly higher for malignant melanoma (O/E = 5.0) and cancers of the buccal cavity (O/E = 11.1), liver (O/E = 7.5), brain or other parts of the CNS (O/E = 7.6), thyroid (O/E = 6.6), bone (O/E = 13.4), and connective tissue (O/E = 8.0). The risk was higher for recipients who were younger at the time of transplantation than for those who were older. Patients receiving TBI with a single dose of ≥10 Gy or ≥13 Gy as a fractionated doses, the risk of second tumors was three to four times compared to patients who did not undergo irradiation [41].

## 31.5 Total Marrow Irradiation/Total Marrow and Lymphoid Irradiation

The attempt to decrease the toxicity and retain the efficacy of TBI has led to the advent of techniques such as "Total Marrow Irradiation" (TMI) and "Total Marrow and Lymphoid Irradiation" (TMLI). It is a natural evolution of organ-sparing techniques in TBI. These techniques allow the radiation oncologist to not just reduce the mean lung dose, but to also spare kidneys, heart, GI tract, oral cavity, and other organs at risk. Liver, brain, and testes can sometimes be included in the target volume [42–44]. The major advantages of TMI/TMLI include reduction in short- and long-term toxicity in the patient and the possibility of a patient with a lowered performance index being able to better tolerate the conditioning regimen.

When increasing the dose of TBI, while lower relapse rates have been seen, there is a concordant increase in toxicity rates and non-relapse mortality [45, 46]. TMLI has allowed for safe dose escalation to 20 Gy in 10 fractions [47]. A Phase II trial showed superior outcomes with TMLI as compared to standard of care [48]. Currently, trials are being conducted to evaluate dose escalation with TMI/TMLI [49], assess its role in reduced-intensity conditioning regimens [50], and how they work with GvHD reduction strategies such as post-transplant cyclophosphamide [51] and T cell immunotherapy [52]. TMI/TMLI is now being considered even for patients with remission, who were classically prescribed TBI [53]. In one study of TMI, it was shown that the incidence of toxicities was lower than conventional TBI, with lowered rates of renal toxicity, hypothyroidism, and cataract formation [54].

A concern with usage of TMI/TMLI is that of extramedullary recurrence. However, a study [55] of 101 patients undergoing TMLI for allogeneic HSCT showed that the site of relapse in the 13 patients who developed recurrences was not dose dependent, and the risk of recurrence was similar to what has been observed with conventional TBI. This suggests that TMLI did not increase the risk of extramedullary relapse, which hints toward the immunosuppressive ability of radiotherapy, along with depletion of leukemic deposits in lymphatic volumes, bone marrow, and sanctuary sites and not the eradication of circulating leukemic cells.

### 31.5.1 Role of Radiotherapy in Leukemias

#### 31.5.1.1 Cranial Irradiation

Cranial irradiation for prevention of relapse in the CNS is a regular part of the treatment of ALL. This is because, traditionally, the systemic treatment for ALL has had poor penetrance through the blood-brain barrier, leading to the CNS serving as a sanctuary site for the malignant cells. Nowadays, only high-risk ALL patients are prescribed PCI. The volume of treatment includes the subarachnoid space in the cranial vault. The inferior margin of the treatment volume should extend to the lower limit of first or second cervical vertebra. The field must also include the cribriform plate and the middle cranial fossa. The posterior globe of the eye should be included to prevent relapse in the posterior retina. Dose regimens include 18 Gy in 9–10 fractions and 12 Gy in 8 fractions.

#### 31.5.1.2 Craniospinal Irradiation

Craniospinal irradiation is carried out in leukemia patients with meningeal spread, either during the initial diagnosis or during relapse. While CNS relapse is a rare event with modern chemotherapy regimens, CSI may still be required in some patients. CSI can be delivered through Cobalt machines or through linear accelerators. In recent years, the role of Tomotherapy has expanded because it allows for a better dose distribution in large treatment fields. Generally, the dose prescription is of 18–30 Gy to the brain and 6–15 Gy to the spine. When analyzing the chronic toxicity, intelligence quotient does not seem to be affected much; however, relative deficiencies in processing speed or working memory have been noted [56].

When carrying out CSI, it is important for the beam divergence between the postero-anterior spinal field and the lateral parallel opposed cranial fields should be matched precisely. “Feathering” of the junction of the spinal and cranial fields can be done to prevent excessive overlap of the dose over the cervical spine. A beam energy of 6 MV is recommended. Intrathecal chemotherapy would also form an integral part of the treatment of CNS leukemia.

#### 31.5.1.3 Testicular Radiotherapy

T cell subtype ALL in boys has a higher chance of involving the testes, with about 2% of the patients being affected. Testicular involvement also serves as a poor prognostic factor. While the microscopic burden of testicular disease has been estimated to be 5–15%, the advent of intermediate and high-dose methotrexate has reduced these rates significantly. Initially, prophylactic testicular radiotherapy was associated with decreased rates of testicular relapse, and it had no impact on overall survival. Modern chemotherapy regimens do not require the usage of prophylactic testicular irradiation.

Testicular relapse tends to be a harbinger of systemic or CNS relapse. In a patient who has had testicular relapse, high-dose chemotherapy and local radiotherapy both should be administered. Doses vary from 24 to 26 Gy being delivered over 2.5–3.5 weeks. While the relapse may be noted in only one testis, it is highly advisable to irradiate both testes since microscopic involvement of the contralateral testis is very frequently observed. It is important that the patient and family are counseled regarding the risk of infertility associated with bilateral testicular irradiation.

Testicular radiotherapy can be carried out through electrons or photons. The patient can be treated in a "frog-leg" position with the penile shaft being taped over the abdomen. One must keep in mind the cremasteric reflex to prevent geographic miss. Anterior inferior oblique photon fields can be used. If the scrotal thickness is less than 2 cm, then 250 kV orthovoltage X-rays can be used or electron beams will work adequately as well. Radiotherapy doses range from 24 to 26 Gy in 1.5–2 Gy per fraction. Testicular boost can also be delivered during a TBI, in which 4 Gy should be given in addition to the TBI dose.

#### 31.5.1.4 Ocular Radiotherapy

Inadequate coverage of the optic nerve and the posterior globe during cranial radiotherapy can put the patient at risk for a choroidal recurrence. This has led to the practice of including the posterior eye in the radiotherapy fields. Isolated relapses in the anterior eye can also be seen. Like testicular relapses, ocular relapse is also a harbinger of systemic relapse. In case of an ocular relapse, radiotherapy to the eye should be carried out to a dose of around 24 Gy. If there is an isolated relapse in the anterior eye, the risk of CNS involvement is much lesser; hence, it can be managed with electron beam radiotherapy along with intensive chemotherapy.

#### 31.5.1.5 Splenic Radiotherapy

There are some conditions which can result in massive splenomegaly. These include CML, CLL, splenic marginal zone lymphomas, and hairy cell leukemia. Splenic radiotherapy has been one option for palliation in such conditions. While now given uncommonly, splenic radiotherapy remains a treatment option for symptomatic splenomegaly. Due to the splenomegaly, patients can present with pain, diaphragmatic irritation, early satiety, and bleeding risk due to platelet sequestration. Leukemic infiltration responds very well to even low doses of radiation. In the elderly patient with multiple comorbidities, splenic radiotherapy can be a much safer treatment than splenectomy.

Generally, the radiotherapy is administered through anteroposterior parallel opposed portals. The whole spleen should be treated with 0.25–1.0 Gy fractions given either daily or 1–3 times per week. The delivery of radiotherapy should be titrated carefully as per response and patient tolerance. The treatment fields might even need to be shrunk as the spleen responds. Blood counts will need to be monitored very carefully. The total dose should be decided as per symptomatic relief, but usually 4–10 Gy is enough for palliation.

In patients with extramedullary hematopoiesis (e.g., in cases of chronic lymphoblastic leukemia or prolymphocytic leukemia), it is prudent to keep in mind the potential for severe neutropenia or thrombocytopenia. In such patients, doses as low as 0.1–0.5 Gy per fraction can be considered, or treatment of only half of the spleen at one time. Splenic irradiation can even lead to abscopal effects. Because of rapid cell lysis in patients undergoing splenic radiotherapy, allopurinol should be prescribed to prevent uric acid nephropathy. Nausea can be managed with anti-emetics.

It is important to monitor the left kidney dose as well, to prevent overdosage during re-irradiation. It is rare for doses greater than 20 Gy to be administered for palliation.

#### 31.5.1.6 TBI in India

TBI requires not just radiotherapy capabilities, but also that the hospital has facilities to carry out stem cell transplantation. Few centers in India exist that have this dual capability. Even when such infrastructure is available, not every institute will have the laboratory infrastructure to facilitate SCT or staff experienced in these techniques. A third point to note is that the cost of these procedures is very high, meaning that only the most financially capable are able to afford such treatment unless the treatment cost is subsidized by public sector facilities or covered by health insurance. There is even a lack of knowledge of such procedures, not just in the general population, but even in the medical fraternity. These factors lead to limited practice of TBI in India [57]. Notwithstanding these shortcomings, TBI facilities exist in many public sector tertiary care centers as well as many private hospitals mainly in larger cities.

**Acknowledgments** Entire team of Division of Radiation oncology, Medanta The Medicity.

**Conflict of Interest** None.

## References

1. Clift RA, Buckner CD, Appelbaum FR, et al. Allogeneic marrow transplantation in patients with acute myeloid leukemia in first remission: a randomized trial of two irradiation regimens. Blood. 1990;76(9):1867–71.
2. Deeg HJ, Sullivan KM, Buckner CD, et al. Marrow transplantation for acute nonlymphoblastic leukemia in first remission: toxicity and long-term follow-up of patients conditioned with single dose or fractionated total body irradiation. Bone Marrow Transplant. 1986;1(2):151–7.
3. Ozsahin M, Pene F, Touboul E, et al. Total-body irradiation before bone marrow transplantation. Results of two randomized instantaneous dose rates in 157 patients. Cancer. 1992;69(11):2853–65.
4. Tutschka PJ, Copelan EA, Klein JP. Bone marrow transplantation for leukemia following a new busulfan and cyclophosphamide regimen. Blood. 1987;70(5):1382–8.
5. O'Donnell MR, Long GD, Parker PM, et al. Busulfan/cyclophosphamide as conditioning regimen for allogeneic bone marrow transplantation for myelodysplasia. J Clin Oncol. 1995;13(12):2973–9.
6. Gaspard MH, Maraninchi D, Stoppa AM, et al. Intensive chemotherapy with high doses of BCNU, etoposide, cytosine arabinoside, and melphalan (BEAM) followed by autologous bone marrow transplantation: toxicity and antitumor activity in 26 patients with poor-risk malignancies. Cancer Chemother Pharmacol. 1988;22(3):256–62.
7. Bradley J, Reft C, Goldman S, et al. High-energy total body irradiation as preparation for bone marrow transplantation in leukemia patients: treatment technique and related complications. Int J Radiat Oncol Biol Phys. 1998;40(2):391–6.
8. Cunningham JR, Wright DJ. A simple facility for wholebody irradiation. Radiology. 1962;78:941–9.
9. Quast U. Physical treatment planning of total-body irradiation: patient translation and beam-zone method. Med Phys. 1985;12(5):567–74.

10. Pla M, Chenery SG, Podgorsak EB. Total body irradiation with a sweeping beam. Int J Radiat Oncol Biol Phys. 1983;9(1):83–9.
11. Van Dyk J, Glavin JM, Glasgow GP. The physical aspects of total and half body photon irradiation: a report of task group 29 radiation therapy committee. American Association of Physicists in Medicine; 1986.
12. Appelbaum FR. The influence of total dose, fractionation, dose rate, and distribution of total body irradiation on bone marrow transplantation. Semin Oncol. 1993;20(4 Suppl 4):3–10; quiz 11.
13. Shank B. Techniques of magna-field irradiation. Int J Radiat Oncol Biol Phys. 1983;9(12):1925–31.
14. Girinsky T, Socie G, Ammarguellat H, et al. Consequences of two different doses to the lungs during a single dose of total body irradiation: results of a randomized study on 85 patients. Int J Radiat Oncol Biol Phys. 1994;30(4):821–4.
15. Lawton CA, Barber-Derus S, Murray KJ, et al. Technical modifications in hyperfractionated total body irradiation for T-lymphocyte deplete bone marrow transplant. Int J Radiat Oncol Biol Phys. 1989;17(2):319–22.
16. Lawton CA, Cohen EP, Murray KJ, et al. Long-term results of selective renal shielding in patients undergoing total body irradiation in preparation for bone marrow transplantation. Bone Marrow Transplant. 1997;20(12):1069–74.
17. Shank B, Brochstein JA, Castro-Malaspina H, et al. Immunosuppression prior to marrow transplantation for sensitized aplastic anemia patients: comparison of TLI with TBI. Int J Radiat Oncol Biol Phys. 1988;14(6):1133–41.
18. Hill-Kayser CE, Plastaras JP, Tochner Z, Glatstein E. TBI during BM and SCT: review of the past, discussion of the present and consideration of future directions. Bone Marrow Transplant. 2011;46(4):475–84. https://doi.org/10.1038/bmt.2010.280.
19. Chaillet MP, Cosset JM, Socie G, et al. Prospective study of the clinical symptoms of therapeutic whole body irradiation. Health Phys. 1993;64(4):370–4.
20. Buchali A, Feyer P, Groll J, et al. Immediate toxicity during fractionated total body irradiation as conditioning for bone marrow transplantation. Radiother Oncol. 2000;54(2):157–62.
21. Thomas ED, Clift RA, Hersman J, et al. Marrow transplantation for acute nonlymphoblastic leukemic in first remission using fractionated or single dose irradiation. Int J Radiat Oncol Biol Phys. 1982;8(5):817–21.
22. Deeg HJ. Acute and delayed toxicities of total body irradiations. Seattle Marrow Transplant Team. Int J Radiat Oncol Biol Phys. 1983;9(12):1933–9. https://doi.org/10.1016/0360-3016(83)90365-6.
23. Parkins CS, Fowler JF, Maughan RL, et al. Repair in mouse lung for up to 20 fractions of X rays or neutrons. Br J Radiol. 1985;58(687):225–41.
24. Travis EL. The sequence of histological changes in mouse lungs after single doses of x-rays. Int J Radiat Oncol Biol Phys. 1980;6(3):345–7.
25. Carruthers SA, Wallington MM. Total body irradiation and pneumonitis risk: a review of outcomes. Br J Cancer. 2004;90(11):2080–4.
26. Sampath S, Schultheiss TE, Wong J. Dose response and factors related to interstitial pneumonitis after bone marrow transplant. Int J Radiat Oncol Biol Phys. 2005;63(3):876–84.
27. Tichelli A, Gratwohl A, Egger T, et al. Cataract formation after bone marrow transplantation. Ann Intern Med. 1993;119(12):1175–80.
28. Benyunes MC, Sullivan KM, Deeg HJ, et al. Cataracts after bone marrow transplantation: long-term follow-up of adults treated with fractionated total body irradiation. Int J Radiat Oncol Biol Phys. 1995;32(3):661–70.
29. Felicetti F, Manicone R, Corrias A, et al. Endocrine late effects after total body irradiation in patients who received hematopoietic cell transplantation during childhood: a retrospective study from a single institution. J Cancer Res Clin Oncol. 2011;137(9):1343–8.
30. Sanders JE, Buckner CD, Leonard JM, et al. Late effects on gonadal function of cyclophosphamide, total-body irradiation, and marrow transplantation. Transplantation. 1983;36(3):252–5.

31. Keilholz U, Korbling M, Fehrentz D, et al. Long-term endocrine toxicity of myeloablative treatment followed by autologous bone marrow/blood derived stem cell transplantation in patients with malignant lymphohematopoietic disorders. Cancer. 1989;64(3):641–5.
32. Sklar CA, Kim TH, Ramsay NK. Thyroid dysfunction among long-term survivors of bone marrow transplantation. Am J Med. 1982;73(5):688–94.
33. DeLeve LD, Shulman HM, McDonald GB. Toxic injury to hepatic sinusoids: sinusoidal obstruction syndrome (veno-occlusive disease). Semin Liver Dis. 2002;22(1):27–42.
34. Shulman HM, Fisher LB, Schoch HG, et al. Veno-occlusive disease of the liver after marrow transplantation: histological correlates of clinical signs and symptoms. Hepatology. 1994;19(5):1171–81.
35. Wingard JR, Nichols WG, McDonald GB. Supportive care. Hematology Am Soc Hematol Educ Program. 2004;2004:372–89.
36. McDonald GB, Sharma P, Matthews DE, et al. The clinical course of 53 patients with venocclusive disease of the liver after marrow transplantation. Transplantation. 1985;39(6):603–8.
37. Barrett A. Total body irradiation (TBI) before bone marrow transplantation in leukaemia: a co-operative study from the European Group for Bone Marrow Transplantation. Br J Radiol. 1982;55(656):562–7.
38. Ellis MJ, Parikh CR, Inrig JK, et al. Chronic kidney disease after hematopoietic cell transplantation: a systematic review. Am J Transplant. 2008;8(11):2378–90.
39. Guinan EC, Tarbell NJ, Niemeyer CM, et al. Intravascular hemolysis and renal insufficiency after bone marrow transplantation. Blood. 1988;72(2):451–5.
40. Kolb HJ, Socie G, Duell T, et al. Malignant neoplasms in long-term survivors of bone marrow transplantation. Late effects working Party of the European Cooperative Group for blood and marrow transplantation and the European Late Effect Project Group. Ann Intern Med. 1999;131(10):738–44.
41. Curtis RE, Rowlings PA, Deeg HJ, et al. Solid cancers after bone marrow transplantation. N Engl J Med. 1997;336(13):897–904.
42. Wong JYC, Liu A, Schultheiss T, Popplewell L, Stein A, Rosenthal J, et al. Targeted total marrow irradiation using three-dimensional image-guided tomographic intensity-modulated radiation therapy: an alternative to standard total body irradiation. Biol Blood Marrow Transplant. 2006;12:306–15. https://doi.org/10.1016/j.bbmt.2005.10.026.
43. Rosenthal J, Wong J, Stein A, Qian D, Hitt D, Naeem H, et al. Phase 1/2 trial of total marrow and lymph node irradiation to augment reduced- intensity transplantation for advanced hematologic malignancies. Blood. 2011;117:309–15. https://doi.org/10.1182/blood-2010-06-288357.
44. Hui SK, Kapatoes J, Fowler J, Henderson D, Olivera G, Manon RR, et al. Feasibility study of helical tomotherapy for total body or total marrow irradiation. Med Phys. 2005;32:3214–24. https://doi.org/10.1118/1.2044428.
45. Bearman SI, Appelbaum FR, Buckner CD, Petersen FB, Fisher LD, Clift RA, et al. Regimen-related toxicity in patients undergoing bone marrow transplantation. J Clin Oncol. 1988;6:1562–8. https://doi.org/10.1200/JCO.1988.6.10.1562.
46. Clift RA, Buckner CD, Appelbaum FR, Bryant E, Bearman SI, Peterson FB, et al. Allogeneic marrow transplantation in patients with chronic myeloid leukemia in the chronic phase: a randomized trial of two irradiation regimens. Blood. 1991;77:1660–5. https://doi.org/10.1182/blood.V77.8.1660.bloodjournal7781660.
47. Stein A, Palmer J, Tsai NC, Al Malki MM, Aldoss I, Ali H, et al. Phase I trial of total marrow and lymphoid irradiation transplantation conditioning in patients with relapsed/refractory acute leukemia. Biol Blood Marrow Transplant. 2017;23:618–24. https://doi.org/10.1016/j.bbmt.2017.01.067.
48. Stein A, Tsai N-C, Palmer J, Al Malki M, Aldoss I, Ali H, et al. Total marrow and lymphoid irradiation (TMLI) in combination with cyclophosphamide and etoposide in patients with relapsed/refractory acute leukemia undergoing allogeneic hematopoietic cell transplantation. In: European Society for Blood and Marrow Transplantation Meeting, Frankfurt; 2019.

49. Wong J. Total marrow irradiation: redefining the role of radiotherapy in bone marrow transplantation. In: Wong J, Hui SK, editors. Total marrow irradiation. 1st ed. New York, NY: Springer Nature; 2020. p. 1–28. https://doi.org/10.1007/978-3-030-38692-4_1.
50. Jensen LJ, Stiller T, Wong JYC, Palmer J, Stein A, Rosenthal J. Total marrow lymphoid irradiation/fludarabine/melphalan conditioning for allogeneic hematopoietic cell transplantation. Biol Blood Marrow Transplant. 2018;24:301–7. https://doi.org/10.1016/j.bbmt.2017.09.019.
51. O'Donnell PV, Luznik L, Jones RJ, Vogelsang GB, Leffell MS, Phelps M, et al. Nonmyeloablative bone marrow transplantation from partially HLA-mismatched related donors using postransplantation cyclophosphamide. Biol Blood Marrow Transplant. 2002;8:377–86. https://doi.org/10.1053/bbmt.2002.v8.pm12171484.
52. Aristei C, Saldi S, Pierini A, Ruggeri L, Piccine S, Ingrosso G, et al. Total marrow/lymphoid irradiation in the conditioning regimen for haploidentical T-cell depleted hematopoietic stem cell transplantation for acute myeloid leukemia. In: Wong J, Hui SK, editors. Total marrow irradiation. 1st ed. New York, NY: Springer Nature; 2020. p. 111–22. https://doi.org/10.1007/978-3-030-38692-4_7.
53. Stein AS, Al Malki M, Yang D, Palmer JM, Tsai N-C, Aldoss I, et al. Total marrow and lymphoid irradiation (TMLI) at a dose of 2000 cGy in combination with post-transplant cyclophosphamide (PTCy)-based graft versus host disease (GHVD) prophylaxis is safe and associated with favorable GVHD-free/relapse-free survival at 1 year in patients with acute myeloid leukemia (AML). In: 62nd Amercian Society of Hematology Annual Meeting and Exposition (San Diego, CA), vol. 136; 2020. p. 41. https://doi.org/10.1182/blood-2020-141469.
54. Shinde A, Wong J. Acute and late toxicities with total marrow irradiation. In: Wong J, Hui SK, editors. Total marrow irradiation. 1st ed. New York, NY: Springer Nature; 2020. p. 187–96. https://doi.org/10.1007/978-3-030-38692-4_14.
55. Kim JH, Stein A, Tsai N, Schultheiss TE, Palmer J, Liu A, et al. Extramedullary relapse following total marrow and lymphoid irradiation in patients undergoing allogeneic hematopoietic cell transplantation. Int J Radiat Oncol Biol Phys. 2014;89:75–81. https://doi.org/10.1016/j.ijrobp.2014.01.036.
56. Hiniker SM, Agarwal R, Modlin LA, et al. Survival and neurocognitive outcomes after cranial or craniospinal irradiation plus total-body irradiation before stem cell transplantation in pediatric leukemia patients with central nervous system involvement. Int J Radiat Oncol Biol Phys. 2014;89:67–74.
57. Shah CA, et al. Hematopoietic stem-cell transplantation in the developing world: experience from a center in Western India. J Oncol. 2015;2015:1–9. https://doi.org/10.1155/2015/710543.

# Palliative Care in Pediatric Oncology

# 32

Chinna Babu Dracham, Divya Khosla, and Rakesh Kapoor

## 32.1 Introduction

Pediatric palliative care (PPC) has evolved as an important aid to cancer children and their families to cope with the physical, psychological, spiritual, and social burdens of disease and treatment. The World Health Organization (WHO) defines PPC as "the prevention and relief of suffering among children with life-limiting or life-threatening disease, as well as their families" [1]. The PPC encompasses similar goals and care domains as in adult palliative care but uniquely focuses on the needs of children and their larger families. Holistic care of pediatric cancer patients includes the care of patients, their parents, siblings, and extended family [2].

Palliative care is provided to patients with severely life-limiting conditions, those who are nudging the end of their lives. The landmark trials on adult palliative care, Temel [3] and Sullivan et al. [4], have shown improvement in survival for patients who were receiving palliative care. The pedagogy of healthcare professionals acquiring knowledge and skills is primarily based on a biological approach and dedicated to curing the illness. But this palliative care field demands both scientific knowledge and emotional preparation to face the end-of-life (EOL) and the family's pain. Improvement in quality of life (QOL) has been associated with early palliative care involvement and observed in both pediatric patients and their families [5]. For adolescents and young adults with cancer, palliative care is associated with less intensive therapy at EOL, improved preparation for EOL, and improved psychosocial outcomes in bereaved parents. Despite the availability of burgeoning literature and innumerable advantages of palliative care implementation in the management of pediatric patients, PPC practice is still poorly executed in pediatric oncology.

C. B. Dracham
Government Cancer Hospital, Kadapa, Andhra Pradesh, India

D. Khosla (✉) · R. Kapoor
Department of Radiotherapy, PGIMER, Chandigarh, India





R. Madan et al. (eds.), *Evidence Based Practice in Pediatric Radiation Oncology*,
https://doi.org/10.1007/978-981-96-4872-6_32

This chapter discusses the evolution and need of PPC in the management of pediatric cancers, barriers to providing PPC, basic principles underlying this integration, and assessment and management of physical symptoms and QOL. Specific symptom management is beyond the scope of this chapter.

## 32.2 The Evolution and Need of PPC

According to a review of global estimates published in 2019, the cancer incidence rates in children and adolescents have been increasing since 1975, with acute leukemia and brain tumors being most commonly diagnosed [6]. This increase in incidence rates has been paced by an increase in survival rates, 5-year survival of 58% in the 1970s to ≥80% in 2016 [7]. Wide variability in disease trajectory and prognosis has been reported across different types of pediatric cancers. In the 1970s, the worst survival rates were reported in acute leukemia; at present, solid tumors particularly rhabdomyosarcoma, bone tumors, neuroblastoma, and central nervous system tumors are associated with poor prognosis [8]. Hematological malignancies are associated with acute onset of life-threatening complications, disease progression, and sudden death occurs mostly in hospitals, whereas solid tumors have a chronic evolution, long course of the disease, and often patients prone to progressive deterioration before death.

According to Cheng BT et al. 2018, a systematic review on palliative care in pediatric oncology reported that only 54.5% of patients received PPC before death and 44.2% of advanced cancer children were referred to PPC only at EOL [9]. Another multinational review from Children's Oncology Group (COG) found that only 60% of pediatric oncology care providers offer PPC services [10]. Furthermore, only 5% of pediatric oncologists and children's families discuss palliative care planning [11]. This suggests that there are many structural barriers that prevent the implementation of standardized PPC approaches in limited resource and high-income countries.

## 32.3 Barriers in Providing PPC

The potential barriers are observed at multiple levels which include (a) shortage of clinicians and care providers capable to deliver PPC, (b) meagre allocation of resources (inadequate funding programs at policy/payment level, restricted reimbursements with health insurance), (c) poor access to essential analgesics and opioids, (d) health system level (lack of workforce and coordination between working groups and PPC providers outside the hospital), (e) ambiguous roles of the care team, (f) organization level (lack of working models for integrating PPC), (g) individual level (gap in knowledge due to lack of experience, time limitations at patient and family level), and (h) non-specific educational and training curriculum for healthcare providers [9]. Due to inadequacy of palliative care and hospice services in pediatric groups, there is discordance between physical, emotional, and psychosocial needs of children, their families, and healthcare providers. The feeling of being alone and having to provide this care themselves, particularly in home-based settings, is very stressful for families. Moreover, PPC is often misperceived as a mutually exclusive service from oncologists by patients and their families and is most commonly associated with EOL care. Due to all these reasons, PPC integration in pediatric oncology practice remains suboptimal.

## 32.4 Basic Principles of PPC

Childhood cancer treatment is lengthy, and major improvements have been achieved in survival over last decades. Children and their families interact with healthcare professionals regularly during the entire disease trajectory. As mentioned above, the PPC has more unique components in comparison to adult palliative care particularly accounting for ethical, developmental, psychosocial, and spiritual issues. Furthermore, parents and siblings have a crucial part in decision-making and retaining legal responsibilities of patients. Even though WHO defines palliative care as aiming to "prevent suffering to families," suggesting that this is solely a parental responsibility is untenable. Several conditions fall under the PPC application and those can be classified into three levels, first as life-threatening (high chances for premature death, but also possibility of long-term survival), second as life-limiting (similar to previous definition, but there is no hope for cure and long-term survival), and third as terminal [12].

In PPC, children and their families should be joined with specific care programs according to the available resources. The PPC can be delivered in three levels, as follows: (1) palliative care provided by all healthcare providers; (2) generalized palliative care provided by an oncologist who trained in PPC; and (3) specialized palliative care provided by a dedicated team of interdisciplinary PPC experts [13]. The level of PPC delivery changes along with disease trajectory. According to severity of disease and complexity of needs, the PPC can be provided in various settings, e.g., in hospital, in pediatric hospice, in ambulatory care, or at home. Current evidence emphasizes on specialized PPC, and it should be performed as a continuous activity between hospital inpatient with consultation, hospice inpatient, and home assistance care with 24/7 telephonic consultation [14]. Home care is a common desire for both children and families, because it ensures a family environment without discomforts. Furthermore, home care allows interaction of family members and friends' network, encourages social inclusion that often affects the families of seriously ill children, reduces healthcare costs, and re-establishing their family cultural background [15]. The healthcare providers must enquire about the family's level of understanding about disease and prognosis, and adapt the communication according to it [16].

General palliative care and supportive care are mandatory for all children diagnosed with cancer. Specialized palliative care should be provided well before the EOL time to children with potential incurable cancer disease, considering their physiological and developmental changes related to growth and prognosis [17].

Indeed, the early integration of PPC support in cancer children helps in improvement of QOL, decrease in symptom burden, development of trusting relationships between children, their families and healthcare professionals, and improved decision-making [12]. There are many dedicated tools to define the complexity of needs and to understand when to seek specialized PPC services. The pediatric palliative screening scale (PaPas) is the tool used to identify cancer children in need of PPC, and assess five domains (disease trajectory, symptom burden, expected outcome and treatment burden, preferences of child and/or family, and estimated life expectancy) [18]. Another tool has been proposed by Kaye et al. 2015 [19] and Jankovic et al. 2019 [20], a consensus on defining eligibility criteria for specialized PPC in children with cancer as "green lights service to consider PPC at diagnosis, during illness, and other complex needs." The ACCAPED scale defines the eligibility criteria to deliver PPC at different levels by measuring the grades of complex medical needs and the risk of life-threatening events [21]. However, using these tools should not replace the specific assessment of each case, and the best approach to understanding the PPC is the "needs of care" of the children and family. Here, we focus on specific domains of PPC at advanced stage disease, whether primary or specialized PPC delivery. Domains included are family-centered communication, assessment and management of physical symptoms, QOL, psychosocial issues, and spiritual concerns of patients and their families.

## 32.5 Family-Centered Communication in PPC

Pediatric cancer is a family illness [22]. Family-centered communication encourages the conversation between patients, families, and healthcare providers that aims to support "more efficient, effective and empathetic pediatric health care" [23]. The communication should be understandable and compassionate, especially when discussing the prognosis of advanced stages of cancer care. The needs of family and concerns should be considered especially level of understanding, family structure, specific culture and family routines, other ongoing conflicts, triggers for emotional distress, financial issues, and spiritual beliefs [24]. This high-quality family-centered communication helps to gain greater trust in the healthcare provider and is associated with family peace, the feeling of being acknowledged and comforted [22]. Families who receive detailed prognostic information can redefine and reframe their short-term and long-term preferences, give maximum time for togetherness, and report less decisional regret [22].

Adolescents and young adults (AYA) with cancer have a better understanding of their disease and priorities of care. The level of involvement in decision-making and the amount of prognostic information asked by AYA patients may change over period of time, so all AYA patients should be asked for their level of involvement before each discussion [25]. Involvement of AYA's and families in decision-making discussions, conversations about goals, and advanced care planning has been associated with reduced suffering, decreased anxiety, realization of EOL wishes, and improved congruence at the time of EOL care [26]. Wiener et al. [27] and Zadeh et al. [28] have reported the methods, tools to assist communication, and example phrases used to engage the AYA patients in discussions about diagnosis, prognosis, and decision-making during advanced care planning. According to recent publications on "advanced care planning and communication using the guide voicing My CHOiCES," the AYAs talk with their family and friends regarding their preferences of care than healthcare providers [29]. The PPC team guidance on navigating the issues of EOL care and bereavement care for a parent of children who die of cancer has been associated with improvement in parents' perception of care [29].

The timely decision of family and preparedness are crucial to ensure coordination during advanced care planning and to prevent difficulties during crisis period. Therefore, this advanced care planning should be initiated before EOL care. Palliative sedation must be incorporated in EOL care for intolerable and resistant symptoms (e.g., pain, delirium, and dyspnea), with the aim of reduction of consciousness [30]. Death is not the end of care, grief after death also has a physical, psychosocial, and spiritual dimension. The PPC team and psychologist should meet with the bereaved family to provide emotional support and help address any questions or feelings of regret.

## 32.6 Assessment and Management of Pain and QOL

The most common physical symptoms during advanced cancer care in children are chronic pain, fatigue, nausea and vomiting, and respiratory distress, followed by cachexia, nutrition problems, and constipation [31]. Treatment of these chronic symptoms must be incorporated into comprehensive care along with anti-cancer treatment. Pharmacological and non-pharmacological therapies should be used in management of pain and other symptoms according to the child's age and developmental stage [12].

Pain is a predominant, complex, and distressing problem that has an immeasurable impact on patients, families, and healthcare professionals. It can be challenging to analyze and quantify pain, particularly in young children. An accurate assessment of pain should be done concerning the type of pain (nociceptive, neuropathic, nociplastic), source and location of pain, and its severity. Proper assessment should include the frequency, duration, description, and severity of pain episodes. The accuracy of pain assessment depends upon age and the cognitive ability of the child. Older children and adolescents can report and quantify their pain. But it becomes very challenging in nonverbal children or patients with neurologic impairment as they cannot report and quantify their pain [32]. So for these children, it is difficult to treat pain appropriately and patients may remain in agony due to pain.

The WHO has defined the utilization of different drugs in a "step ladder pattern" and classified the drugs into four categories—non-opioids like non-steroidal anti-inflammatory drugs (NSAIDS), weak and strong opioids, adjuvants, and local anesthetics [33, 34]. The routes of administration are ranging from oral, subcutaneous, and venous to sublingual, transmucosal, transcutaneous, and aerosol. Non-drug therapies are physical, behavioral, and cognitive, which primarily work by involving child's sensory system, behavior, and thought. Various techniques are used in the management including attention, distraction, relaxation, imagery, and behavioral change [35].

Olagunju AT et al. reported that increased somatic symptom burden and mood disturbances in children were associated with poor parental emotional functioning [36]. Historically, physical symptoms and psychosocial issues in pediatric patients have been measured by parent's proxy reports because of a lack of validated tools for their age range and concern about children's ability to understand the tools. However, there is concordance between parent's proxy report and patient's self-report in symptom assessment and QOL. In contrast to children's self-reports, parents generally overestimate, while clinicians tend to underestimate both the severity and prevalence of physical symptoms in children [37]. Patient Reported Outcomes (PROs) measurement information system has demonstrated good acceptability and feasibility from children and AYAs undergoing cancer treatment and in cancer survivors.

## 32.7 Conclusion

The PPC should be initiated early in the course of the disease for ease of communication and shared decision-making with the family, and caregivers of children and adolescents suffering from cancer. Parents and caregivers should be motivated to express their objectives and desires so that physicians can tailor treatment and care according to a patient and their family's preferences. The two important components in delivering good palliative care are patient- and family-centered communication and shared decision-making. Appropriate and effective anticipatory guidance should be provided to the families about the diagnosis, course of disease, treatment, and supportive care. Palliative care should be offered parallel to the therapies intended to treat the advanced stage of cancer.

## References

1. World Health Organization. Integrating palliative care and symptom relief in paediatrics. 2018. https://apps.who.int/iris/handle/10665/274561.
2. Jones BL, Contro N, Koch KD. The duty of the physician to care for the family in pediatric palliative care: context, communication, and caring. Pediatrics. 2014;133(Suppl 1):S8–S15.
3. Temel JS, Greer JA, Muzikansky A, Gallagher ER, Admane S, Jackson VA, et al. Early palliative care for patients with metastatic non-small-cell lung cancer. N Engl J Med. 2010;363(8):733–42.
4. Sullivan DR, Chan B, Lapidus JA, Ganzini L, Hansen L, Carney PA, et al. Association of Early Palliative Care Use with survival and place of death among patients with advanced lung cancer receiving care in the Veterans Health Administration. JAMA Oncol. 2019;5(12):1702–9.
5. Weaver M, Wichman C, Darnall C, Bace S, Vail C, MacFadyen A. Proxy-reported quality of life and family impact for children followed longitudinally by a pediatric palliative care team. J Palliat Med. 2018;21(2):241–4.

6. Bhakta N, Force LM, Allemani C, Atun R, Bray F, Coleman MP, et al. Childhood cancer burden: a review of global estimates. Lancet Oncol. 2019;20(1):e42–53.
7. Donnelly DW, Gavin AT. Mortality among children and young people who survive cancer in Northern Ireland. Ulster Med J. 2016;85(3):158–63.
8. Ward E, DeSantis C, Robbins A, Kohler B, Jemal A. Childhood and adolescent cancer statistics, 2014. CA Cancer J Clin. 2014;64(2):83–103.
9. Cheng BT, Rost M, De Clercq E, Arnold L, Elger BS, Wangmo T. Palliative care initiation in pediatric oncology patients: a systematic review. Cancer Med. 2019;8(1):3–12.
10. Johnston DL, Nagel K, Friedman DL, Meza JL, Hurwitz CA, Friebert S. Availability and use of palliative care and end-of-life services for pediatric oncology patients. J Clin Oncol. 2008;26(28):4646–50.
11. Kaye EC, Woods C, Kennedy K, Velrajan S, Gattas M, Bilbeisi T, et al. Communication around palliative care principles and advance care planning between oncologists, children with advancing cancer and families. Br J Cancer. 2021;125(8):1089–99.
12. Benini F, Papadatou D, Bernadá M, Craig F, De Zen L, Downing J, et al. International standards for pediatric palliative care: from IMPaCCT to GO-PPaCS. J Pain Symptom Manage. 2022;63(5):e529–43.
13. Quill TE, Abernethy AP. Generalist plus specialist palliative care—creating a more sustainable model. N Engl J Med. 2013;368(13):1173–5.
14. Brock KE, Snaman JM, Kaye EC, Bower KA, Weaver MS, Baker JN, et al. Models of pediatric palliative oncology outpatient care-benefits, challenges, and opportunities. J Oncol Pract. 2019;15(9):476–87.
15. Chong PH, De Castro Molina JA, Teo K, Tan WS. Paediatric palliative care improves patient outcomes and reduces healthcare costs: evaluation of a home-based program. BMC Palliat Care. 2018;17(1):11.
16. Sisk BA, Friedrich A, Blazin LJ, Baker JN, Mack JW, DuBois J. Communication in pediatric oncology: a qualitative study. Pediatrics. 2020;146(3):e20201193.
17. Cuviello A, Raisanen JC, Donohue PK, Wiener L, Boss RD. Defining the boundaries of Palliative Care in Pediatric Oncology. J Pain Symptom Manage. 2020;59(5):1033–42.
18. Song IG, Kwon SY, Chang YJ, Kim MS, Jeong SH, Hahn SM, et al. Paediatric palliative screening scale as a useful tool for clinicians' assessment of palliative care needs of pediatric patients: a retrospective cohort study. BMC Palliat Care. 2021;20(1):73.
19. Kaye EC, Rubenstein J, Levine D, Baker JN, Dabbs D, Friebert SE. Pediatric palliative care in the community. CA Cancer J Clin. 2015;65(4):316–33.
20. Jankovic M, De Zen L, Pellegatta F, Lazzarin P, Bertolotti M, Manfredini L, et al. A consensus conference report on defining the eligibility criteria for pediatric palliative care in Italy. Ital J Pediatr. 2019;45(1):89.
21. Lazzarin P, Giacomelli L, Terrenato I, Benini F, Behalf of the ACCAPED Study Group. A tool for the evaluation of clinical needs and eligibility to pediatric palliative care: the validation of the ACCAPED scale. J Palliat Med. 2021;24(2):205–10.
22. Snaman J, McCarthy S, Wiener L, Wolfe J. Pediatric palliative care in oncology. J Clin Oncol. 2020;38(9):954–62.
23. Levetown M, American Academy of Pediatrics Committee on Bioethics. Communicating with children and families: from everyday interactions to skill in conveying distressing information. Pediatrics. 2008;121(5):e1441–60.
24. Papadatou D, Kalliani V, Karakosta E, Liakopoulou P, Bluebond-Langner M. Home or hospital as the place of end-of-life care and death: a grounded theory study of parents' decision-making. Palliat Med. 2021;35(1):219–30.
25. Brand SR, Fasciano K, Mack JW. Communication preferences of pediatric cancer patients: talking about prognosis and their future life. Support Care Cancer. 2017;25(3):769–74.
26. Lyon ME, Jacobs S, Briggs L, Cheng YI, Wang J. A longitudinal, randomized, controlled trial of advance care planning for teens with cancer: anxiety, depression, quality of life, advance directives, spirituality. J Adolesc Health. 2014;54(6):710–7.

27. Wiener L, Zadeh S, Battles H, Baird K, Ballard E, Osherow J, et al. Allowing adolescents and young adults to plan their end-of-life care. Pediatrics. 2012;130(5):897–905.
28. Zadeh S, Pao M, Wiener L. Opening end-of-life discussions: how to introduce voicing my CHOiCES™, an advance care planning guide for adolescents and young adults. Palliat Support Care. 2015 Jun;13(3):591–9.
29. Kassam A, Skiadaresis J, Alexander S, Wolfe J. Differences in end-of-life communication for children with advanced cancer who were referred to a palliative care team. Pediatr Blood Cancer. 2015;62(8):1409–13.
30. Sanderson A, Hall AM, Wolfe J. Advance care discussions: pediatric clinician preparedness and practices. J Pain Symptom Manage. 2016;51(3):520–8.
31. Wolfe J, Orellana L, Ullrich C, Cook EF, Kang TI, Rosenberg A, et al. Symptoms and distress in children with advanced cancer: prospective patient-reported outcomes from the PediQUEST study. J Clin Oncol. 2015;33(17):1928–35.
32. Stapelkamp C, Carter B, Gordon J, Watts C. Assessment of acute pain in children: development of evidence-based guidelines. Int J Evid Based Healthc. 2011;9(1):39–50.
33. Wolfe J, Grier HE, Klar N, Levin SB, Ellenbogen JM, Salem-Schatz S, et al. Symptoms and suffering at the end of life in children with cancer. N Engl J Med. 2000;342(5):326–33.
34. Splinter W. Novel approaches for treating pain in children. Curr Oncol Rep. 2019;21(2):11.
35. Tutelman PR, Chambers CT, Stinson JN, Parker JA, Fernandez CV, Witteman HO, et al. Pain in children with cancer: prevalence, characteristics, and parent management. Clin J Pain. 2018;34(3):198–206.
36. Olagunju AT, Sarimiye FO, Olagunju TO, Habeebu MY, Aina OF. Child's symptom burden and depressive symptoms among caregivers of children with cancers: an argument for early integration of pediatric palliative care. Ann Palliat Med. 2016;5(3):157–65.
37. Dupuis LL, Johnston DL, Baggott C, Hyslop S, Tomlinson D, Gibson P, et al. Validation of the symptom screening in pediatrics tool in children receiving cancer treatments. J Natl Cancer Inst. 2018;110(6):661–8.

MIX
Papier aus verantwortungsvollen Quellen
Paper from responsible sources
FSC® C105338

If you have any concerns about our products,
you can contact us on
**ProductSafety@springernature.com**

In case Publisher is established outside the EU,
the EU authorized representative is:
**Springer Nature Customer Service Center GmbH**
**Europaplatz 3, 69115 Heidelberg, Germany**

Printed by Libri Plureos GmbH
in Hamburg, Germany